LIVE THE TRUTH

THE MORAL LEGACY OF JOHN PAUL II IN CATHOLIC HEALTH CARE

LIVE THE TRUTH

THE MORAL LEGACY OF JOHN PAUL II IN CATHOLIC HEALTH CARE

The Twentieth NCBC
Workshop for Bishops

Edward J. Furton, Editor

Nihil Obstat
Rev. Msgr. Francis A. Barszczewski, S.T.L.
Censor Librorum

Imprimatur
✠ Justin Cardinal Rigali
Archbishop of Philadelphia
March 14, 2006

The *Nihil Obstat* and *Imprimatur* are a declaration that
a book or pamphlet is considered to be free from doctrinal
or moral error. It is not implied that those who granted the
Nihil Obstat and Imprimatur agree with the contents,
opinions, or statements expressed therein.

Cover Design: Mark Bradford and Tom Gannoe

ISBN 0-935372-49-0

Library of Congress Cataloging-in-Publication Data

Workshop for Bishops of the United States and Canada (20th : 2005
: Dallas, Tex.)
  Live the truth : the moral legacy of John Paul II in Catholic health
care / the Twentieth NCBC Workshop for Bishops ; Edward J.
Furton, editor.
     p. ; cm.
  Includes bibliographical references.
  Includes two papers in Spanish with English translations.
  ISBN 0-935372-49-0
  1. Pastoral medicine—Catholic Church—Congresses. 2. Religion
and medicine—Congresses. 3. Values clarification—Congresses. 4.
Medical ethics—Congresses. I. Furton, Edward James. II. National
Catholic Bioethics Center. III. Title.
  [DNLM: 1. John Paul II, Pope, 1920-2005. 2. Bioethical Issues—
Congresses. 3. Catholicism—Congresses. 4. Religion and Medi-
cine—Congresses. WB 60 W926L 2006]
  RA975.C37L58 2006
  174'.957—dc22
                                              2006012356

In memory of Pope John Paul II

1920–2005

Contributors

SARAH-VAUGHAN BRAKMAN, PH.D.
Assistant Professor of Philosophy and
Director of the Ethics Program (1999–2005)
Villanova University
Villanova, Pennsylvania

PETER J. CATALDO, PH.D.
Ethicist and Director of Research
National Catholic Bioethics Center
Philadelphia, Pennsylvania

FRANCIS L. DELMONICO, M.D.
Medical Director
New England Organ Bank
Newton, Massachusetts

Director of Renal Transplantation
Massachusetts General Hospital
Boston, Massachusetts

REV. RAYMOND J. DE SOUZA
Chaplain, Newman House
Queen's University
Kingston, Ontario

RICHARD M. DOERFLINGER
Associate Director for Policy Development
Secretariat for Pro-Life Activities
United States Conference of Catholic Bishops
Washington, D.C.

REV. KEVIN L. FLANNERY, S.J., S.T.D.
Dean of the Faculty of Philosophy and
Ordinary Professor of the History of
Ancient Philosophy
Pontifical Gregorian University
Rome, Italy

EDWARD J. FURTON, PH.D.
Ethicist and Director of Publications
National Catholic Bioethics Center
Philadelphia, Pennsylvania

JOHN M. HAAS, PH.D., S.T.D.
Ethicist and President
National Catholic Bioethics Center
Philadelphia, Pennsylvania

Dr. Oscar J. Martínez-González
Dean of the School of Bioethics
Anahuac University
Mexico City

Gilbert Meilaender, Ph.D.
Richard and Phyllis Duesenberg Professor
of Christian Ethics
Valparaiso University, Indiana
Member of the President's Council on Bioethics
Washington, D.C.

Rev. Gonzalo Miranda, L.C.
Dean of the School of Bioethics
Regina Apostolorum Pontifical University
Rome, Italy

Sr. Renée Mirkes, O.S.F., Ph.D.
Director of the Center for NaProEthics
Pope Paul VI Institute
Omaha, Nebraska

Rev. Albert S. Moraczewski, O.P., Ph.D
Ethicist and President Emeritus
National Catholic Bioethics Center
Philadelphia, Pennsylvania
Former Professor of Pharmacology
Baylor College of Medicine
Houston, Texas

Rev. Tadeusz Pacholczyk, Ph.D.
Ethicist and Director of Education
National Catholic Bioethics Center
Philadelphia, Pennsylvania

Very Rev. Russell E. Smith, S.T.D.
Episcopal Vicar for Health Care Ministries
Diocese of Richmond, Virginia
Past President
National Catholic Bioethics Center
Philadelphia, Pennsylvania

Anthony R. Tersigni, Ed.D., FACHE
President and Chief Executive Officer
Ascension Health
St. Louis, Missouri

Contents

—•—

Principles

Application

Appendices

FROM THE VATICAN

Dear Bishop Wuerl,

The Holy Father was pleased to learn that on January 24–28, 2005, the Twentieth Workshop for Bishops sponsored by The National Catholic Bioethics Center will be held in Dallas, Texas. He asks you to convey his cordial greetings to the Bishops from Canada, Central America, Mexico, the Philippines, and the United States who have assembled for this year's meeting of study and prayer. He also takes this occasion to express his gratitude to the Knights of Columbus for their consistent support of this important pastoral initiative, and to The National Catholic Bioethics Center for its efforts to contribute to the Church's judgment on the complex ethical issues emerging in the medical and life sciences.

His Holiness trusts that this year's workshop, dedicated to a study of the moral teachings proposed by the papal magisterium in recent decades, will provide renewed inspiration and direction to Bishops in their ministry as heralds of the Gospel and teachers of "the faith which is to be believed and put into practice" (see *Lumen Gentium*, n. 25). He is confident that their careful study and discernment of the principles guiding a sound ethical evaluation of new trends in medical research and clinical practice will promote an ever more fruitful dialogue with health-care professionals in the service of the human person, so that the integral good and the inviolable dignity of each individual will be better defended and promoted. As is tragically evident, the loss of a philosophically and theologically sound understanding of man has led, in many of our most technologically advanced societies, to an alarming lack of respect for God's gift of life from the first moment of conception to natural death. For its part, the Church's moral teaching, grounded in divine revelation and in the dictates of right reason, proposes a consistent anthropological vision which can offer much to the spiritual renewal of society, above all by its rejection of a utilitarian mentality which effectively denies the moral worth of particular human beings and does not shrink from using one class of persons for the presumed benefit of others. A clear proclamation and consistent application of Catholic moral doctrine is consequently an essential element of the Church's prophetic witness to the Gospel in contemporary culture.

It is the Holy Father's hope that the Workshop will pay particular attention to the delicate moral issue of personal and institutional cooperation with evil. The significant challenges facing Catholic health care institutions in changing social and economic situations must in no case detract from their fundamentally religious mission and corporate witness to the faith. For this reason, "established policies in complete conformity with the Church's moral teaching need to be firmly in place in Catholic health care facilities" (*Address to the Bishops of the Provinces of Portland in Oregon, Seattle, and Anchorage*, June 25, 2004, n. 5). If, in order to survive and to realize the great goods to which they are committed, such facilities must sometimes cooperate with other institutions which do not share their moral convictions, this cooperation must protect the right of individuals and institutions not to be party to immoral procedures involving violations of human dignity. "To refuse to take part in committing an injustice is not only a moral duty; it is also a basic human right" (*Evangelium vitae*, n. 74), which must be respected in every circumstance.

With these sentiments His Holiness assures the Bishops assembled in Dallas of a special remembrance in his prayers. Commending them, the organizers and presenters, and all associated with the Workshop, to the loving intercession of Mary, Mother of the Church, he cordially imparts his Apostolic Blessing as a pledge of wisdom, strength, and peace in the Lord.

With personal good wishes for the workshop, I remain

Yours sincerely in Christ,

+ Angelo Card. Sodano

ANGELO CARDINAL SODANO
Secretary of State
January 18, 2005

Welcome from Bishop Wuerl

As chairman of the board of The National Catholic Bioethics Center, it is my privilege and joy to welcome all of you to this twentieth workshop, which will focus on the moral legacy of Pope John Paul II in Catholic health care. This series of workshops began twenty-five years ago.

As you know, The National Catholic Bioethics Center offers a unique service to bishops as we carry out our episcopal ministry. This workshop continues a tradition of appreciation for and support of the episcopal teaching office. This year our theme has a direct pastoral significance, since we deal with the vision of human life and concomitant moral action that flows from our Catholic heritage rooted in the Gospel and articulated in the magisterium, most especially by our Holy Father.

Together with the other members of the board of directors and the officers of the Center, I offer you not only a welcome but an invitation to enjoy the scholarship provided us over the next several days. I encourage you to participate in the discussion and dialogue that are a hallmark of these workshops.

Over the years, this workshop has come to be for many of us an integral part of our own personal continuing education. It reflects our efforts as bishops to respond to the challenge of ongoing formation, particularly in an area as challenging and changing as medical-moral ethics. As a bishop, I have long been grateful for the work of The National Catholic Bioethics Center in preparing and presenting the material of these workshops.

Una bienvenída muy carinosa a nuéstros hermános, los obíspos del Caríbe, America Centrál y Mexico. Es un placér a saludárles en el nombre del Centro Nacional Católico Bioético y a celebrar nuestra solidáridád en el ministério episcopál.

Une bienvenue affectueuse à nos chers frères les évêcques francophones du Canada. Je vous prie d'accepter mes salutations pour cette opportunité d'exprimer notre solidarité dans notre ministère episcopal à l'occasion de cette reunion.

Our gathering and participation in this workshop is also a reflection of that solidarity in ministry that our Holy Father, Pope John Paul II, called for in the Post-Synodal Apostolic Exhortation *Ecclesia in America*. Here we are reminded that

> the bishops, remembering that "each of them is the visible, principal and foundation of the unity of his particular Church" cannot but feel duty bound to promote communion in their dioceses, so that the drive for a new evangelization in America may be more effective. (36)

Our Holy Father continues,

> Experiences of episcopal communion, more frequent since the Second Vatican Council as a result of the growth of Bishops' Conferences, should be seen as encounters with the living Christ, present in the brothers gathered in his name (cf. Mt. 18.20). (37)

This workshop serves, then, not only the purpose of bringing us together to enhance our teaching and pastoral ministry, but also to strengthen and manifest our own solidarity in episcopal ministry.

As you can see from the program, we have attempted to engage a variety of speakers who will deal with the issues in a way that will provide a solid overview. The program also includes those breakout sessions devoted to applying these principles in concrete situations and, in a particular manner, to reflect on issues as they affect the Church's effort to carry out her ministry, particularly her health-care ministry, today.

It has been my privilege to be associated with the Center and its workshops for a quarter of a century. It has always been one of the highlights of the program to receive the encouragement of our Holy Father. At every workshop since the first one, our Holy Father, Pope John Paul II, has indicated his appreciation of the efforts of the Center and his regard for the bishops who attend the workshop by sending a personal message. I am deeply honored to read these words of greetings from our Holy Father.

Just as the Holy Father has lent his moral support to the workshops, so the Knights of Columbus from the very beginning in 1980 have supported and made possible by their largess each and every one of the workshops. Therefore, a particular word of gratitude is in order to the Knights of Columbus, who through a grant make possible our gathering and this opportunity to explore the challenges and opportunities of episcopal ministry as we face the challenge of our theme.

The gracious generosity of the Knights is something we all appreciate, and I take the liberty of speaking for each of us gathered at this workshop to express profound and sincere thanks to Mr. Carl Anderson, the Supreme Knight and, through him, to all of our brother Knights of Columbus.

As you can see from the program that you received at registration, we have an exceptionally well prepared workshop, thanks to the efforts of The National Catholic Bioethics Center under the direction of Professor John M. Haas, its very competent and capable president. Since 1997, it has been a joy for me to work with John Haas not only in the preparation of these workshops but in the day-to-day activities of the Center that he so competently directs.

MOST REV. DONALD W. WUERL, S.T.D.
Bishop of Pittsburgh
Chairman of the Board of Directors
The National Catholic Bioethics Center
January 24, 2005

Greetings from the Knights of Columbus

On behalf of Carl Anderson, the Supreme Knight, and the more than 1.7 million members of the Knights of Columbus, I welcome you to the Twentieth Workshop for Bishops, sponsored by The National Catholic Bioethics Center.

Carl Anderson could not be here today. He was invited, along with Archbishop Dermot Martin, to offer a Catholic perspective on economics at the World Economic Summit in Davos, Switzerland. This is the first time in our 123 year history that a Supreme Knight has been invited to that convention. He will soon be making an intervention.

I know the work that you, the bishops, do at these workshops in grappling with the moral issues that now confront us. You really must become mini-scientists for a few days in order to understand how these new technologies affect all of us. Certainly the Knights of Columbus are with you in this endeavor. We are happy to be associated with The National Catholic Bioethics Center.

Today is the March for Life in Washington. Saturday was the anniversary of *Roe v. Wade*. We have reason to be optimistic today that either incrementally, or in toto, we can reverse *Roe v. Wade* and *Doe v. Bolton*. We at the Knights believe it is time for a more aggressive approach to these ill-conceived decisions. We need to speak out forcefully against them.

On today's anniversary of *Roe v. Wade*, Carl Anderson said:

> The year 2005 will be a pivotal year in the long battle to replace the culture of death, enabled by *Roe v. Wade*, with a culture of life. Roe has long been recognized as fundamentally flawed as a matter of constitutional law even by abortion proponents. And today, with the benefits of three decades of scientific research in human biology, it is readily apparent to all that its science was equally flawed.

We face today a new totalitarianism, in which attacks upon the human body are justified in the name of progress. More than ever, we need to understand the science that is tipping our world on its ear faster than we can determine its meaning for the moral life of our nation.

I wish you well in this work and ask God's blessings on this conference.

DEACON KENNETH N. RYAN
Supreme Treasurer of the
Knights of Columbus
January 24, 2005

In Appreciation of
Rev. Albert S. Moraczewski, O.P.

Rev. Albert S. Moraczewski, O.P., was the founder of the National Catholic Bioethics Center and is currently President Emeritus and Distinguished Scholar in Residence. His invaluable contributions to the Center and to research in Catholic bioethics were honored formally on the first day of the Workshop. This letter, from Rev. Carlos Azpiroz Costa, O.P., Master of the Dominican Order, was written on the occasion of the dedication of the Center's library to Fr. Moraczewski later in 2005.—Ed.

It is indeed with great joy that I have heard about the planned reception in The National Catholic Bioethics Center, during which the library of the Center will be dedicated in honor of Fr. Albert Moraczewski, O.P. To the words of esteem and gratitude that will be expressed on this occasion by Cardinal Justin Rigali, the present Archbishops and Bishops and other distinguished guests, including the numerous friends and disciples of Fr. Albert Moraczewski, I add my own words of thanks, respect, and support.

Fr. Albert Moraczewski, being the son of a Polish army doctor who served in France during World War I, received in his family a concern for the poor and sick and a profound understanding of the significance of the Hippocratic Oath that grants an ethical basis for all the medical professions. This, together with the intellectual formation that he has received as a Dominican friar and priest, enabled him very quickly to see the importance of the Church's attention ot the ethical formation of doctors, nurses, and scientists developing medical techniques. The establishment of the Pope John XXIII Center for Medical and Moral Research, which is now known as The National Catholic Bioethics Center, is a fruit of the genial intuition and the untiring service and devotion of Fr. Moraczewski. We know that today advances in medical techniques raise daily new and complex moral issues. It is important that these questions be studied with a competence in the principles of ethics and a thorough understanding of the matter itself. The scholarly work of Fr. Moraczewski and of the Center that he had strived to build is a great gift to the Church, and Fr. Moraczewski is respected in the Holy See for his work.

To this appreciation for the academic service of Fr. Moraczewski, I would like to add a very personal note of gratitude. It has come to my knowledge that Fr. Albert is very aware of the need to support the Master of the Dominican Order and his Council with his prayers. As he advances in age, and his scholarly work is reduced, he continues to support the Church and the Dominican Order with his daily prayers and sacrifices. For this, I can only express my sincere thanks.

I, in my turn, promise to remember both Fr. Albert and the Center that he founded in my prayers, as I remain sincerely yours in St. Dominic,

REV. CARLOS A. AZPIROZ COSTA, O.P.
Master of the Order of Preachers
Convento Santa Sabina
Rome

Principles

WHAT IS AT STAKE IN BIOETHICS?

Gilbert Meilaender

In asserting what he called "the legitimacy of the modern age," the philosopher Hans Blumenberg argued that self-assertion is the appropriate posture for human beings in the world.[1] By such self-assertion he meant to point to the curiosity for knowledge, our urge for technical mastery over nature (and over our own bodies), and our refusal to be drawn by anything that transcends the human. We need, Blumenberg argued, to set aside much of the hand-wringing that accompanies worry about our Promethean urge for mastery. We ought to stop thinking of the gods as powers who seek to stifle us and to keep us from making too much progress in the relief of suffering and the enhancement of human life. It is, of course, just such disquieting attempts at mastery that are often at stake in the questions of bioethics.

Portions of this paper were published under the title "Bioethics and the Character of Human Life" in *The New Atlantis* 1 (Spring 2003): 67–78.

[1] Hans Blumenberg, *The Legitimacy of the Modern Age* (Cambridge, MA: MIT Press, 1983).

When the Hastings Center was founded in 1969 as the first bioethics "think tank" in the United States, it planned research in four areas of concern: death and dying (and efforts to overcome the limits of our finitude); behavior control (and the relation between human activities and the happiness attendant upon them); genetic screening, counseling, and engineering (including questions of kinship, procreation, and attitudes toward future generations); and population policy and family planning (which, at least implicitly, asked about the relation of our own time to future generations). If we add explicit attention to moral problems raised by human experimentation, the list could still serve well today as a brief itemization of the central concerns of bioethics.

The reason these issues have been and continue to be central, and no doubt the reason bioethics has been an object of such lively public interest and concern, is obvious: These topics are not driven simply by concern for public policy regulations; rather, they involve some of the most important aspects of our humanity and raise some of the deepest questions about what it means to be human. In order to uncover those questions, I will attend not to the policy issues themselves but to the way they engage the meaning of our humanity, forcing upon us questions that lie in the background whenever we consider any of these problems. Acknowledging from the outset that much more might be said about any of the matters I take up, I will consider briefly four aspects of our humanity that are at stake in bioethics.

The Unity and Integrity of the Human Being

> The *body* is no longer perceived as a properly personal reality, a sign and place of relations with others, with God, and with the world. It is reduced to pure materiality: it is simply a complex of organs, functions, and energies to be used according to the sole criteria of pleasure and efficiency.[2] — JOHN PAUL II

The beginning of wisdom in bioethics may lie in the effort to think about what human beings are and why it matters morally how we think about what they are. From several different angles, medical advance has tempted us to lose sight of any sense in which the embodied human being is an integral,

---

[2] *The Gospel of Life* (Boston: Pauline Books & Media, 1995), n. 23.

organic whole, and has encouraged us to think of human beings as no more than collections of parts.

Suppose, for example, that we simply string together, in random order, sentences taken from different pages of a book—from, let us say, *The Gospel of Life*. No doubt each sentence, taken by itself, would be clear enough; yet the whole would be almost unintelligible. Why? What would have been lost? Would not the answer be that we would have lost the unity and integrity of the author?

One of the great blessings of the computer age, we are sometimes told, is that one can move sentences or whole paragraphs with ease. One need not work out a thesis or an argument. Just write—and then move the pieces around later. It is as if the argument were somehow built up from below—from words, phrases, and sentences moved around, combined, and recombined. As if a thesis would just emerge without an organizing intelligence, an authorial perspective, at work from the outset.

In our age of rapid advances in genetic knowledge, an analogous image has been used to characterize our humanity. Consider, for example, the following passage from biologist Thomas Eisner:

> As a consequence of recent advances in genetic engineering, [a biological species] must be viewed as ... a depository of genes that are potentially transferable. A species is not merely a hard-bound volume of the library of nature. It is also a loose-leaf book, whose individual pages, the genes, might be available for selective transfer and modification of other species.[3]

I have provided a humble illustration of this by inviting us to consider what it would be like to read a collection of sentences spliced together randomly from *The Gospel of Life*. And, letting our imaginations roam just a bit, we might also splice in sentences from Tolstoy's *Anna Karenina* and Kant's *Critique of Pure Reason*—producing thereby something we may not even know how to name. To think of a book this way would

---

[3] Thomas Eisner, "Chemical Ecology and Genetic Engineering: The Prospects for Plant Protection and the Need for Plant Habitat Conservation," Symposium on Tropical Biology and Agriculture, St. Louis, Missouri, July 15, 1985. Cited in Mary Midgley, "Biotechnology and Monstrosity," *Hastings Center Report* 30.5 (September–October 2000): 11.

be to ignore the presence of an authorial hand. It would treat a book as if it were just the sum of a number of words, sentences, or paragraphs. Part of what is at stake in bioethics today is that we might try to think of human beings (or the other animals) in this way: as collections of genes, or as collections of organs possibly available for transplant. What is lost, however, is a sense of ourselves as integrated, organic wholes.

Even if we think of the human being as an integrated organism, the nature of its unity remains puzzling in a second way. The seeming duality of person and body has played a significant role in bioethics. As the language of "personhood" gradually came to prominence in bioethical reflection, attention has often been directed to circumstances in which the duality of body and person seems pronounced. Suppose a child is born who, throughout his life, will be profoundly retarded. Or suppose an elderly woman has now become severely demented. Suppose because of trauma a person lapses into a permanent vegetative state. How shall we describe such human beings? Is it best to say that they are no longer persons? Or is it more revealing to describe them as severely disabled persons? Similar questions arise with embryos and fetuses. Are they human organisms that have not yet attained personhood? Or are they the weakest and most vulnerable of human persons?

Related questions arise when we think of conditions often, but controversially, regarded as disabilities. Perhaps those who are deaf and have learned to sign create and constitute a culture of their own, a manualist as opposed to an oralist culture. If so, one might argue that they are disabled only in an oralist culture, even as those who hear would be disabled if placed in the midst of a manualist culture. So long as the deaf are able to function at a high level within that manualist culture, does it matter what way they function? Notice that the harder we press such views, the less significant becomes any normative human form. A head, or a brain, might be sufficient, if it could find ways to carry out at a high level of mastery the functions we think are important. But then, of course, in the words I quoted from John Paul II, the body would no longer be perceived "as a properly personal reality" but, rather, as "a complex of organs, functions and energies."

Such puzzles are inherent in the human condition, and they are sufficiently puzzling that we may struggle to find the right language in which to discuss that aspect of the human being which cannot be reduced to body. Within the unity of the human being a duality remains, and I will here use the language of "spirit" to gesture toward it. As embodied spirits (or inspirited bodies), we stand at the juncture of nature and spirit, tempted by reductionisms of various sorts. We have no access to the spirit—the person—apart from the body, which is the locus of personal presence; yet we are deeply ill at ease in the presence of a living human body from which all that is personal seems absent. It is fair to say, I think, that in reflecting upon the duality of our nature, we have traditionally given a kind of primacy to the living human body. Thus, uneasy as we might be with the living body from which the person seems absent, we would be very reluctant indeed to bury that body while its heart still beat.

In any case, the problems of bioethics force us to ask what a human being really is and, in doing so, to reflect upon the unity and integrity of the human person. We must think about the moral meaning of the living human body—whether it exists simply as an interchangeable collection of parts, whether it exists merely as a carrier for something else (the personal realm of mind or spirit), whether a living human being who lacks cognitive, personal qualities is no longer one of us or, rather, is simply the weakest and most needy one of us. This is one aspect of our humanity that is at stake in bioethics.

Finitude and Freedom

> Human nature ... could be reduced to and treated as a readily available biological or social material. This ultimately means making freedom self-defining and a phenomenon creative of itself and its values. Indeed, when all is said and done man would not even have a nature; he would be his own personal life-project. Man would be nothing more than his own freedom.[4] — JOHN PAUL II

In one of his essays collected in *The Medusa and the Snail*, the late Lewis Thomas explored the deeply buried origins of our word "hybrid." It comes from the Latin *hybrida*, the name for the offspring of a wild boar and a domestic sow. But in its more distant origins the word, as Thomas puts it, "carries its own disapproval inside." Its more distant etymological ancestor is the Greek *hubris*, insolence against the gods. That is, buried somewhere in the development of our

---

[4] *The Splendor of Truth* (Boston: St. Paul Books & Media, 1993), n. 46.

language is a connection between two beings unnaturally joined together and human usurping of the prerogatives of the gods. Thomas summarizes his excursion into etymology as follows:

> This is what the word has grown into, a warning, a code word, a shorthand signal from the language itself: if man starts doing things reserved for the gods, deifying himself, the outcome will be something worse for him, symbolically, than the litters of wild boars and domestic sows were for the Romans.[5]

That is only one side of the matter, however. For Thomas can also write in a provocative paragraph:

> Is there something fundamentally unnatural, or intrinsically wrong ... in the ambition that drives us all to reach a comprehensive understanding of nature, including ourselves? I cannot believe it. It would seem to be a more unnatural thing ... for us to come on the same scene endowed as we are with curiosity ... and then for us to do nothing about it or, worse, to try to suppress the questions. This is the greater danger for our species, to try to pretend ... that we do not need to satisfy our curiosity.[6]

Using some old religious language, we might say that Thomas sees how, given the duality of our nature, we may go wrong in either of two ways: pride or sloth. As prideful beings, we may strive to be all freedom—acknowledging no limits to our creativity, supposing that our wisdom is sufficient to master the world. As slothful beings, we may timidly fear freedom and ignore the lure of new possibilities. Either is a denial of something essential to being human, a reduction of the full meaning of our humanity. Clearly, Thomas is inclined to fear most the dangers of sloth, but that may be only the mark in him of a passing modernity.

In any case, the duality of body and person—explored briefly in my first point above—is clearly related to what we may call a duality of finitude and freedom. The human being is the place where freedom and finitude meet; hence, it will always contravene something significant in our humanity to act as if we were *really* only free personal spirit or only finite body. Yet, because of the two-sidedness of our nature, we can look at a human being from each of these angles.

---

[5] Lewis Thomas, "The Hazards of Science," in *The Medusa and the Snail* (New York: Viking Press, 1979), 65–75.

[6] Ibid..

Drop me from the top of a fifty-story building and the law of gravity takes over, just as it does if we drop a stone. We are finite beings, located in space and time, subject to natural necessity. But we are also free, able sometimes to transcend the seeming limits of nature and history. As I fall from that fifty-story building, there are truths about my experience that cannot be captured by an explanation in terms of mass and velocity. Something different happens in my fall than in the rock's fall, for this falling object is also a subject characterized by self-awareness. I can know myself as a falling object, which means that I can to some degree "distance" my*self* from that falling object. I cannot simply be equated with it. I am that falling object, yet I am also free from it.

What is true of our nature is, to some extent, also true of our history. I am the person constituted by the story of my life. I cannot simply be someone else with a different history. Yet I can also, at least to some degree, step into another's story, see the world as it looks to him—and thus be free from the limits of my history. The crucial question, of course, is whether there is any limit to such free self-transcendence—whether we are, in fact, wise enough and good enough to be free self-creators or whether we should acknowledge destructive possibilities in our culture's inclination to think of human beings as nothing other than the freedom to make and remake themselves.

Understanding our nature as both finite and free, we can appreciate how hard it may be to evaluate advances in medicine, claims about the importance (or even obligatoriness) of research, attempts to enhance our nature in various ways, or efforts to master death. If we simply oppose the forward thrust of scientific medicine, we fail to honor human freedom. The zealous desire to know, to probe the secrets of nature, to combat disease—all that is an expression of our freedom from the limits of the "given." Yet, of course, if we can never find reason to stop in this restless attempt at mastery, we may fail to honor the finite limits of our wisdom and virtue. Human freedom, as John Paul II has put it, "finds its authentic and complete fulfillment precisely in the acceptance" of God's law.[7] Thus, it may trivialize freedom to think of it as limitless.

There is probably no cookbook that gives the recipe for knowing how best to honor—simultaneously—both our freedom and our finitude. That there ought to be limits to our

---

[7] *Splendor of Truth*, n. 35.

freedom does not mean that we can easily state them in advance. But a truly human bioethics will recognize not only the creative but also the destructive possibilities in the exercise of our freedom. Thus, from a second and slightly different angle, we can see a part of what is at stake in bioethics.

The Relation between the Generations

> Procreation brings it about that the man and the woman ... know each other reciprocally in the "third," sprung from them both. Therefore, this knowledge becomes a discovery.[8] — JOHN PAUL II

Because we are not only free but are also embodied spirits, the biological bond that connects the generations has moral meaning for us. We occupy a fixed place in the generations of humankind. Both Jews and Christians inculcate a command that calls upon us to honor our father and mother. It is, after all, a puzzling duty: to show gratitude for a bond in which we find ourselves without ever having freely chosen it. Yet, of course, insofar as the child is a "gift," we might say that father and mother have also not chosen this bond. They too simply find themselves in it. A truly limitless freedom to make and remake ourselves, to pursue our projects in the world, would divorce us from the lines of kinship and descent that locate and identify us. Would that be the fulfillment of our nature? Or alienation from it?

It is, I think, fair to say that several different aspects of medical advance—in reproductive technologies, in psychopharmacology, in genetic screening, and one day perhaps in techniques for genetic enhancement or cloning—have made it more difficult for both parents and children simply to honor and affirm the bond between the generations and accept as a gift the lines of kinship that locate and identify them.

We are given a captivating image of the child as gift in Galway Kinnell's poem, "After Making Love We Hear Footsteps":

> For I can snore like a bullhorn
> Or play loud music
> or sit up talking with any reasonably sober Irishman
> and Fergus will only sink deeper
> into his dreamless sleep, which goes by all in one
>   flash,

---

[8] General audience of March 12, 1980, in *The Theology of the Body: Human Love in the Divine Plan* (Boston: Pauline Books & Media, 1997), 81.

but let there be that heavy breathing
or a stifled come-cry anywhere in the house
and he will wrench himself awake
and make for it on the run—as now, we lie together,
after making love, quiet, touching along the length of
    our bodies,
familiar touch of the long-married,
and he appears—in his baseball pajamas, it happens,
the neck opening so small he has to screw them on,
which one day may make him wonder
about the mental capacity of baseball players—
and flops down between us and hugs us and snuggles
    himself to sleep,
his face gleaming with satisfaction at being this very
    child.

In the half darkness we look at each other
and smile
and touch arms across his little, startlingly muscled
    body—
this one whom habit of memory propels to the ground
    of his making,
sleeper only the mortal sounds can sing awake,
this blessing loves gives again into our arms.[9]

This image, of the child as a gift that is the fruition not of an act of rational will but an act of love, can be contrasted with an image of the child as the parents' project or product. For the latter way of thinking, having a child becomes a project we undertake to satisfy our purposes and make our life complete. And, of course, our desire may be not simply for a child but for a child of a certain kind—of a certain sex, with certain characteristics or capacities. Human cloning, were it possible, would from one angle bring to completion this image of the next generation as a product of rational will, undertaken to fulfill our desires. From another angle, of course, cloning might be thought to break entirely the bond between the generations, since in the instance of cloning we do not even know how to name the relation between progenitor and offspring.

Pondering how best to think about the relation between the generations, we are driven once again to questions about when we should use our freedom to seek mastery or control and when, by contrast, we should accept certain limits inherent in human bodily life. The twentieth century began with

---

[9] Galway Kinnell, *Mortal Acts, Mortal Words* (Boston, MA: Houghton Mifflin, 1980), 5.

considerable confidence in the possibility of eugenic control of the relation between the generations. That confidence suffered eclipse in the face of revelations of Nazi eugenic experiments, but it has reemerged in quite different ways. Today, any state-sponsored eugenic ideology would surely face considerable opposition, but instead we have "privatized" eugenic decisions.

Here again, there is no simple recipe for making decisions. Parents must indeed exercise reason and will to shape their children's lives. They do not and should not simply accept as given whatever disabilities, sufferings, or (even just) disappointments come their children's way. Still, as every child realizes at some point, the conscientious parent's effort to nurture and enhance can be crushing. It can make it difficult to accept the child who has been given, impossible to say simply "it's good that you exist."[10] And we must say that if we are to see in the child not simply our own image but, as John Paul II writes, "the image of God's glory."[11]

The implications for the bond between the generations become still more far-reaching when we consider that research may make possible alteration of the human germ line. More than fifty years ago, without any precise knowledge of such intervention, C. S. Lewis contemplated such eugenic efforts, and he noted the salient point that relates to my theme here: "What we call Man's power over Nature turns out to be a power exercised by some men over other men with Nature as its instrument."[12]

Alterations in the human germline would be an awesome exercise of human freedom and, if used in the struggle against disease, might promise (over time) a cure not only for individual sufferers but also for the human species. Yet, of course, the exercise of freedom is also an exercise of power, and just as—synchronically—parents need to allow the mystery of humanity to unfold in the lives of their children, so also—diachronically—one generation needs to allow others their freedom. How we sort out these competing goods will reveal much about how we understand the character of human life and will express our own insight into what is at stake in bioethics.

---

[10] Josef Pieper, *About Love* (Chicago: Franciscan Herald Press, 1974), 19.

[11] *Gospel of Life*, n. 84.

[12] C. S. Lewis, *The Abolition of Man* (New York: Macmillan, 1947), 69.

Suffering and Vulnerability

Although martyrdom represents the high point of the witness to moral truth, and one to which relatively few people are called, there is nonetheless a consistent witness which all Christians must daily be ready to make, even at the cost of suffering and grave sacrifice.[13] — JOHN PAUL II

Part of the sadness of human life is that we sometimes cannot and other times ought not do for others what they fervently desire. With respect to the relief of suffering, the great quest of modern research medicine, this is certainly true. Some relief we are unable to provide, a fact that only gives greater impetus to our efforts to discover causes and cures. It is precisely the fact of our inability to help in the face of great suffering that fuels the research "imperative" of which we are all beneficiaries. Nevertheless, it is important to ask how overriding this "imperative" is—whether there are means to the possible relief of suffering which we ought not take up, and whether it would be good if we were not vulnerable to suffering.

So great is our modern concern to overcome suffering, we may almost forget that there are perspectives from which this goal is deliberately made secondary. For anyone drawn to Stoic philosophy, for example, bodily suffering could not finally be of overriding significance. It can harm us only if we are deceived into supposing that anything other than one's own inner self-mastery really counts. Consider Seneca's story of the sage Stilbo.[14] His country was captured, his children and wife were lost; yet, "as he emerged from the general desolation alone and yet happy, [he] spoke as follows to Demetrius, called Sacker of Cities because of the destruction he brought upon them, in answer to the question whether he had lost anything: 'I have all my goods with me!'" And Seneca's comment demonstrates the power of Stoicism:

> There is a brave and stout-hearted man for you! The enemy conquered, but Stilbo conquered his conqueror. "I have lost nothing!" Aye, he forced Demetrius to wonder whether he himself had conquered after all. "My goods are all with me!" In other words, he deemed nothing that might be taken from him to be a good.[15]

---

[13] *Splendor of Truth*, n. 93.

[14] Seneca, "Epistle IX: On Philosophy and Friendship," in *Ad Lucilium: Epistulae Morales I*, trans. Richard M. Gummere (London: William Heinemann, 1925), 42–57.

[15] Ibid.

While it may be hard sometimes not to be repelled by the harshness of such Stoic vision, it is equally hard not to recognize the nobility of an outlook that makes how we live more important than how long. And if it seems to denigrate too much the goods of everyday life, we can detect a similar nobility in another ancient worldview that does not think these ordinary goods of no account.

Discussing some sermons of St. Augustine, first preached in the year 397 but newly discovered only in 1990, Peter Brown notes that Augustine was often required to preach at festivals of the martyrs. At Augustine's time the cult of the martyrs continued to be of profound importance to average Christians, for persecution was still a recent memory. The martyrs were the great heroes, the "muscular athletes" and "triumphant stars" of the faith. But, Brown suggests, one can see Augustine quite deliberately making the feasts of the martyrs "less dramatic, so as to stress the daily drama of God's workings in the heart of the average Christian."[16] For that average believer did not doubt that God's grace had been spectacularly displayed in the courage of the martyrs. What he was likely to doubt, however, was whether such heroism could possibly be displayed in his own less dramatic and more humdrum day-to-day existence. So Augustine points "away from the current popular ideology of the triumph of the martyrs to the smaller pains and triumphs of daily life."

An example of how he does this is instructive. "God has many martyrs in secret," Augustine tells his hearers. "Sometimes you shiver with fever: you are fighting. You are in bed: it is you who are the athlete." Brown comments:

> Exquisite pain accompanied much late-Roman medical treatment. Furthermore, everyone, Augustine included, believed that amulets provided by skilled magicians ... did indeed protect the sufferer—but at the cost of relying on supernatural powers other than Christ alone. They worked. To neglect them was like neglecting any other form of medicine. But the Christian must not use them. Thus, for Augustine to liken a Christian sickbed to a scene of martyrdom was not a strained comparison.[17]

Here again—though in a way of life that will be, in some respects, quite different from Stoicism—one sees an outlook for

---

[16] Peter Brown, *Augustine of Hippo: A New Edition with an Epilogue* (Berkeley, CA: University of California Press, 2000), 454.

[17] Ibid.

24

which relief of suffering, however desired and desirable, is not the overriding imperative of life. To the degree that John Paul II has accurately described our own "cultural climate" as one which "considers suffering the epitome of evil, to be eliminated at all costs," we can hardly claim to have made much moral progress since the time of Augustine.[18]

The Stoics remind us that an authentically human life may prize goodness more than happiness and, indeed, that true virtue may be achieved precisely when we seem most vulnerable to suffering. The ancient Christians remind us that one might value competing goods (such as faithfulness to God) more highly than relief of suffering.

In the modern world we may admire such views, but we tend to keep our distance from them. The quest for health, the attempt to master nature in service of human need and to refuse to accept the body's vulnerability to suffering, has characterized the modern period. If such a world offers less occasion for the display of nobility, it does not despise the sufferings of countless ordinary people—and that is no small gain. The research that makes such gains possible is greatly to be desired, but is it also imperative? Many questions of bioethics, especially of research, invite us to try to determine the difference between the desirable and the imperative.

One of the now classic essays in bioethics, first published in 1969, was Hans Jonas's "Philosophical Reflections on Experimenting with Human Subjects."[19] It articulated at the very outset of the development of bioethics a difference between the desirable and the imperative. Jonas noted that sometimes it is imperative that a society avoid disaster; hence, we conscript soldiers to fight. The fact that we do not (ordinarily) conscript experimental subjects indicates that, however much we value the improvements to life made possible by medical research, we do not think of ourselves as having an obligation to make such improvements. Research brings betterment of our lives; it does not save our society.

Because this is true, we seek volunteers, not conscripts, in the cause of medical progress. And because this is true, far from using those who might be most readily available as handy research subjects, we should be most reluctant to use them.

---

[18] *Gospel of Life*, n. 15.

[19] Reprinted in Hans Jonas, *Philosophical Essays* (Englewood Cliffs, NJ: Prentice-Hall, 1974), 105–131.

Indeed, Jonas defended "the inflexible principle that utter helplessness demands utter protection." That is, the vulnerability that ought to concern us most is not our own vulnerability to illness and suffering but, rather, the vulnerability of those whose very helplessness might make them seem all too readily available to us in our never-ending struggle to make progress. If utter helplessness demands utter protection, we will have to ask ourselves whether it is right to build our medical progress upon the sacrificed lives of those—such as so-called "spare" embryos—who seem expendable because doomed to die anyway.

Finally, we must also ask ourselves whether there might be research that is neither imperative nor desirable. If goodness is to be prized more than happiness, the endless quest to remake and enhance human life, to overcome vulnerability, may destroy other, equally important goods of an authentically human life. We recognize this truth, for example, in our role as parents. Conscientious parents want with all their hearts to give their children what they need, to make them happy. They also know, however, that some goods cannot be given but must be developed and achieved in the child's own life. We cannot simply give our children the happiness that comes from finding a vocation, a spouse, or inner strength. Trying to give such goods would, in effect, subvert and undermine them. So, too, we have to ask whether there might be research aims which, however well-intentioned, would seek to bestow traits of character and skill that have no value apart from the process whereby they are developed and achieved. We are, that is, forced to ask hard questions about projects aimed at "enhancing" human nature.

Where do such ambivalent reflections lead? Bioethics directs our attention to *bios*—to human bodily life in all its vulnerability and with all the goods (biological, rational, cultural, spiritual) that characterize it. For that life we seek health, and in that life we seek to avoid suffering. These are great goods of bodily life, but they sometimes compete with other, equally human goods. Relief of suffering is surely of great importance; yet it remains only one desideratum of a truly human life. At a few times and places it may seem imperative; at many times and places it is desirable; in some times and places, because we judge other, competing goods to be even more fundamental to human life, it may be neither imperative nor desirable. This too is part of what is at stake in bioethics.

26

The Myth of Prometheus

> There exists in contemporary culture a certain Promethean attitude which leads people to think that they can control life and death by taking the decisions about them into their own hands.[20] — JOHN PAUL II

When Jean-Jacques Rousseau published what we call his "first discourse," which discussed whether the arts and sciences have contributed to the betterment of human life, he chose as its frontispiece an image of Prometheus bringing fire to earth. To a satyr standing nearby, who reaches out to embrace and kiss the fire, Prometheus cries out: "Satyr, you will mourn the loss of the beard on your chin, for it burns when touched."

That captures quite well the ambivalence the story of Prometheus is usually thought to carry. Fire brings light and warmth, making possible all the useful arts and sciences that enhance human life—but it burns if you get too close and embrace it. On the one hand, the exercise of human freedom through scientific and technological advance is of great benefit; yet, on the other hand, we need to find a safe way to gain those benefits for ourselves without simultaneously getting burned.

This way of reading the myth expresses the duality of our nature as finite and free, and I have, to some degree, drawn on such an understanding in my discussion of what is at stake in bioethics. Nevertheless, there is, I think, a danger in allowing ourselves to draw this lesson from the Prometheus myth. The lesson, at least as we often understand it, tends to hold up before us a yellow light. Not green—since, after all, we know the myth, and we do not want to be moved by hubris. But also not red—since, after all, the technology that makes fire possible is a great good, and we want to garner its benefits.

But yellow. And what does a yellow light mean? It means, "proceed with caution." That is to say, keep on going. Keep on proceeding. Do not stop. And, moreover, proceed with a very good conscience, because we know that we are being cautious, thoughtful, and morally concerned. Such people never find a good enough reason to stop.

Quite often, of course, proceeding with caution is perfectly sound advice. But it also gives us a good conscience about our mastery of nature, and it never suggests that we

---

[20] *Gospel of Life*, n. 15.

might do anything other than continue to advance. The ability to stop, to refuse to characterize our freedom as limitless, is also at stake in bioethics. This means, of course, that it is our humanity that is at stake; for without the ability to recognize that we are not gods, without a willingness to accept limits to our freedom, we cannot remain human. Seeking to be more than human, we must inevitably become less; for, as John Paul II has written, "when the sense of God is lost, there is also a tendency to lose the sense of man."[21]

---

[21] Ibid., n. 21.

EVANGELIUM VITAE AND THE STRUGGLE FOR A CULTURE OF LIFE

John M. Haas

One of the most distinctive characteristics of the pontificate of John Paul II was certainly his concern with culture. In almost all his encyclicals, apostolic exhortations, and formal addresses, he called for a new evangelization of culture. Very early in his pontificate, he established the Pontifical Council for Culture. In his great encyclical on the "life issues," *Evangelium vitae*, he delineated the attributes of a culture of death and a culture of life, terms which have now come to be incorporated into contemporary social discourse and debate.

According to George Weigel, the late Pope's biographer, John Paul II adopted a "cultural priority," or a "culture-first approach," in his petrine ministry.[1] In dealing with two totalitarian regimes in his homeland, the Pope knew how critically important culture was to preserving the national identity of his country. John Paul II was also keenly aware of the writings of the Marxist Antonio Gramsci and of Gramsci's belief that the Communist revolution could most effectively be brought

---

[1] George Weigel, "John Paul II and the Priority of Culture," *First Things* 80 (February 1998): 19–25.

about by permeating the political and cultural institutions of society with a Marxist system of values, attitudes, and beliefs. Gramsci, an educational theorist who died in 1937, had been committed to revolution through cultural means.

Both the Marxist philosopher Gramsci and the Catholic philosopher Wojtyla were aware of the importance of cultural institutions for transforming a society. The Marxist, of course, saw culture as a reflection of the underlying economic and material structures of a society, while the Catholic saw culture as an expression of humanity's deepest beliefs and spiritual aspirations. The word *culture,* after all, is derived from *cultus,* "worship," and John Paul II saw clearly that what a society worships will be reflected in its political and social institutions, in its art, its poetry, and its music.

The most lapidary definition of culture that I have found in the writings of Pope John Paul II is contained in an address he gave in Los Angeles during his second pastoral visit to the United States. In his meeting with the bishops on September 16, 1987, the Holy Father asked:

> But how is the American culture evolving today? Is this evolution being influenced by the Gospel? ... Your music, your poetry and art, your drama, your painting and sculpture, the literature that you are producing—are all those things which reflect the soul of a nation being influenced by the spirit of Christ for the perfection of humanity?[2]

Here we have a wonderfully concise definition of culture: "all those things which reflect the soul of a nation."

Some have considered *Evangelium vitae* to be a significant advance in Catholic moral thought as it grappled with the growing practices of abortion and euthanasia. In harsh language, the Pope speaks of "an extremely serious and mortal danger: that of confusion between good and evil." He speaks of a threat to civilization itself. He argues that "among all the crimes which can be committed against life, procured abortion has characteristics making it particularly serious and deplorable."[3]

But these insights are a matter of morality, not of faith. In *Evangelium vitae,* the Pope repeatedly points out that the pro-

---

[2] National Catholic News Service, *Pope John Paul II "Building up the Body of Christ": Pastoral Visit to the United States* (San Francisco: Ignatius Press, 1987), 188.

[3] John Paul II, *Evangelium vitae* (March 25, 1995), n. 58.

hibition against the direct killing of the innocent is of the natural law. At the very beginning of the encyclical he states:

> Even in the midst of difficulties and uncertainties, every person sincerely open to truth and goodness can, by the light of reason and the hidden action of grace, come to recognize in the natural law written in the heart (cf. Rom 2:14–15) the sacred value of human life from its very beginning until its end, and can affirm the right of every human being to have this primary good respected to the highest degree. Upon the recognition of this right, every human community and the political community itself are founded.[4]

In *Evangelium vitae,* the Pope points out that abortion is murder and an unspeakable crime, hardly theological concepts, and that it ought to be called by its proper name.[5] He also goes to lengths to show that the evil of abortion has been a constant teaching of the Church and is hardly a development. He quotes the *Didache.* He quotes Athenagoras, an early Greek Father of the Church, and Tertullian, a theologian of the West. Through this he shows that the universal Church, East and West, from the very beginning taught that abortion, infanticide, and euthanasia were heinous crimes. Consequently, the teaching contained in *Evangelium vitae* can hardly be seen as a development of Catholic thought.

Rather, *Evangelium vitae* is more correctly to be seen as a profound cultural critique of contemporary liberal societies. In this encyclical we see the Pope struggling with the fact that a profound cultural shift has occurred. The encyclical attempts to ascertain how it is possible that human actions which until very recently were considered crimes have now come to be viewed as human rights. The Pope points out that this tragic development is fundamentally not a political but a "cultural crisis":

> A new cultural climate is developing and taking hold, which gives crimes against life a *new and—if possible—even more sinister character,* giving rise to further grave concern: broad sectors of public opinion justify certain crimes against life in the name of the rights of individual freedom, and on this basis they claim not only exemption from punishment

---

[4] Ibid., n. 2

[5] See *Evangelium vitae,* n. 65: "Depending on the circumstances, [euthanasia] involves the malice proper to suicide or murder." See also n. 58.

but even authorization by the State, so that these things can be done with total freedom ... [which is] a disturbing symptom and a significant cause of grave moral decline. Choices once unanimously considered criminal and rejected by the common moral sense are gradually becoming socially acceptable.[6]

His dismay at this cultural shift is apparent throughout the encyclical. He says elsewhere:

It is not only that in generalized opinion these attacks tend no longer to be considered as "crimes"; paradoxically they assume the nature of "rights," to the point that the State is called upon to give them *legal recognition and to make them available through the free services of health-care personnel.*[7]

One cannot read this encyclical without recognizing the United States as a prime example of what the Pope has called a culture of death. The cultural determinants of most societies are so generally accepted and pervasive that it is almost impossible for people to recognize them. There are, indeed, certain unexamined presuppositions of contemporary American culture which direct the manner in which our common life is ordered and determine the manner and substance of our debates about public policy. The Pope names them for us and calls on us to examine them.

First of all, there is a disordered understanding of freedom. He writes, "To claim the right to abortion, infanticide and euthanasia, and to recognize that right in law, means to attribute to human freedom a *perverse and evil significance*: that of an *absolute power over others and against others.*"[8] Other determinants of liberal democratic societies to which the Pope refers are radical individualism, which gives rise to such a perverse sense of freedom; moral relativism; utilitarianism; and secularism.

In the encyclical the Pope points out that it is the duty of religious individuals of all persuasions to place themselves at the service of life, and that this will lead to a "practical ecumenism":

Service of the *Gospel of life* is ... an immense and complex task. This service increasingly appears as a valuable and

---

[6] *Evangelium vitae*, n. 4 (emphasis added).

[7] Ibid., n. 11 (emphasis added).

[8] Ibid., n. 20 (emphasis added).

fruitful area for positive cooperation with our brothers and sisters of other Churches and ecclesial communities, in accordance with the *practical ecumenism* which the Second Vatican Council authoritatively encouraged.... It also appears as a providential area for dialogue and joint efforts with the followers of other religions and with all people of good will. *No single person or group has a monopoly on the defence and promotion of life. These are everyone's task and responsibility* ... [to] prevent a setback of unforeseeable consequences for civilization.[9]

In its struggle against the anti-life forces and in its defense of life and marriage and family, the Catholic Church has at times forged a very effective alliance with evangelical Christians. But this "serious and mortal danger" which we now face in common did not appear suddenly. As the Pope says, "with tragic consequences, a long historical process is reaching a turning point."[10]

One of the most significant factors in that "long historical process" is, in my estimation, Protestantism. I call attention to this with some hesitancy because of what the Pope said about practical ecumenism and because I came to know and love Jesus Christ as a Protestant. Furthermore, as I said, there are some Protestants who are our staunchest allies in the struggle against the culture of death. But if we would earnestly reflect on the cultural critique provided by the Pope in this encyclical in order more effectively to counter the culture of death, then it seems it is necessary to understand what has contributed to it. I believe one of the reasons the struggle for life is so difficult in the United States is because American culture has been shaped so definitively by Protestantism that the entire debate is generally framed in its terms. Even the secularist opponents of our Protestant brothers and sisters largely couch the debates in Protestant terms. Despite the fact that the Catholic Church is the largest religious body in the United States, the cultural influences are overwhelmingly those of Protestantism.

The Pope spoke of individualism, subjectivism, and moral relativism giving rise to the culture of death. Yet the rise of western subjectivism and individualism can be seen to a large extent in the Protestant movement of the sixteenth century, which tended to repudiate communal life, tradition, and

---

[9] Ibid., n. 91 (emphasis added).

[10] Ibid., n. 18.

hierarchical authority by appealing to its formulae of *sola scriptura*, *sola gratia*, and *sola fides*. The individual Christian was saved when he responded to the Word of God in faith. Luther mistranslated Romans, as we all know, to insist that we are saved "by grace through faith alone." The "alone" was his hermeneutical addition.

Through faith the Christian could also claim the right to individual interpretation of Scripture. The theoreticians of the Protestant movement developed the notion of a spiritual church over against the visible church of the flesh. Christian faith became spiritualized, subjective and individual. Even the communal sacraments of baptism and communion no longer actually and in fact incorporated one into the Body of Christ and deepened one's membership in that Mystical Body. They became mere public testimonies to the fact that a person had already been saved due to the gift of faith given by God to that particular individual.

Also repudiated in some ways—and this really needs to be acknowledged—was the capacity of the intellect to raise itself to God. Luther, with his doctrine of the total depravity of man, feared that an erroneous regard for reason over against faith would place one's salvation in jeopardy. In his *Commentary on Galatians* he wrote, "Every Christian is a true priest; for first he offers up and kills his own reason ... the evening sacrifice is to kill reason."[11] He went so far elsewhere as to refer to reason as "the Devil's greatest whore."[12]

The general understanding of religion in the United States is that it is irrational, dealing with emotion or perhaps moral sensibility but not with truth or the intellect. In 1984, in *Time* magazine, Roger Rosenblatt wrote an opinion piece titled "Defenders of the Faith," which is highly characteristic of widespread American understanding of religion. Arguing for the separation of Church and state Rosenblatt wrote, "Fundamentally, religions oppose rational processes." He then went on to quote Martin Luther, not fairly, but in Luther's own words: "Reason is the greatest enemy that faith has. It never

---

[11] John Dillenberger, ed., *Martin Luther: Selections from His Writings* (Garden City, NJ: Anchor Books, 1961), 131.

[12] Martin Luther, "Last Sermon in Wittenberg, Second Sunday in Epiphany, 17 January 1546," *Dr. Martin Luther's Werke: Kritische Gesamtsusgabe* (Weimar, Germany: Herman Boehlaus Nachfolger, 1914), band 51, 126.

comes to the aid of spiritual things, but ... struggles against the divine Word."[13] Rosenblatt continued:

> Governments depend wholly on rational processes.... When religions and governments clash, therefore, it is a collision not simply of institutions but of entirely different ways of apprehending experience.... All this connects with the American debate on church versus state in a fundamental way.... Keeping church and state apart was a way of separating reason and passion, or reason and faith, another check and balance ... the premises of church and state are not merely opposed but actively antagonistic.... In short, church and state are natural enemies, not because one is superior to the other ... but because they make antipodal and competing claims on the mind.[14]

The Pope countered this particular erroneous cultural understanding of religion and the relationship between faith and reason in his encyclical *Fides et ratio*, showing that there was no incompatibility between faith and reason in the Catholic intellectual tradition. Yet I remember the absolute incredulity of the CEO of a prominent biotechnology firm, Advanced Cell Technology, when I told him that the Pope had written a work on the compatibility between science and religion, reason and faith. He had been raised in a strict Protestant home and thought the nature of religion was to be set over against reason and science. He told me that this was the reason he left his religion behind when he decided to pursue a career in science.

One of the reasons that the debate over embryonic stem cells is so difficult to wage is the public perception that the position of the Catholic Church on the status of the human embryo is an article of faith. In the course of the debates, I have heard the Church's position on embryonic stem cell research referred to as "dogma." If one is Catholic, it is thought, then one must accept the humanity of the embryo "on faith." In fact, the Catholic presidential candidate in the last election said precisely that.

Nothing could be further from the truth, of course. The ontological reality of the embryo can be established by science. But the cultural perception of religion in this country is that if a Christian holds a particular moral position, it must be

---

[13] Roger Rosenblatt, "Defenders of the Faith," *Time* magazine (November 12, 1984).

[14] Ibid.

because it has been mandated by the Bible or by an irrational religious authority.

If one adopts a position of *sola scriptura*, then the scriptures become the sole source for the moral life. Evangelical Christians were initially slow to join the pro-life movement because of an absence of scriptural references to abortion. Once they were able to find scriptural texts that supported the pro-life position, however—such as, "Thou didst know me in my mother's womb"—they joined the struggle with considerable zeal.

If the dominant perception in our society is that moral beliefs are derived solely from scripture and religious belief and are ultimately articles of faith, however, then it is thought that those who hold those moral positions have nothing to say to those who do not share their faith. This has been a very effective way of disenfranchising Christians and excluding them from national public policy debates. Somehow Catholics must be able, in charity, to acknowledge that this current state of cultural affairs is to a large degree the result, in my opinion, of Protestant theological errors regarding the nature of faith and reason, and that these errors have come to shape our cultural thinking about the relationship of reason and religion.

In the radical Protestant neo-orthodoxy of Karl Barth of the 1930s and 1940s, even religion was to be repudiated, because it was seen as a human creation, a human institution, a construct of the intellect. Religion did not bring the human person to God but rather placed his relationship with God in jeopardy. In a perverse sort of historical development, this radical neo-orthodoxy of Barth prepared the way for the radically secular, religion-less Christianity of the 1960s and 1970s. It spawned works such as Gibson Winter's *The New Creation as Metropolis*, Harvey Cox's *The Secular City*, and Thomas J. J. Altizer's *The Death of God*, which found no place in contemporary experience for the transcendent or the supernatural.

I believe there is a secularizing tendency built into much of Protestantism, and the Protestant experience has profoundly shaped American culture. Once encounter with God was confined to scripture and one's own religious experiences, then religion had no role to play in the realm of the profane. One can actually see the theory worked out in praxis in many places in Europe. If one visits the Catholic town of Fribourg, Switzerland, one finds the fountains in public squares surmounted by statues of the saints. One of the most impressive is a stone sculpture of Jesus and the woman at the well on top of a pillar in one of the major fountains in one of the town squares. Niches on public buildings shelter statues of the Blessed Virgin or St. Peter. Yet in Berne, in the neighboring Protestant canton, one finds the niches are now either empty or filled with magistrates and soldiers. Fountains are now decorated with sculpted bears or knights. Religion was quite literally taken from the public square by the Protestants. Now many of them want back in.

Also, the Protestant principle of *sola scriptura* linked to a belief in the private interpretation of scripture surely was, and continues to be, a powerful impetus toward the widespread subjectivism and individualism of our day, even if people are unaware of the historical roots of this individualism. This doctrine of the private interpretation of scripture is sometimes known as the "internal testimony of the Holy Spirit." The Westminster Confession states succinctly, "Our full persuasion and assurance of the infallible truth and divine authority [of scripture], is from the inward work of the Holy Spirit bearing witness by and with the Word in our hearts."[15]

What began as a belief in the charism of the individual interpretation of scripture worked its way out culturally, I believe, to the subjectivism and individualism of our own day. Today, an objective moral order is often denied, and social life is frequently reduced to attempting to adjudicate the claims of individuals or individualized, self-interested groups. In his criticism of the judicial activism leading to the legalization of abortion, Robert Bork pointed out that "radical individualism is the only explanation for the Supreme Court creation, out of thin air, of a general and undefined right of privacy."[16]

This supposed constitutional right was first articulated in 1965, in *Griswold v. Connecticut*, which challenged a law against the sale and distribution of contraceptives. In this decision the Court claimed that the law violated the privacy of the marital bedroom. But it was not long until the principle led to striking down a Massachusetts law against making contraceptives available to single people. Then, of course, in 1973, this supposed constitutional right to privacy was extended to mothers who sought medical assistance in the aborting of their own children.

---

[15] Westminster Confession, chapter I, n. 5.

[16] Robert H. Bork, *Slouching towards Gomorrah* (New York: Regan Books, 1996), 103.

The judicial defense of the application of this supposed principle of privacy led to ever more stark articulations of the radical subjectivism, relativism, and individualism characteristic of our society. It reached its apotheosis in *Planned Parenthood v. Casey*, in the infamous "mystery" passage written by Justice Kennedy: "At the heart of liberty is the right to define one's own concept of existence, of meaning, of the universe, and of the mystery of human life."

Could any passage from the writings of one of our higher cultural institutions more powerfully illustrate the extreme subjectivism and individualism that have come to define American culture and, tragically, to establish a tyranny of the powerful over the weak? As the Pope writes in *Evangelium vitae*, "To claim the right to abortion, infanticide and euthanasia, and to recognize that right in law, means to attribute to human freedom a *perverse and evil significance*: that of an *absolute power over others and against others.*"[17] Later in the encyclical he writes, "When a parliamentary or social majority decrees that it is legal ... to kill unborn human life, is it not really making a 'tyrannical' decision with regard to the weakest and most defenceless of human beings?"[18] Democracy is, of course, one of our greatest cultural achievements. Yet we have distorted even it by our radical subjectivism and moral relativism. In the United States it has become an instrument of tyranny of the strong against the weak and vulnerable.

The Holy Father passes harsh judgment on the situation which obtains in this country:

> The State is no longer the "common home" where all can live together on the basis of principles of fundamental equality, but is transformed into a *tyrant State*, which arrogates to itself the right to dispose of the life of the weakest and most defenseless members, from the unborn child to the elderly, in the name of a public interest which is really nothing but the interest of one part. The appearance of the strictest respect for legality is maintained ... in accordance with what are generally seen as the rules of democracy. Really, what we have here is only the tragic caricature of legality; the democratic ideal, which is only truly such when it acknowledges and safeguards the dignity of every human person, *is betrayed in its very foundations.*

---

[17] *Evangelium vitae*, n. 20 (emphasis added).

[18] Ibid., n. 70.

The Holy Father goes on ominously, "When this happens, the process leading to the breakdown of a genuinely human co-existence and the disintegration of the State itself has already begun."[19]

By the Pope's own analysis, I think one would have to say that any political candidates or holders of public office who pledge support to the agendas of organizations such as Planned Parenthood or the National Abortion Rights Action League, regardless of their religious affiliation, are contributing to the disintegration of the State. They are party to tyranny and constitute an objective threat to a truly democratic social order, which has no value whatsoever unless it is grounded in the moral order. However, even Catholic politicians and public servants have been blinded to this fact, so strong are the dominant cultural determinants of radical individualism, subjectivism, and moral relativism.

The Pope insists that we must counter these cultural influences, particularly by discovering again the essential link between freedom and objective moral truth. He writes:

> No less critical in the formation of conscience is *the recovery of the necessary link between freedom and truth*. As I have frequently stated, when freedom is detached from objective truth it becomes impossible to establish personal rights on a firm rational basis; and the ground is laid for society to be at the mercy of the unrestrained will of individuals or the oppressive totalitarianism of public authority.[20]

There are, again, philosophical and cultural bases for the phenomenon of a supposed freedom detached from truth. We live in a society in which freedom has no perceived limits. In a society dominated by a radical secularism, which is the same as a practical atheism, there is a refusal to accept human freedom as created and embodied and therefore limited. Despite the name, the Age of Reason was a time of profound skepticism, not only about religion and received traditions but about reason itself. David Hume called into question even a necessary link between cause and effect. I think it was no historical accident that Hume was a product of Calvinist Scotland.

Skepticism can also be seen in Immanuel Kant, who wrote in his *Critique of Pure Reason* of the impossibility of coming to know the actual objective realities one encounters. One

---

[19] Ibid., n. 20 (emphasis added).

[20] Ibid., n. 96.

cannot, according to Kant, come to know *das Ding an sich,* "the thing itself." It is the mind which imposes reality, as it were, on our inchoate sense experience. Furthermore, the will became the determining human faculty for human action, not the intellect. Again, I think it no historical accident that Kant was raised in the context of German Pietism. The skepticism, subjectivism, and secularism that John Paul II pointed to as attributes of a culture of death do have deep historical roots.

The Pope told us that we must be cognizant of the ways in which culture has shaped our thinking and our morality. We as a Church in this country have worked on political and moral solutions to the challenges of the anti-life policies of our society without sufficiently addressing the cultural issues. It should be apparent by now in our recent national history that it does not matter whether or not, for example, we can argue coherently from the scientific evidence and from logic for the personhood of the unborn child. The effective use of the syllogism, or even the scientific evidence, will not change public policy, for the cultural decay is far too deep. Innocent human life no longer has an intrinsic value which is perceived and protected. Rather, innocent life has worth only if those in power ascribe worth to it or view it as being useful in some way or another.

In 1996, in the case *Compassion in Dying v. State of Washington,* the U.S. Ninth Circuit Court of Appeals found that there was a constitutional right for a citizen to seek the assistance of a physician in killing himself. In defense of physician-assisted suicide, the justices took full cognizance of the cultural realities surrounding them and repeatedly appealed to the right to abortion established in *Roe v. Wade.* They said, in essence, "If a citizen is free to kill an unborn child who does not ask to die, then surely one is free to kill those who expressly ask to die." While these are not words taken from the opinion, they certainly express the thinking contained in it. Occasionally it requires a statement as stark and unvarnished as that one to manifest just how far our cultural decline has gone. And, of course, we see it everywhere in popular culture. An abortionist wrote recently in *Boston Magazine,* "I appreciate that life starts early in the womb, but also believe that I'm ending it for good reasons."[21]

---

[21] As told to Cheryl Alkon, "Confessions of an Abortion Doctor," *Boston Magazine* (December 24, 2004), http://www.bostonmagazine. com/ArticleDisplay.php?id=495.

As the Pope said, "with tragic consequences, a long historical process is now reaching a turning-point." The cultural foundations for the culture of death were laid long ago in the radical subjectivism, individualism and anti-rationalism of certain elements of the Protestant movement, through the radical notions of freedom of the French Revolution and the Enlightenment, in the skepticism of the so-called Age of Reason, and in the atheism and materialism of Marx, Freud, Darwin, Nietzche, Kinsey, and other shapers of modern culture.

Another determinant of the culture of death mentioned by the Pope is philosophical utilitarianism or pragmatism. This is indeed a philosophical school of thought compatible with Anglo-American societies that are democratic, commercial, industrial, and technological. As presented by John Stuart Mill and Jeremy Bentham, morality is determined by the greatest good for the greatest number—which has at least a surface appeal to democratic values. When the utilitarians are asked what constitutes the greatest good, we are told, "Whatever maximizes pleasure and minimizes pain."

Utilitarianism is clearly the approach most commonly taught in the medical ethics courses in our medical schools, and it has been influential in shaping public health policy. For example, those who have argued most strongly for federal funding for embryonic stem cell research have used thoroughly utilitarian argumentation. Embryos left over from in vitro fertilization procedures should be allowed to be destroyed so that we may use their stem cells. They are going to die anyway, so the argument goes, so we should be able to use them for research that could bring healing to millions—"the greatest good for the greatest number."

It becomes almost immediately obvious that utilitarianism leads to great danger for the weak and the vulnerable. The Pope saw this clearly, and writes in *Evangelium vitae*:

> Euthanasia is sometimes justified by the utilitarian motive of avoiding costs which bring no return and which weigh heavily on society. Thus it is proposed to eliminate malformed babies, the severely handicapped, the disabled, the elderly, especially when they are not self-sufficient, and the terminally ill.[22]

At the deepest level of the culture of death, one encounters another determinant of our current pluralistic

---

[22] *Evangelium vitae*, n. 15.

democratic societies, to which allusion has already been made—secularism:

> In seeking the deepest roots of the struggle between the "culture of life" and the "culture of death," we cannot restrict ourselves to the perverse idea of freedom mentioned above. We have to go to the heart of the tragedy being experienced by modern man: *the eclipse of the sense of God and of man,* typical of a social and cultural climate dominated by secularism, which, with its ubiquitous tentacles, succeeds at times in putting Christian communities themselves to the test.[23]

There is even here a way in which the sharp contrast between faith and reason, the sacred and the profane, in some Christian traditions helped spawn secularism, a loss of the sense of the divine in the world. If reason is suspect and cannot bring us to any knowledge of God, then those who do not have the gift of faith are, as it were, godless. Those who are not believers then come to think that religion has no social role to play, since it has to do only with one's individual, subjective experiences of whether or not one is saved. They then attempt to build a social order without adverting to a Creator God and an objective moral order.

In the face of today's militant secularism, it is instructive to notice that within the Catholic intellectual tradition, the virtue of religion is a natural moral virtue under the cardinal virtue of justice. The awareness of a Creator God who is just and who punishes those who are wicked and rewards the good can be known from the use of natural reason. There are sound arguments for the existence of God; to acknowledge that God exists is profoundly more reasonable than to maintain that he does not exist.

The dominance of Protestant thought, however, led to a repudiation of natural theology and philosophical arguments for the existence of God. Religion came to be understood only in terms of divine revelation and the supernatural reality of grace. Religion no longer had a role to play in the natural life of man. Once more, religion was not so much driven out of the public square as carried out by certain Christians themselves.

In the United States, we face in the culture of death an increasingly militant secularism. The Pope writes:

---

[23] Ibid., n. 21 (emphasis added).

The eclipse of the sense of God and of man inevitably leads to a *practical materialism*, which breeds individualism, utilitarianism and hedonism. Here too we see the permanent validity of the words of the Apostle: 'And since they did not see fit to acknowledge God, God gave them up to a base mind and to improper conduct' (*Rom* 1:28)...[24]

The Pope is so overwhelmed by the array of the forces of the culture of death in what he calls "the advanced societies" that he is led almost to sound a note of despair. He writes, "Faced with the countless grave threats to life present in the modern world, one could feel overwhelmed by sheer powerlessness: good can never be powerful enough to triumph over evil!"[25]

He does not despair, of course, but he does call us to a course of action to remedy this situation. How does one go about the attempt to transform culture in the face of such odds?

In *Veritatis splendor*, particularly the middle section, the Pope uses the full arsenal of his philosophical prowess to show the inadequacies of certain moral methodologies. But he does not rely merely on his intellectual acumen. In the third section of *Veritatis splendor*, he reveals what he calls the "secret" of the Church's educative power. He says that it is

> not so much in doctrinal statements and pastoral appeals to vigilance, as in *constantly looking to the Lord Jesus.* Each day the Church looks to Christ with unfailing love, fully aware that the true and final answer to the problem of morality lies in him alone. In a particular way, it is *in the Crucified Christ* that *the Church finds the answer.*[26]

The Pope takes exactly the same approach in *Evangelium vitae* when calling us to action in what appears as almost a hopeless situation in the struggle against the culture of death:

> I would like to pause with each one of you to *contemplate the One who was pierced* and who draws all people to himself (cf. *Jn* 19:37; 12:32). Looking at "the spectacle" of the Cross (cf. *Lk* 23:48) we shall discover in this glorious tree the fulfillment and the complete revelation of the whole *Gospel of life.* He who had come "not to be served but to serve, and to give his life as a ransom for many" (*Mk* 10:45), attains on the Cross the heights of love.[27]

---

[24] Ibid., n. 23 (emphasis added).

[25] Ibid., n. 29.

[26] John Paul II, *Veritatis splendor*, n. 85 (emphasis added).

[27] *Evangelium vitae*, n. 50 (emphasis added).

Notice that the Pope does not simply call on us "to look to Jesus," but specifically to the crucified Christ. The culture of death is characterized by the disposition of the powerful to use the weak for their own benefit, whether it is to terminate a tenuous life to save resources, or to harvest tissue and organs from aborted babies, or to destroy embryos to garner stem cells for research. The culture of death is characterized by the disposition *not* to be at the service of the other, but rather to place the weak and vulnerable at the service of ourselves:

> In the materialistic perspective [writes the Pope] ... *interpersonal relations are seriously impoverished.* The first to be harmed are women, children, the sick or suffering, and the elderly. The criterion of personal dignity—which demands respect, generosity and service—is replaced by the criterion of efficiency, functionality and usefulness: others are considered not for what they "are," but for what they "have, do and produce." This is the supremacy of the strong over the weak.[28]

As the Holy Father said, the only true antidote to this situation is Jesus Christ crucified. Ultimately, the only truly effective weapon we have against the arrayed forces of the culture of death is the One who offered his life in service to others. Throughout his pontificate, the Pope reminded us that the nature of human fulfillment is to live for the benefit of others. Jesus, who not only reveals God but also reveals man to himself, shows us on the cross the true nature of human fulfillment: it is a life given in the service of others.

The Pope points out repeatedly in *Evangelium vitae* that human life is inviolable because it is sacred. He tells us that "The *sacredness* of life gives rise to its *inviolability*."[29] Elsewhere he writes, "Human life is thus given a sacred and inviolable character, which reflects the inviolability of the Creator himself."[30] In fact, every violation of an innocent human life has something of the character of sacrilege, since the human person has been created in the image and likeness of God, and through the incarnation, in the words of the Council, "the Son of God has united himself in some fashion with every person."[31] The Pope writes, "It is precisely in the 'flesh' of every person

---

[28] Ibid., n. 23 (emphasis added).

[29] Ibid., n. 40 (emphasis added).

[30] Ibid., n. 53.

[31] *Gaudium et spes*, n. 22.

that Christ continues to reveal himself and to enter into fellowship with us, so that *rejection of human life*, in whatever form that rejection takes, *is really a rejection of Christ.*"[32]

The Church will, of course, continue to manifest a culture of life and be the harbinger of a civilization of love in her charitable works, in her health care, and in the countless acts of self-sacrifice of her members. Health care has been one of the areas in which the Church has most generously and remarkably worked for a culture of life. The Church's health care ministry is found in every part of the country, and no one provides more non-reimbursed care to indigent patients than Catholic health care. Yet at the heart of this generosity must be a sense of the sacredness of human life. Regrettably in a society as secularized as our own, there is little sense of the sacred.

If the sacred is the source of the dignity and inviolability of the human person, it is obvious that its eclipse in a society will place weak and vulnerable persons at risk. As the Pope said, "at the heart of every culture lies the attitude man takes to the greatest mystery: the mystery of God."[33] And it is the Catholic Church alone which fully manifests the mystery of God revealed in Jesus Christ, since she is the Body of Christ and brings us into contact with Christ himself in the sacraments, particularly the Holy Eucharist. The Church must be the principal agency for the transformation of culture, by bringing men and women into the presence of the sacred itself, into the presence of Jesus Christ. And as she offers the holy sacrifice of the Mass, the Church brings men, women, and children not simply to Jesus but specifically to Jesus Christ crucified. Only as we encounter the Man for Others in the sacrifice of the Mass, and only as we receive and are transformed by Him, will we be able to work truly effectively for a culture of life and a civilization of love.

---

[32] *Evangelium vitae*, n. 104 (emphasis added).

[33] Ibid., n. 96.

Placing Oneself "In the Perspective of the Acting Person"

Veritatis splendor and the Nature of the Moral Act

Rev. Kevin L. Flannery, S.J.

The section of John Paul II's encyclical letter *Veritatis splendor* that deals with the moral act contains nothing new, nor does it claim to be doing anything but presenting—in a modern context, of course—the teaching of Thomas Aquinas.[1] This is evident near the beginning of the section, at n. 74, where reference is made to the traditional question "regarding the sources of morality" (*de fontibus moralitatis*). These "sources of morality"—i.e., object, intention, and circumstances of human acts—are all three treated in questions 6 to 21 of the *prima secundae*

---

[1] John Paul II, *Veritatis splendor* (August 6, 1993), AAS 85 (1993): 1133–122, nn. 71–83 (chapter II, section 4, "The Moral Act"). In this article, translations are by the Holy See, with occasional emendations by the author.

of the *Summa theologiae*, sometimes referred to as the treatise *De actibus humanis*. Further into the argument of *Veritatis splendor*—that is, having first explained that many contemporary theories go astray by putting too much emphasis on intention and circumstances (the latter including "in particular the consequences" [n. 74])—the Holy Father tells us (n. 78), "The morality of the human act depends primarily and fundamentally on the 'object' rationally chosen by the deliberate will, as is borne out by the acute analysis, still valid today, made by Saint Thomas" [*in acuta etiam nunc valida sancti Thomae investigatione*]; he cites *Summa theologiae* (*ST*) I-II, Q. 18.6.

In the sentence immediately following this tribute to Thomas (and mention of the "deliberate will"), we read the following words: "For this reason [*proinde*], in order to be able to grasp the object of an act which specifies that act morally, it is necessary to place oneself in the perspective of the acting person." It might appear to some that this latter remark constitutes a shift away from the more traditional approach—sometimes (inaccurately) dismissed as excessively "physicalist"—and toward a more modern approach that looks to the reasons why we do things rather than to the objective characterization of the things we do. But there are no grounds for such an interpretation in the text of *Veritatis splendor*. For one thing, the conjunction with which the sentence in question begins—*proinde*, "for this reason"—leaves no doubt that the Holy Father is expounding the Thomistic idea, set out in the previous sentence, that the morality of an act depends on the object "rationally chosen by the deliberate will." Moreover, the sentence in question is a faithful representation of *ST* I-II, Q. 18.6, where Thomas says that a human act receives its characterization as good or bad from the end, which is the object of the interior act of the will, and from the object of the exterior act, which depends on the interior act of the will for its very characterization as moral.[2] Thus, according to Thomas (and also

---

[2] *In actu autem voluntario invenitur duplex actus, scilicet actus interior voluntatis, et actus exterior, et uterque horum actuum habet suum obiectum. Finis autem proprie est obiectum interioris actus voluntarii, id autem circa quod est actio exterior, est obiectum eius. Sicut igitur actus exterior accipit speciem ab obiecto circa quod est; ita actus interior voluntatis accipit speciem a fine, sicut a proprio obiecto. Ita autem quod est ex parte voluntatis, se habet ut formale ad id quod est ex parte exterioris actus, quia voluntas utitur membris ad agendum, sicut instrumentis; neque actus exteriores habent rationem moralitatis, nisi inquantum sunt voluntarii* (*ST* I-II, Q. 18.6c). Since refer-

the encyclical), even though there is such a thing as an "exterior" act, it can only be understood as a human act at all in a "non-physicalist" way, i.e., by placing oneself "in the perspective of the acting person."

So we sense in this encyclical that we stand on the terra firma of traditional teaching: and that is a good thing. In such delicate and important matters—matters that concern not only our own day but also future generations—the Church cannot be seen to be speaking from a platform that will be toppled when the ideological ground shifts. She must establish solid doctrinal connections with future generations by means of similar connections with the past—in particular with those thinkers whose role it was in history to establish the principles of sound philosophy and (as the instruments of God's grace) of sound theology. Otherwise, her teaching will have no more permanence than an editorial in the *New York Times* or the "mission statement" of a trendy university.

What I would like to do here, therefore, is to take a quick run through some of the salient points of the theory of human action found in the very dense early questions of the *prima secundae* of Thomas's *Summa theologiae*; that is, I would like to look at the arguments on which the "action theory" of *Veritatis splendor* is based. Having gone through these points of Thomas's theory, I will then discuss two concrete ethical questions and how they are answered by applying the ideas found in Thomas and, therefore, at least by implication, in the encyclical *Veritatis splendor*. The first is whether it is licit to withdraw food and water from patients whose abilities to communicate are much diminished or even nonexistent; the second is whether AIDS victims ought to use condoms. Under this second question, I will also consider the question whether a bishop ought to speak in favor of the distribution of condoms in order to prevent the spread of AIDS.

---

ence is to this article in Thomas, it is clear that in *Veritatis splendor*, n. 78 (and elsewhere in the encyclical), the term "object" refers not just to that which specifies the basic unit of action performed (as in, for instance, *ST* I-II, Q. 18.2) but to the object of the interior act and the object of the exterior act. Accordingly, in what follows, when I mean the object of the external act, I say this explicitly; I also use expressions like "the species as given by the object of the external act" or simply "the basic species" when I have in mind the basic unit of action performed.

I

Probably the most important idea in the analysis of human action is mentioned, appropriately enough, in the first question, first article, of the *prima secundae*.[3] There Thomas draws a distinction between an action considered as an action, i.e., as an act of the will, and the same action's end (or object). The object of the will is the end, "just as the object of sight is color," he says. Even if we can speak of sight as, in a sense, the object of sight—we *see* that we are seeing—what we see is, in the first instance, something visible and only secondarily that we are seeing it. A similar thing can be said about willing. There is such a thing as willing to will. Every time we deliberately do something, we rouse up the will by means of the will itself. But there has to be *something*, some concrete action, that we will to will to do. This is the act *as specified* by its object. The object, we might say, brings everything to a point, completing the act as an act. The upshot of this doctrine, which comes in fact from Aristotle, is that the things we do are delimited—delimited by the objects that give them their "species" (what they are).[4] When we will to do something, insofar as we will to do that thing (whatever it is), we do not will to do anything that lies beyond the bounds of the species fixed by the object.

A key question for us is going to be: What are the factors that determine that something is within and other things outside of what a person is doing? Clearly, the species of human acts are not like physical species, which we determine by identifying the stable characteristics, as distinct from those that are more fleeting (the accidents). Under the genus of animals, for instance, we find the species of birds; an animal belongs in

---

[3] *Nam obiectum voluntatis est finis, sicut obiectum visus est color, unde sicut impossibile est quod primum visibile sit ipsum videre, quia omne videre est alicuius obiecti visibilis; ita* impossibile est quod primum appetibile, quod est finis, sit ipsum velle. See also *ST* I-II, Q. 3.4 ad 2.

[4] See, for instance, Aristotle's *De anima*, iii, 10, 433a15, where he says that "every desire is for something." In his commentary on this remark, Aquinas says, "It is clear ... that 'every desire is for something'—for it would be nonsense to say that someone desires something in order to desire; for to desire is a certain motion tending towards another thing" (*In De anima* [editio Leonina], lb. 3, cap. 9, ll. 50–53). See also Aristotle's *De anima* i, 1, 402b14–16. For the idea that the object gives an act its (basic) species, see *ST* I-II, Q. 18.2: *Primum autem quod ad plenitudinem essendi pertinere videtur, est id quod dat rei speciem. Sicut autem res naturalis habet speciem ex sua forma, ita actio habet speciem ex obiecto; sicut et motus ex termino.*

this species if it has (or, at least, normally would have) wings, if it has lungs instead of gills, if its young are born from eggs. A circumstance such as whether the animal was born in 2000 rather than 1995 will make no difference to its species. In the realm of morals, on the other hand, circumstances may indeed change an act's species. Suppose that a man knows that lighting his pipe will signal the killing of another man. The act of lighting his pipe becomes in these circumstances an action of an entirely different species than it would have been otherwise: it is no longer an innocent act aimed at pleasure but an act of murder (or, at least, complicity in murder). And if the man to be murdered is the president of the country, the act of lighting the pipe becomes also an assassination, which changes the species yet again, since an assassination has a different bearing on the common good than a nonpolitical murder. None of this is to say that the species of a moral act is not quite definite and delimited: if a murder is a murder, it is not *not* a murder. On the other hand, it is also clear that determining the species of a human action is a business quite a bit more delicate than determining the species of an animal.

It is by no means, however, an impossible task. There are ways of organizing and analyzing the various factors (including the circumstances) that go into determining the species of a human act. To begin with, there are identifiable within the moral universe certain set patterns of behavior such as "giving to someone what is his" (and not taking things that are not one's own), "communicating a truth" (and not communicating a falsehood), "having intercourse with one's wife" (and not with the wife of another), or "performing an operation on a patient for his health" (and not doing something to worsen his health). *Veritatis splendor* refers to such patterns when it speaks of someone's choosing a "concrete kind of behavior [that] is 'according to its species'—or 'in itself'—morally good or bad, licit or illicit."[5] (The species here is the species as given by the object of the exter-

---

[5] *Veritatis splendor*, n. 77. It is apparent in n. 80 that the Pope includes in the class of things that are *secundum suam speciem* good or bad more things than Thomas would include among the class of the *bonum* or *malum ex genere* (see SI-II, Q. 18.2). (Thomas occasionally uses the expression *bonum* or *malum ex genere* but regards it as equivalent to speaking about the species of an act; see *ST* I-II, Q. 18.2: *Et dicitur malum ex genere, genere pro specie accepto, eo modo loquendi quo dicimus humanum genus totam humanam speciem*). At *Veritatis splendor*, n. 80, the Pope cites *Gaudium et spes*, n. 27, which speaks in this regard of "[w]hatever is hostile to life itself, such as any kind of

nal act.) When one performs an action that falls among the positive versions of these patterns, the action, at least under that consideration, is moral. When one deliberately and knowingly performs an action that falls among the negative versions of these patterns—taking something not one's own, communicating a falsehood, having intercourse with the wife of another, doing something to worsen a patient's health—it can immediately be declared immoral. An action that is immoral in its species in this way can never be made good by the end for which it is done. On the other hand, an act good in its basic species can be bad, if the end is bad. Thomas uses the example of a man who gives alms but for vainglory [*ST* 1-2.18.6 obj./ad 2]; another example is someone who tells the truth in order to wound.

There are, however, circumstances in which what would otherwise be an act evil in its basic species is not evil at all. What are these circumstance? They have to do with what the agent knows or does not know about what he is doing—which is another reason why, in determining the morality of an action, one must place oneself in the perspective of the acting person. Thomas lists the relevant circumstances; the list can also be found in Aristotle and in Cicero, in slightly different versions.[6] An agent may be ignorant, says Aristotle, "of who he is, or of what he is doing, or of that regarding which or on whom he is acting; sometimes also of what he is using (i.e., what instrument), or of why he is doing it (e.g., for safety's sake), or of how he is doing it (either gently or with too much force)." Let us say that a man is lying with a woman who is not his wife, although he believes she is his wife. This circumstance changes the very nature (the very species) of his basic act: his act is not an act of adultery. Circumstances can also have a bearing on the morality of acts that are not evil in their basic species. Take the man with the pipe. If he thinks that lighting the pipe is to signal the president's being spirited off into safety (i.e., if he does not know the true end of

---

homicide, genocide, abortion, euthanasia and voluntary suicide; whatever violates the integrity of the human person, such as mutilation, physical and mental torture and attempts to coerce the spirit; whatever is offensive to human dignity, such as subhuman living conditions, arbitrary imprisonment, deportation, slavery, prostitution and trafficking in women and children; degrading conditions of work which treat laborers as mere instruments of profit, and not as free responsible persons."

[6] *ST* I-II, Q. 7.3. In Cicero, see *De inventione* 1.26; in Aristotle, *Nichomachean Ethics*, iii, 1, 1111a3-6.

his action), his lighting the pipe is no longer murder or assassination. Similar things can be said about the other circumstances.

Although all these types of circumstance involve ignorance, however, not every type of ignorance exonerates. Take a person who is ignorant of what the moral law requires in the sense that, due to passion or habituation, he simply does not consider it; or let us say that he has negligently declined to inform himself of what the moral law, in its more universal precepts, requires. If such a person does something that is contrary to these precepts, he is culpable not only for not knowing the law or bearing it in mind but also for the action that any such ignorance leads him to perform.[7] Thomas is quite insistent that the circumstances that change the moral character of an act correspond to those "enumerated" by Aristotle and Cicero.[8] If the ignorance involved does not fall among these, the agent is responsible for the corresponding action. That is, not only is the acting person culpable for not informing himself, but his culpability extends to *the act he performs* on the basis of such ignorance. All other factors remaining equal, such an act is to be judged like any other voluntary action.

This may strike some who have followed recent debates in moral theology as incorrect. Does not Thomas say that someone with an erroneous conscience is morally bound to follow that conscience? Yes, he does, in article 5, question 19 of the *prima secundae*. But he also says, in the very next article, that the will of one who so acts is evil [*mala*]. He acknowledges that a man who lacks the circumstantial knowledge that a particular woman is not his wife, if she asks him to "render the debt"

---

[7] *Hoc igitur modo dicitur ignorantia, sive cum aliquis actu non considerat quod considerare potest et debet, quae est ignorantia malae electionis, vel ex passione vel ex habitu proveniens, sive cum aliquis notitiam quam debet habere, non curat acquirere; et secundum hunc modum, ignorantia universalium iuris, quae quis scire tenetur, voluntaria dicitur, quasi per negligentiam proveniens* (ST I-II, Q. 6.8). The body of article begins in this way: *ignorantia habet causare involuntarium ea ratione qua privat cognitionem, quae praeexigitur ad voluntarium, ut supra dictum est. Non tamen quaelibet ignorantia huiusmodi cognitionem privat.* Thomas is speaking here of ignorance that makes an *act* involuntary, and he is saying that certain types of ignorance, such as negligent ignorance of the universal precepts of the law, do not do this. Thus, the culpability in such cases attaches not just to the acts that *lead* to negligence but also to the acts that otherwise would be excused, due (say) to circumstantial ignorance.

[8] *Et ratio huius annumerationis sic accipi potest* (ST I-II, Q. 7.3c).

and have intercourse with her, does not sin if he has intercourse with her. But, he also says,

> if erroneous reasoning says that a man is *obliged* to lie
> with the wife of another, the will going along with this
> erroneous reasoning is evil because this error originates
> in ignorance of the law of God, which he is obliged to
> know.[9]

This is all perfectly consistent with the teaching of *Veritatis
splendor,* one of whose major themes is the role of conscience
in the moral life (see chapter II, section 2, nn. 54–64, "Conscience and Truth"). The encyclical cites Thomas a number of
times in this regard, although it actually quotes Bonaventure:

> Conscience is like God's herald and messenger; it does
> not command things on its own authority, but commands
> them as coming from God's authority, like a herald when
> he proclaims the edict of the king. This is why conscience
> has binding force. (n. 58)

When a conscience is erroneous, it is obviously not "God's
herald and messenger"; it may have binding force (*ST* 1-2.19.5)
but that does not make acts performed in accordance with it
good.

This approach is also consistent with the *Catechism of the
Catholic Church,* which notes that ignorance of the moral law

> can often be imputed to personal responsibility. This is
> the case when a man "takes little care [*parum curat*] to
> find out what is true and good, or when conscience is by
> degrees almost blinded through the habit of committing
> sin." In such cases, the person is culpable for the evil he
> commits.[10]

Such "vincible" ignorance can possibly be attributed to those
who dedicate even considerable time to the study of ethics but

---

[9] *ST* I-II, Q. 19.6c. That Thomas's position depends on the Aris-
totelian/Ciceronian exhaustive enumeration of circumstantial ignorance is apparent here in *ST* I-II, Q. 19.6 when he says, *Haec autem
quaestio dependet ab eo quod supra de ignorantia dictum est,* a reference
to *ST* I-II, Q. 6.8, which, as we have seen, depends largely on the
Aristotelian/Ciceronian understanding of circumstances. See on this
general issue Richard Schenk, "Perplexus Supposito Quodam: Notizien
zu einem Vergessenen Schlüsselbegriff Thomanischer Gewissens-
lehre," *Recherches de Théologie Ancienne et Médiévale* 57 (1990): 62–95.

[10] *Catechism of the Catholic Church,* n. 1791 (quoting *Gaudium et
spes,* n. 16).

who do not accept the various precepts of the moral law as true [*Catechism of the Catholic Church*, nn. 1783–1785], for this latter is a type of (culpable) ignorance as well. (A person who does not *believe* that something is true does not know it, and not to know something is to be ignorant of it.) Thus, a moral theologian's "knowledge of his field" does not remove the evil from the sins he commits in following his erroneously formed conscience.

To return, though, to Thomas Aquinas, there is one more factor (not strictly speaking a "circumstance") that can excuse an otherwise evil action, and that is force (*violentia* in Latin, *bia* in Greek). If a person is carried away by the wind and is thrown against another person, provided he has not cooperated in any way, he is not culpable for any harm done. Similarly, if someone takes one's hand and forces it to do what it otherwise would not do, what is done is in no sense voluntary. As far as the forced person is concerned, he has performed no human—that is, no moral—act. But in order to escape from the realm of the moral in this way, an action, with respect to the aspect under consideration, can contain nothing of the will of the person involved. This is a logically necessary proposition. As soon as one's will is involved, one becomes liable to moral judgment, since the moral realm simply *is* the realm of the voluntary. One cannot put something into the moral without its being voluntary—this is why, in order to identify correctly the species of an act, one must place oneself in the perspective of the acting person; but, similarly, one cannot admit that something is voluntary without putting it into the moral: the two things, the moral and the voluntary, coincide.[11]

So, even in the famous case of the precious cargo thrown overboard, found in Aristotle [*Nichomachean Ethics*, iii, 1, 1110a8–10] and cited by Thomas [*ST* 1-2.6.6c], in the end we must say that the act is voluntary. Of course, in a certain sense, jettisoning the cargo is involuntary: in calm waters, the owner of the cargo would never have done it. But as it is, he picks the cargo up by the handles, moves to the ship's edge, and lets it drop. Since his will is clearly involved here, one has no choice but to consider the act a moral act. Aristotle, in the same discussion, cites an even tougher example: that of a person who is subject to pressure by a tyrant who holds his parents and children and threatens to kill them all unless the person commits

---

[11] See Kevin L. Flannery, "The Field of Moral Action according to Thomas Aquinas," *The Thomist* 69.1 (January 2005): 1–30.

some heinous deed [*Nichomachean Ethics*, iii, 1, 1110a5–8]. One would surely feel pity for the person who commits such a deed— one might pardon him—but the deed cannot *not* be a voluntary act, since what the person was forced to do was to make a choice, and choices depend on the will. Even the act of pardon, borne of the same compassion that urges us to say that the act has nothing of the voluntary in it, testifies to the fact that it does. We do not extend pardon to those whose acts are completely involuntary; we acknowledge that they are not to blame.

To conclude this section, therefore, in order to escape the realm of the moral, an action has to contain nothing of the voluntary at all. Of course, in making a pastoral assessment (in the confessional, for example), one must take into account mitigating circumstances that might reduce culpability; but such taking into account will not alter the definition of the moral as the voluntary, and vice versa, or the general analysis of human action. The moral realm *is* "the perspective of the acting person."

II

These, then, are some of the key principles found in the early questions of the *prima secundae*. I would like now to discuss, more briefly than they merit, the two ethical questions mentioned above. My intention is not to give an exhaustive treatment of either, but only to demonstrate how the principles I have set out bear on them: i.e., how the principles can be applied to give a coherent account to others of why the Church takes the positions it does with respect to two very politically contested issues.

I begin with the withdrawal of food and water from patients whose abilities to communicate are much diminished or even nonexistent. Allow me to make two preliminary points. First, it is not strictly relevant to this question whether or not the patient is technically in a "vegetative state." In the Theresa Schindler-Schiavo case, which attracted wide attention, some experts declared her to be in a permanent vegetative state, although there is reason to believe that she was not.[12] If she had been, however, the moral issue would have been the

---

[12] See, for example, Robert Johansen, "Starving for a Fair Diagnosis," *National Review Online* (March 16, 2005), http://www.nationalrev iew.com/comment/johansen200503160848.asp; and the affidavit of William Polk Cheshire, Jr., M.D. (filed March 23, 2005), http://www. miami.edu/ethics/schiavo/032305%20Cheshire%20affidavit.pdf.

same—that issue being whether food and water can be withdrawn from patients whose care is burdensome (or fairly burdensome) and whose interaction with others is minimal or even nonexistent. Second, as far as Catholic doctrine is concerned, given the Holy Father's March 2004 statement that withdrawal of food and water, "if done knowingly and willingly, [is] true and proper euthanasia by omission," there can be little doubt that Catholics and Catholic hospitals are obligated to administer food and water until it is clear that the food and water could not possibly be of nutritional (or hydrational) value to the patient.[13] Still, we are interested here in understanding how the teaching of *Veritatis splendor* helps us give a coherent account of the position that the Holy Father has set out. We cannot simply repeat it, but are obligated rather to explain how it is the necessary consequence of a sound moral theory.

The first substantive thing to call to attention are the various fixed patterns of basic behavior that are involved in the practical reasoning surrounding the case. Thomas, of course, is never frightened by the complexity of an issue into parroting a scholastic adage or repeating a pious maxim; faced with

---

[13] See John Paul II, "Address to the Participants in the International Congress on Life-sustaining Treatments and Vegetative State: Scientific Advances and Ethical Dilemmas," (March 20, 2004), http://www.vatican.va/holy_father/john_paul_ii/speeches/2004/mar ch/documents/hf_jp-ii_spe_20040320_congress-fiamc_en.html. In number 4, the Pope says that the administration of food and hydration "should be considered, in principle, ordinary and proportionate, and as such morally obligatory, insofar as and until it is seen to have attained its proper finality, which in the present case consists in providing nourishment to the patient and alleviation of his suffering." In the same paragraph he says, "Death by starvation or dehydration is, in fact, the only possible outcome as a result of their withdrawal. In this sense it ends up becoming, if done knowingly and willingly, true and proper euthanasia by omission." See also the joint statement of the Pontifical Academy for Life and the World Federation of Catholic Medical Associations, issued subsequent to the same Congress (March 20, 2004): "The possible decision of withdrawing nutrition and hydration, necessarily administered to [vegetative state] patients in an assisted way, is followed inevitably by the patients' death as a direct consequence. Therefore, it has to be considered a genuine act of euthanasia by omission, which is morally unacceptable," http://www.vatican.va/roman_curia/pontifical_academies/acdlife/documents/rc_pont-acd_life_doc_20040320_joint-statement-veget-state_en.html.

complexity, his first instinct is to begin organizing. In any concrete moral question, he looks first to the most basic unit of human action; he considers also whether such an action is part of a larger system of rational human activity (such as medicine or marriage); and then, as we have seen, he asks whether other circumstances might have a bearing on the morality of the action. He does all this because he realizes that adequate moral analysis demands understanding—in all its articulation—everything that is within the will of the agent (or possible agent), for, as we have seen, whatever is within the will has a bearing on the morality of the action.

In the case of feeding and hydrating, the basic unit of action, the species as fixed by the object of the external act, is "giving sustenance to a hungry and thirsty person," as opposed to withholding such sustenance. If this sounds simple, it is supposed to do so. Since acting according to the moral law is acting according to reason, if we want to understand the moral law, we must begin with the most simple things that rational creatures, blessed with intellects and wills, understand themselves to *do*. They give food (or not), they make love to their spouse (or with someone not their spouse), they tell the truth (or they lie).[14] The positive members of these pairs—giving food, making love to one's spouse, telling the truth—*are* positive because they contain the rationality of this particular type of human action. Their negative counterparts are parasitic on them, which is to say that they can only be spoken of because we first understand the positive members: adultery, for instance, presupposes marriage, but marriage does not presuppose adultery. And since the intelligibility of these basic patterns is on the positive side, they also represent morally acceptable options, since to act morally is to act in a way that is intelligible.

In the case of the administration of food and water, we have an action that is both a very basic pattern of human

---

[14] See *ST* I-II, Q. 14.6c: *Huiusmodi autem principia quae in inquisitione consilii supponuntur, sunt quaecumque sunt per sensum accepta, utpote quod hoc sit panis vel ferrum; et quaecumque sunt per aliquam scientiam speculativam vel practicam in universali cognita, sicut quod moechari est a Deo prohibitum, et quod homo non potest vivere nisi nutriatur nutrimento convenienti. Et de istis non inquirit consiliator.* The *consiliator* does not inquire into the goodness of such actions, since they are first principles: that by means of which we come to know whether other, more complex patterns of behavior are good or bad. They give us our basic ideas of good and bad action.

behavior (something we do *qua* human beings) and also an element in a more deliberately organized human practice, that of medicine. It is an argument for the rationality of an action performed by a doctor that it is in accordance with good medicine—i.e., medicine based on sound principles, such as the principles that life is a good in itself and that a doctor ought to do no harm. Thus, one can make an argument for the basic goodness of administering food and water by looking to what humans do *qua* humans and also by looking to what doctors do *qua* doctors.[15]

So much for analysis of the species as given by the object of the external act. What then about circumstances? For we have said that the analysis of human action must include also these. Considered on its own, the positive member of the pair "administering food and water / withdrawing food and water," so far "passes muster." We set aside the possible circumstance that a caregiver might not know what he is doing, since that sort of consideration has the effect of taking the action out of the realm of morality altogether. But there are some circumstances that can change the essentially good act of providing food and water into a bad one. Suppose, for instance, that a certain type of food is bad for the patient and could injure his health. In this case providing that food cannot be justified by pointing to the essential goodness of providing food: the species of the act is no longer merely providing food; the act is an act of deliberately damaging the patient's health.

But there is no way that withdrawing food and water—i.e., withdrawing them completely and willingly in such a way that

---

[15] Medicine is, in a sense, a subsidiary science: its efforts to preserve human health depend on principles (such as that life is a good in itself) that are not the sole property of medicine; but this does not mean that such principles are not also part of medicine. All this is said in interpretation of a remark in the Pope's address of March 2004. He says there that "the administration of water and food, even when provided by artificial means, always represents a natural means of preserving life, not a medical act" (John Paul II, "Address to the Participants in the International Congress on Life-Sustaining Treatments and Vegetative State: Scientific Advances and Ethical Dilemmas," n. 4). In the very next sentence, the Holy Father says that the administration of food and water "should be considered, in principle, ordinary and proportionate." I take it that the point is that the administration of water and food is not *merely* a medical act, such as would allow it to count as "extraordinary means" and, therefore, sometimes to be omitted.

their lack causes death—could ever be made moral by the presence of a circumstance (excluding, as I have said, circumstances of ignorance that take the act out of the moral realm altogether). This could not happen because, as Thomas never tires of repeating, *bonum causatur ex integra causa*. The principle comes down to him from pseudo-Dionysius and means basically that *any* bad element in the breakdown of a human action ruins the whole: "the good comes of a wholly good cause."[16]

There is a possible doubt or objection I must resolve before going on to the second question (the use of condoms to prevent AIDS). Someone could argue that failing to administer food and water does not enter the will of the acting person, since it is an omission and not the positive commission of an act. After all, when a person's life is being prolonged by truly extraordinary means—by means, for instance, of periodic electric shocks to the heart—it is permitted to stop the shocks, even knowing that the person will die as a consequence, since omitting to do something that is maintaining life is different from actively bringing about death.[17] Why can we not just say that withdrawing food and water is permitted because it is an omission, like ceasing to administer shocks? Granted, administering shocks is an extraordinary means, feeding is ordinary; but why should the ordinary/extraordinary distinction be so important, if the ethical depends on what a person wills to do?

The answer to this question is that the ordinary/extraordinary distinction *is* very much tied up with what a person has in his will. Extraordinary means are employed when things occur that are beyond the ordinary functioning of the human organism: when diseases or injuries occur. In such instances, the medical problem is already present when the doctor arrives on the scene. It is not due to his will (or so we presume) that the patient has the problem he has. By ceasing to employ extraordinary means, the doctor is allowing a pathology, for which he is not responsible, to run its "natural" course. By withdrawing food and water, on the other hand, the doctor is *creating* a pathology that did not exist previously: he is willfully bringing about starvation and dehydration.

---

[16] *ST* I-II, Q. 18.4 ad 3; Q. 19.6 ad 1; *in EN* lb.2 cap.7 II.9–12 (Marietti: §320); and especially *ST* II-II, Q. 110.3c.

[17] If the patient does not die once the shocks cease, one cannot administer a lethal dose of arsenic, for example.

A persistent objector might reply, "But doesn't the doctor who, for instance, turns off a respirator *want* the patient to die?" The answer is no—or, more precisely, if he does want the patient to die, he ought not to act. Foreseeing an effect is not equivalent to having it within one's will. In the case we are considering, i.e., in which a doctor ceased to administer electric shocks to the heart, the doctor can truthfully say that he wanted the patient to live but it was impossible. But a doctor cannot *always* say this. If he knows that the use of even extraordinary means stands a good chance of bringing the patient past the crisis: if he knows, for instance, that after two or three days in intensive care a patient will very likely recover but otherwise will not; if he pulls the patient out of intensive care, he is responsible for the patient's death: he clearly wanted it to occur. But in other cases, to omit such extraordinary means is simply to permit an already existing pathology to run its course.

III

This brings us to the second question, whether AIDS victims ought to use condoms. As we have already seen, the assessment of human actions necessarily includes consideration of very basic patterns of behavior, such as giving food to a human person or conveying information, etc. One cannot avoid consideration of these basic patterns, since what we choose to do ultimately comes down to them; they are the species—*what we do*—as given by the object of the external act. Other factors, such as the reason why we do what we do, also come into the species of an act—and necessarily so. But, even so, what human beings do most immediately are things like give food to other human persons and convey information. We cannot exclude these basic descriptions of what we choose to do from the realm of the moral.[18]

---

[18] See *ST* I-II, Q. 18.2c: ...*bonum et malum actionis, sicut et ceterarum rerum, attenditur ex plenitudine essendi vel defectu ipsius. Primum autem quod ad plenitudinem essendi pertinere videtur, est id quod dat rei speciem. Sicut autem res naturalis habet speciem ex sua forma, ita actio habet speciem ex obiecto; sicut et motus ex termino. Et ideo sicut prima bonitas rei naturalis attenditur ex sua forma, quae dat speciem ei, ita et prima bonitas actus moralis attenditur ex obiecto convenienti; unde et a quibusdam vocatur bonum ex genere; puta, uti re sua.* See, too, *ST* I-II, Q. 9.1c: ... *voluntas bona et mala sunt actus differentes secundum speciem. Differentia autem speciei in actibus est secundum obiecta, ut dictum est. Et ideo bonum et malum in actibus voluntatis proprie attenditur secundum obiecta.*

In the case before us, there are a number of such basic patterns involved. Obviously, there is an act of sexual intercourse. In order to simplify matters, we can presume that the person involved is a man and that he intends to have intercourse with his wife; in this way, we do not have to deal with adultery or fornication, which is not our interest at the moment. In addition to the act of sexual intercourse, there is an act by means of which the likely sequence of a natural process is impeded: an artificial barrier is placed between the man's sperm and his wife's ova, toward which the sperm naturally tend (even if it turns out that there are no ova outside the ovaries when they arrive at their destination). Since the natural process being impeded is no incidental process—we are not talking about wearing ear plugs—but pertains rather to the intelligibility of marriage itself, impeding this process is a moral negative. The whole story is right there. Since an act which deliberately impedes procreation is intrinsically disordered, it can never be permitted. If one spouse has AIDS and the other does not, the couple ought not to engage in intercourse, with a condom or not, since to do so without a condom risks spreading the disease and to do so with a condom is to engage in an immoral sexual act.[19]

But does not this not come down to "physicalism," such as the Holy Father excludes when he writes in *Veritatis splendor*, "By the object of a given moral act, then, one cannot mean a process or an event of the merely physical order, to be assessed on the basis of its ability to bring about a given state of affairs in the outside world"?[20] We can show that it does not by proceeding further into the question of whether the use of con-

---

[19] This paragraph does not address the issue whether a sterile couple, one spouse of which has AIDS, might use a condom during sexual intercourse. The present author holds that condom use would be immoral also in cases such as this; his position depends on canon law (CIC 1061, §1) and doctrinal teaching in authentic interpretation of the natural law (*Decretum circa impotentiam quae matrimonium dirimit* [May 13, 1977], *AAS* 79 [1977]: 426).

[20] *Veritatis splendor*, n. 78 (*Ergo nefas est accipere, velut obiectum definiti actus moralis, processum vel eventum ordinis tantum physici, qui aestimandus sit prout gignat certum rerum statum in mundo exteriore*). In any case, it is clear from the words "to be assessed on the basis of its ability to bring about a given state of affairs in the outside world" that the *type* of physical account rejected is that in which one looks just to consequences, ignoring such factors as object, intention, and circumstances.

traceptive devices can ever be licit. There are a number of instances in which such use might be moral, even according to principles accepted by the Church's magisterium. One example is the use of substances that are contraceptive (i.e., would impede conception) but for a reason other than contraception—to impede ovulation, for instance, so that a woman (who has no intention of engaging in intercourse) might participate more successfully in a sporting event.[21] Here, although "physically" the act of taking the contraceptive is identical to that of a woman wishing to avoid pregnancy, the intention (the will) is quite different. This changes the species of the act accordingly: it is now not an act of impeding sperm from arriving at ova but simply of preventing ovulation. To impede ovulation does not in itself go against the intelligibility of marriage; it does not impinge on the relevant basic pattern of behavior, having intercourse with one's spouse.

Another example is the use of contraceptives in situations where rape is a strong possibility. The sort of scenario often posited is one in which religious sisters must regularly cross through a war zone in order to care for the suffering, knowing full well that if they are captured they will be raped. In such a situation, the use of contraceptives would be permitted on the grounds that it is purely defensive, analogous to the blows a woman lands, with full justice, on an attacker in order to repel him.[22] Since the religious sisters have no intention of engaging in intercourse, the act of taking the contra-

---

[21] Whether this would constitute "doping" is obviously a question that, in the present context, we need not consider.

[22] See P. Palazzini, F. Hürth, and F. Lambruschini, "Una Donna Domanda: Come Negarsi Alla Violenza?" *Studi Cattolici* 5 (1961): 62–72; Marcellino Zalba, "Sobre la Píldora Anti-Estupro: Extraña Sorpresa Entre Moralistas de Vanguardia," *Burgense* 35 (1994): 209–217; Germain Grisez, *The Way of the Lord Jesus*, vol. 3: *Difficult Moral Questions* (Quincy, Illinois: Franciscan, 1997), 86–94, 251–255; Kevin L. Flannery, "Marriage, Mental Handicap, and Sexuality," *Studies in Christian Ethics* 17 (2004): 24–26. It is presupposed that the contraceptive means is not actually abortifacient (as many "contraceptives" are). I might add that the issue of sexual abuse within marriage is another issue entirely. Here we ought not to speak of rape, since man and wife are in fact one body; moreover, what is called for where such abuse is a strong possibility is not contraception but separation of the man and his wife. The possibility of using of contraceptives in war zones is related to the teaching that it is moral to employ means to prevent conception after a rape has occurred. See National Conference of Catholic Bishops, *Ethi-*

ceptives cannot go against the intelligibility of marriage, since one goes against the intelligibility of marriage (in this particular respect) by intending to engage in intercourse from which procreation has been deliberately excluded. The sisters' intention is simply to repel possible attacks on their bodies, including possible attacks on their ova. Thus, the morality of the act is determined not in a physicalist way—by looking just to the physical event—but by looking to what is intended.

But how do we know that this *is* their intention? And, presuming that it is, why can we not just say that the man infected with AIDS has as his intention not the violation of marriage but simply the avoidance of disease in his wife? The answers to both these questions are present in what Thomas, drawing on Aristotle, says about force (as explained previously). The difference between the sisters and the AIDS-carrying husband is that the husband *wants* to engage in intercourse: that intention is within his will. By contrast, according to our presuppositions, none of the sisters, who "physically" take contraceptives, wants to do the same. What occurs is forced on them: they are in no way responsible for it. If the substance they have taken turns out to have a contraceptive effect, that is a consequence of their adopting legitimate means to protect their bodies. They are like Aristotle's person carried away by the wind, who contributes nothing to the wind's force. The husband with AIDS, on the other hand, is more like the man who throws his goods into the sea. We might suppose that (in a sense) he does not *want* to contracept: he only does so because he wants to protect his wife. But what he does he does voluntarily, for he uses his will to do something that he could have refrained from doing, i.e., having (contracepted) intercourse with his wife.[23] That the act is voluntary is proved by the fact that it can be par-

---

cal and Religious Directives for Catholic Health Care Services, rev. ed. (Washington, DC: NCCB, 1995), 36: "A female who has been raped should be able to defend herself against a potential conception from the sexual assault. If, after appropriate testing, there is no evidence that conception has occurred already, she may be treated with medications that would prevent ovulation, sperm capacitation, or fertilization. It is not permissible, however, to initiate or to recommend treatments that have as their purpose or direct effect the removal, destruction, or interference with the implantation of a fertilized ovum."

[23] Important here is the clause I included above when introducing the issue of force. There I said that "in order to escape from the realm of the moral [by reason of force], an action, *with respect to the*

doned. What the husband does is, therefore, within the moral realm; and since it is disordered in its species—and in particular by the species as given by the object of the external act—it is immoral.

There are other ways of arguing against the use of condoms by those infected by AIDS. One could point out, for instance, that no one really knows whether condoms are 100 percent effective in preventing AIDS, and that subjecting one's wife to such a species of Russian roulette can hardly be called an act of love. But such an argument would not go to the core of the moral issue. Even if a pharmaceutical company produces someday a condom that is provably fail-safe with respect to AIDS, its use within marriage would still be immoral, since its use would knowingly impede the possible fecundity of a freely chosen act of intercourse. The *species* of the act as given by the external object is intrinsically immoral. It is clear that the act would be voluntary, since the man could have done otherwise. And when something is within one's will in this way, we have no choice but to regard it as a moral act and to evaluate it accordingly.

Before closing, I would like to introduce one sub-question. I do so because it is topical, connected with what I have been arguing, and important. Could a bishop support the distribution of condoms to AIDS victims on the grounds that, in many cases, the AIDS-carriers will be engaging in intercourse anyway and intercourse with a condom is a lesser evil than intercourse without?

The moral issue here is somewhat different from the one we have been considering. I take it as sufficiently established by what I have already said, that the act of using a condom, even in marital intercourse, to reduce the possibility of spreading AIDS is intrinsically disordered. Similarly, I do not think I *need* to establish in the present context that any act of homosexual "intercourse" is intrinsically disordered. The question before us, then, does not concern the morality of these acts but rather the morality of a bishop's *cooperation* in them by favoring

---

aspect under consideration, can contain nothing of the will of the person involved." In the present case, the relevant aspect is willful sexual relations. The sisters do not have within their wills any act of sexual intercourse (although they do will to cross through the war zone); the AIDS-carrying husband does have within his will an act of sexual intercourse.

the distribution of condoms. Would such a bishop be cooperating formally? Would he—as the standard phrase would have it—be "mixing his intention" with the intention of the perpetrator(s) of immoral acts? In other words, if he does publicly advocate the distribution of condoms, does the immorality of the acts with which he cooperates come also into *his* will?

Whenever one needs to determine whether an action comes into the will of an agent, one needs to go back to the criteria for the voluntary that Thomas takes from Aristotle. In this case, the relevant criterion is force: does the bishop have no other choice except to favor the distribution of condoms? If he does have other choices, by speaking in favor of condom distribution he formally cooperates in immoral activity: they enter into his will.

In considering what to say about, for example, governmental distribution of condoms, a bishop is not forced—even by the principle of the lesser evil—to speak in favor of such distribution. He has the option—which turns out, therefore, to be the only moral option—of saying that the only effective means of preventing the spread of AIDS is chastity. (He could also add that this is the only effective way of avoiding sexual sin.) It is true that the use of a condom impedes the AIDS virus from being transmitted in some cases; but the bishop has no information about the long-term effects of official promotion of condom use on the spread of the disease or on the rate of promiscuity. And common sense will tell him that such promotion will not have a positive effect on the rate of promiscuity or probably, therefore, on the spread of AIDS.

The bishop, therefore, is not forced by the principle of the lesser evil to speak in favor of condom use, since there is no way that he could know what the lesser evil is in this case. Since, then, his action is not forced (nor is he ignorant, in the pertinent sense, of what he is doing), for him to come out publicly in favor of condom distribution is formal cooperation in immoral acts: they enter into his will.

The classical moral manuals use a standard example to depict the difference between material and formal cooperation.[24] If a thief asks you to turn over the keys of the safe, otherwise he will kill you, you can give him the keys since you are forced to do this in order to effect (as you hope) the lesser

---

[24] See, for instance H. Noldin and A. Schmitt, *Summa theologiae moralis* (Innsbruck, Austria: F. Rauch, 1939–1940), v. 2, p. 117, §117.

evil. Suppose that a young man knows that his roommate has AIDS and knows too that the latter is heading over to his girlfriend's (or boyfriend's) house in order to have intercourse. He hears the roommate cursing that he cannot find his condoms. This young man is in a different situation from that of the bishop we have been considering. He can tell his roommate where the condoms are; indeed, he is obliged to do so in order to avoid the greater evil. The immoral act that follows does not enter into his will.

The same cannot be said of the bishop—for the reasons I have given.

IV

In conclusion, then, the understanding of the moral act put forward in the encyclical *Veritatis splendor* is taken largely from Thomas Aquinas—although, of course, Thomas himself draws on a rich tradition of philosophers and theologians, both pagan and Christian. We do well to attend to what Thomas says about the moral act, not only because it is traditional and, therefore, more likely to hold up to scrutiny by others outside our particular slice of history, limited as it is both temporally and culturally, but also because it has the ring of truth. As we work through the distinctions Thomas proposes, we see that they correspond to the way that moral universe is divided up, how it all works.

Thomas's theory has as its governing principle the idea that only the voluntary, issuing from the collaboration of will and intellect, admits of moral evaluation, so if something is forced on one or performed in ignorance of essential circumstances, it can be neither praised nor blamed. Conversely, if something is neither forced on one nor performed while one is burdened with such ignorance, it must enter into the moral universe. We cannot refuse to say whether it is good or bad. This principle stands behind the encyclical's assertion that in moral analysis one must place oneself in the perspective of the acting person. This perspective is an intentional perspective: it is the realm of the will, as opposed to the realm of consequences considered independently of how and why they are intended. The point of human life is to take that which falls within this perspective and to order it, in all its concrete detail, to God.

Essential Moral Principles in Health Care in the Thought of John Paul II

Sarah-Vaughan Brakman

In this article, I review selected moral principles central to moral evaluation in Catholic bioethics, with particular attention to the way in which John Paul II's work on moral theology in *Veritatis splendor* has clarified and strengthened the foundation of these principles.[1] This review will serve as a useful heuristic for the rest of this volume, giving us a common base of reference and language. It also gives us an opportunity to see how the principles play out in regard to contemporary challenges in medicine and health care.

The principles I review here are those of double effect, totality and integrity, and informed consent. Prior to their consideration, I provide a brief overview of natural law with refer-

---

[1] John Paul II, *The Splendor of Truth* (*Veritatis splendor*) (Washington, DC: U.S. Catholic Conference, 1993). In this chapter, the original italics appear in all quotations from the encyclical, except where noted.

ence to the personalist approach of Pope John Paul II, for each of these principles must be understood within the tradition. This is important to emphasize, as the principles (especially double effect and informed consent) also appear in secular analyses in bioethics, with the unfortunate and all too frequent result of misunderstanding and misapplication. After the theoretical presentation, I discuss each of the principles in turn and consider specific instances of their application. I also look at how the principles have been incorporated by the United States Conference of Catholic Bishops into the *Ethical and Religious Directives for Catholic Health Care Services* (ERDs).[2]

Natural Law and the Dignity of the Human Person

> Acting is morally good when the choices of freedom are *in conformity with man's true good* and thus express the voluntary ordering of the person towards this ultimate end: God himself. — JOHN PAUL II, *Veritatis splendor,* n. 72

In the first line of Book I of the *Nichomachean Ethics,* Aristotle tells us that "every art and every inquiry, and similarly every action and pursuit, is thought to aim at some good."[3] Aristotle believes that every act and every entity has an end, or purpose, that is inscribed in its nature. The end is called the *telos* in Greek. He goes on to say, "if there is an end for all that we do, this will be the good achievable by action, and if there is more than one, these will be the goods achievable by action."[4] The excellent achievement, or fulfillment of the end, is called the *good* for that thing. The end of the acorn is to become an oak tree. The good of the pen is to write. The good pen writes well. The good meal is nutritious, tasty, and satisfying.

When we ask about the *moral* good, though, we are asking about what makes for a good act or a good person. This moral perspective is known as "teleological," since it holds that the good act or good person is one that aims at a particular end. To know what the good is for human beings, we need

---

[2] U.S. Conference of Catholic Bishops, *Ethical and Religious Directives for Catholic Health Care Services,* 4th ed. (Washington, DC: USCCB, 2001).

[3] Aristotle, *Nicomachean Ethics,* in *The Basic Works of Aristotle,* ed. Richard McKeon (New York: Random House, 1941), book I, chapter 1, 1094a.

[4] Ibid., book I, chapter 7, 1097a.

look to the end of human actions, which according to Aristotle is true human happiness. To understand what is meant by human happiness, we need to look to the nature of man himself. Aristotle tells us that rationality is the distinctive characteristic of human nature, and "the function of man is an activity of soul which follows or implies a rational principle."[5] Aristotle understood that the life of reason must also have other goods, however, to fulfill the complete nature of humans, for we are not only rational beings, but emotional and embodied beings as well. The external goods which must be sufficiently met, then, include friends, health, family, and money.[6]

Thomas Aquinas brought together these Aristotelian insights as well as some Stoic elements and provided them with the proper theological grounding. Aquinas showed that we know that we act rightly when we act in such a way that the end of our nature, rationality and its attendant goods, is respected and promoted. He said:

> Hence the first precept of law is that good is to be done and pursued, and evil is to be avoided. All the other precepts of the law of nature are based on this, so that all the things that are to be done or evils to be avoided belong to the precepts of the natural law which the practical reason naturally apprehends as human goods.[7]

Aquinas defined the natural law as "nothing other than the light of understanding infused in us by God, whereby we understand what must be done and what must be avoided. God gave this light and this law to man at creation."[8] In *Veritatis splendor*, John Paul II says that this is called the natural law "not because it refers to the nature of irrational beings but because the reason which promulgates it is proper to human nature."[9]

The central question here is, of course, What is the good and what is the evil? Our rationality tells us that the good refers to those elements of which we must have a sufficiency in order to thrive as a species and as individuals. On this list, then, are goods that address the basic areas of human na-

---

[5] Ibid., book I, chapter 7, 1098a.

[6] Ibid., book I, chapter 8, 1099b.

[7] Thomas Aquinas, "Summa Theologiae: The Treatise on Law," in *St. Thomas Aquinas on Politics and Ethics*, ed. and trans. Paul E. Sigmund (New York: W.W. Norton, 1988), question 94, no. 2, 49.

[8] *Veritatis splendor*, n. 12.

[9] Ibid., n. 42.

ture—rationality, yes, but also our embodiment and the ful-fillment of our emotional and spiritual life. The basic (or fundamental) human goods include life, health, basic nutrition, shelter, knowledge, sociality (friendship), procreation, and the rearing of children.[10] A good act, then, is one that protects or promotes these basic human goods. An evil act is one that directly violates one or more of them.

Morality, then, is founded on an explicit philosophical and theological anthropology, which grounds the good in a particular understanding of human nature. In the words of the noted Catholic bioethicist Edmund Pellegrino,

> This anthropology grounds the notion of human dignity as something intrinsic to being human and not something that can be lost if we lose consciousness, suffer disfigurement or a physical disability. A Christian anthropology gives meaning to humans as finite creatures, not self-created; stewards, not absolute masters of their lives.[11]

What makes an act good or evil, therefore, is the specific kind of act it is; that is, does it promote the good (for humans), is it neutral to the good (for humans), or does it directly violate a good (for humans). The concept of the specific *kind* of act refers to what is known as the moral object of an act. The moral object is the primary source of moral status of any given act.[12] John Paul II says, "An act is ... good if its object is in conformity with the good of the person with respect for the good morally relevant for him."[13]

In the same section in *Veritatis splendor*, however, he goes on to say that

> Christian ethics, which pays particular attention to the moral object, does not refuse to consider the inner "teleology" of action, inasmuch as it is directed to promoting

---

[10] In fact, there is great debate about what belongs on the list, especially whether "life" itself is a more fundamental good than the others or whether it is first among equals.

[11] Edmund D. Pellegrino, "Secular Bioethics and Catholic Medical Ethics: Moral Philosophy at the 'Margins,'" in *The Bishop and the Future of Catholic Health Care: Challenges and Opportunities*—Proceedings of the Sixteenth Workshop for Bishops, ed. Daniel P. Maher (Boston: Pope John Center, 1997), 39.

[12] Peter J. Cataldo, "The Moral Fonts of Action and Decision Making," in *Catholic Health Care Ethics: A Manual for Ethics Committees*, eds. Peter J. Cataldo and Albert S. Moraczewski, O.P. (Boston: National Catholic Bioethics Center, 2001), 2/2–2/3.

[13] *Veritatis splendor*, n. 78.

the true good of the person; but it recognizes that it is really pursued only when the essential elements of human nature are respected.[14]

This quote is particularly wonderful, for by it John Paul II tells us so much about the truth of morality for the Catholic tradition. While recognizing that the nature of morality is to promote certain ends, so that it is, in one sense, teleological in structure, he is agreeing that it does so not by some sort of weighing or measuring of consequences (this theory is known as consequentialism) or even by solely balancing goods and evils (this theory, espoused by some Catholic theologians and directly critiqued by John Paul II in *Veritatis splendor,* is known as proportionalism).[15] Natural law morality has absolute prohibitions against certain kinds of actions because the acts by their nature do not respect or promote the essential elements of human nature. This is what is meant by "inner teleology."

In addition to the moral object, two other elements are central to the structure of a moral act. The second element is intention. Intention refers to why the act is being done and is thus, as Peter Cataldo says, "the subjective aspect of aiming toward an ultimate end, or subordinate ends, or toward the particular means selected for possibly attaining one or more of those ends."[16] Intention is central to the moral structure of actions and, therefore, to the moral evaluation. Someone's intention for acting tells us what that person wills by the action. When a physician orders the removal of life-sustaining treatment, we need to know whether her intention is the immediate death of the patient or the alleviation of the patient's suffering and protection of his dignity. The third and final element is circumstances—the particularity of where and how an action is carried out. The moral integration of all three elements—object, intention, and circumstances—is necessary for an act to be considered good.[17]

Critiques of natural law have been made by Catholic and non-Catholic theologians alike. The usual charge is that in natural law one argues from biological fact, or mere mechanistic

---

[14] Ibid., n. 78.

[15] Proportionalist views in the field of medical ethics were most notably advanced by Richard McCommick, S.J., who wrote extensively in defense of this approach and criticized John Paul II for mischaracterizing the claims of proportionalist arguments.

[16] Cataldo, "Moral Fonts of Actions and Decision Making," 2/2.

[17] Ibid., 2/3.

truths of the world, to moral values. John Paul II himself provides the strongest and clearest formulation of this critique:

> a morally negative evaluation of such acts [contraception, direct sterilization, autoeroticism, premarital sexual relations, homosexual relations, and artificial insemination] fails to take into adequate consideration both man's character as a rational and free being and the cultural conditioning of all moral norms.[18]

He directly argues against this charge in *Veritatis splendor* by showing that it overlooks the essence of the nature in question—that is, the essence of human nature. He claims that the human body is not "a raw datum, devoid of any meaning and moral values until freedom has shaped it in accordance with its design." The body is not a mere container but is central to the essence of the person. John Paul II frames it thus:

> The spiritual and immortal soul is the principle of unity of the human being, whereby it exists as a whole.... It is in the light of the dignity of the human person—a dignity which must be affirmed for its own sake—that reason grasps the specific moral value of certain goods towards which the person is naturally inclined. And since the human person cannot be reduced to a freedom which is self-designing, but entails a particular spiritual and bodily structure, the primordial moral requirement of loving and *respecting the person as an end and never as a mere means* also implies, by its very nature, respect for certain fundamental goods, without which one would fall into relativism and arbitrariness.[19]

We see in this response the clear influence of Kant upon John Paul II's philosophy. Indeed, the best-known formulation of Kant's categorical imperative states, "Act so that you treat humanity, whether in your own person or in that of another, always as an end and never as a means only."[20] The emphasis on the dignity of *persons* for determining an action's moral worth is shared by both scholars.

At the same time, we see in this quotation John Paul II's clear disagreement with Kant's definition of what it means to be a person. For Kant, rationality is the sole key to personhood.[21]

---

[18] *Veritatis splendor,* n. 47.

[19] Ibid., n. 48 (emphasis added).

[20] Immanuel Kant, *Foundations of the Metaphysics of Morals,* trans. Lewis White Beck (New York: Macmillan, 1986), 47.

[21] Kant, *Metaphysics of Morals,* 57.

In his view, humans who lack the capacity for rationality are not persons and, therefore, are not entities of intrinsic moral worth. (Indeed, he refers to them as "things" in the moral sense.)

Kant's conception of personhood has had a tremendous influence on secular thinking about many bioethical issues, from euthanasia and abortion to stem cell research and cloning. Rejecting Kant and the Cartesian dualism on which Kant's work rests, John Paul II's anthropology is informed by classical philosophy (natural law) and modern phenomenology (personalism). For John Paul II, human nature is by definition a rational, spiritual, embodied nature. As William E. May says, "The truth that human persons are *bodily* beings and that human bodily life is a good *of* the person, intrinsic to the person, and not merely a good *for* the person, extrinsic to the person, is at the heart of a sound bioethics, Catholic or otherwise."[22]

For Kant, furthermore, the subjective experiences and particular knowledge of a rational being have no moral worth, whereas for John Paul II, respect for subjectivity is central to respect for persons. This particular point brings us to a brief consideration of personalism, the philosophical approach most closely associated with John Paul II. Personalism is characterized by a different emphasis in morality from that of natural law. It starts at the level of *subjectivity*, which refers to our lived experience, our self-consciousness. Notice, however, that this is not the same thing as *subjectivism*. Subjectivism is a moral viewpoint that there are no universal truths, that morality is, fundamentally, determined by the individual. Subjectivity, on the other hand, is a focus on the experiences and consciousness of individuals, i.e., subjects. Personalism focuses on the concrete individuality that all humans share. Painting in very broad strokes, we see that where natural law focuses on the objective universal goods and the characteristics that define humanity in general, personalism centers on the subjectivity of the person and on how an individual's actions and choices shape who he is. In comparing the two approaches as they are represented in *Veritatis splendor*, Janet Smith says,

> The Aristotelian definition of man adopted by Aquinas, defined man not only as a rational animal, but also as a social animal. His individual good was dependent upon

---

[22] William E. May, "John Paul II, *Veritatis splendor* and Bioethics," in *John Paul II's Contribution to Catholic Bioethics,* ed. Christopher Tollefsen. Philosophy and Medicine, no. 84 (Dordrecht, The Netherlands: Springer, 2004), 36 (original emphasis).

the common good.... [Personalism in *Veritatis splendor*] portrays man in his deepest ontological core as being one who should make a "gift of himself." Talk of "gift of self" is nearly always linked to the imitation of Christ.[23]

One of the most important topics of discussion in *Veritatis splendor,* which shows not only the complementarity of the traditions of natural law and personalism but also Kantian sensibilities, is the role of the conscience in moral decision making. John Paul II says,

> The relationship between man's freedom and God's law is most deeply lived out in the "heart" of the person, in his moral conscience.... The way in which one conceives the relationship between freedom and law is thus intimately bound up with one's understanding of the moral conscience.[24]

John Paul II reaffirms the dignity of human freedom but argues most directly against theoretical positions that unhinge human freedom from human nature and the law and hold freedom "exalted almost to the point of idolatry." He clarifies: "To the affirmation that one has a duty to follow one's conscience is unduly added the affirmation that one's moral judgment is true merely by the fact that it has its origin in the conscience."[25]

Human freedom depends on truth, "a dependence which has found its clearest and most authoritative expression in the words of Christ: 'You will know the truth, and the truth will set you free' (Jn 8:32)."[26] Authentic human freedom is expressed in the recognition of the good and the subsequent willing of the act which respects that good (Kant) and moreover promotes it (Aquinas).

The proper role of conscience, and the true relationship between freedom and nature, are central to all the principles I discuss in the following pages. Let me turn first to a discussion of the principle of double effect.

---

[23] Janet E. Smith, "Natural Law and Personalism in *Veritatis splendor*," http://www.aodonline.org/aodonline-sqlimages/SHMS/Faculty/SmithJanet/Publications/MoralPhilosophy/NaturalLawandPersonalism.pdf, 10. First published in *Veritatis Splendor: American Responses,* ed. Michael E. Allsopp and John J. O'Keefe (Kansas City, MO: Sheed & Ward, 1995), 194–207; reprinted in *John Paul II and Moral Theology,* ed. Charles E. Curran and Richard A. McCormick, S.J., Readings in Moral Theology, no. 10 (Mahwah, NJ: Paulist Press, 1998), 67–84.

[24] John Paul II, *Veritatis splendor,* n. 54.

[25] Ibid., n. 32.

[26] Ibid., n. 34.

The Principle of Double Effect

> Hence human activity cannot be judged as morally good merely because it is a means for attaining one or another of its goals, or simply because the subject's intention is good.... If the object of the concrete action is not in harmony with the true good of the person, the choice of that action makes our will and ourselves morally evil, thus putting us in conflict with our ultimate end, the supreme good, God himself. — JOHN PAUL II, *Veritatis splendor,* n. 72.

Double effect is one of the most widely invoked principles, not only in Catholic health care but in secular medicine as well. Not surprisingly, then, it is often misapplied. The principle itself is actually a set of four subprinciples, or propositions, each one necessary and jointly sufficient for the principle to be correctly invoked.[27] The history of double effect can be traced through Aquinas, in his discussion of the permissibility of killing an unjust aggressor, but it was really the Salmanticenses of the sixteenth and seventeenth centuries who developed the principle, with the greatest credit going to the nineteenth-century Jesuit theologian Jean ·Pierre Gury.[28]

The purpose of the principle is to determine whether an action or proposal that involves both a good and an evil effect is itself morally licit; there is sometimes confusion, however, over whether these effects are moral or what are called premoral (or physical) effects. Albert Moraczewski, O.P., has clarified this nicely:

> In the case of the pregnant woman who has cancer, say of the cervix, the good, intended effect is the saving of her

---

[27] Peter Cataldo and Orville Griese, for example, believe there are five conditions of the principle, the fifth being that "the good effect can only be achieved concomitant with, but not by means of, the bad effect" (Peter Cataldo, "The Principle of Double Effect," *Ethical Principle in Catholic Health Care,* ed. Edward J. Furton [Boston: National Catholic Bioethics Center, 1999], 83). This means that there is no alternative possible in the situation which does not also risk the bad effect. I see this not as a fifth condition, but rather as a precursor to invoking the principle. If one can attain the good effect without risking the evil effect, then that is the action that one should take. Also, this condition is implied or closely related to the second condition. See also Orville Griese, "The Principle of the Double Effect," in *Catholic Identity in Health Care: Principles and Practice* (Braintree, MA: Pope John Center), 1987, 246–299.

[28] F. J. Connell, "Double Effect, Principle of," *New Catholic Encyclopedia* vol. 4 (New York: McGraw-Hill, 1967), 1020–2.

life. Life is a physical good, not in itself a moral good, although as such it is an ontological good (i.e., the good of simply existing). The foreseen and unintended death of the child is of itself a physical evil. If, however, a person freely chooses to directly destroy that life, the *intention and action* following thereupon are morally evil. The loss of life in itself abstracted from any morally evil intention and action is nonmoral.[29]

We may never directly and intentionally do evil, but in some cases we may allow evil to occur as a result of our actions, when we are in direct pursuit of the good. Let us consider each of the four conditions of double effect:

1. *The act to be performed is in itself good (determined by its object) or at least neutral (i.e., it cannot be intrinsically evil).* As Pope John Paul II says, "consequently, circumstances or intentions can never transform an act intrinsically evil by virtue of its object into an act 'subjectively' good or defensible as a choice."[30] The often-repeated example is of adultery committed to save a life, as in a minor scene from the classic movie *Casablanca,* in which a young wife fleeing the Nazis asks if it would be wrong to sleep with an official to obtain exit visas to save her husband's life and her own, especially if she did it out of love for her husband. That we cannot do evil even for a good intention is founded in the incommensurability of the fundamental human goods—we cannot trade off or weigh these goods against each other. To violate one is to act wrongly.

2. *The good effect must be intended (or willed), and the evil effect, although it may be foreseen, must be unintended.* The person acting must intend the good effect directly. The evil may be foreseen as a logical result, but it cannot be the reason for or direct purpose of the action. The Secret Service agent who jumps in front of a bullet aimed at the President is fully aware that her action will probably kill her, but if this is not her intention—if the reason for her sacrifice is her sworn duty to protect the life of the President—then the act has moral worth. If the person is disappointed that she did not die, then obviously this condition has not been met.

---

[29] Albert S. Moraczewski, O.P., "The Double Effect," in Cataldo and Moraczewski, *Catholic Health Care Ethics,* 3D/1 (original italics).

[30] *Veritatis splendor,* n. 81.

3. *The evil effect may not be the means to the good effect.* This proposition speaks to the issue of causality. Both the good and the evil effect must result from the act. It cannot be the case that the evil was necessary to achieve the good. Moreover, the good effect flows from the action "at least as immediately (in the order of causality, though not necessarily in the order of time) as the bad effect."[31] An example is the fire bombings of Dresden, Germany, in World War II, which some have even called a war crime. In this case, evil (the terror attack on an already suffering civilian population in the service of no stated military goal) was done so that good (further demoralization of the Nazis and indirect threatening of Russia) could come, which was a violation of natural law.

4. *The good to be achieved must be proportionate to the evil that is risked.* This condition speaks to the moral permissibility of even risking evil through one's actions. This is not a weighing of goods and evils. It is a call to understanding when such risks are prudent or foolhardy in a given situation:

> In forming this decision many factors must be weighed and compared, with care and prudence proportionate to the importance of the case. Thus, an effect that benefits or harms society generally has more weight than one that affects only an individual; an effect sure to occur deserves greater consideration than one that is only probable; an effect of a moral nature has greater importance than one that deals only with material things.[32]

As an example, directive 49 of the ERDs states that "for a proportionate reason, labor may be induced after the fetus is viable." The health of the fetus may be risked when the health of the mother is at stake; the life of the fetus may be risked when the life of the mother is at stake. In another type of example, risking the harms of surgery in the pursuit of health is usually proportionate. Sometimes risking such harms is not proportionate, however, as when one chooses extensive elective cosmetic surgery for aesthetic enhancement, knowing that there is a small but real risk to one's life and, in some cases, a substantial risk to one's overall health.

---

[31] Connell, "Double Effect."

[32] Ibid.

It is, in fact, to this last condition of double effect that proportionalists appeal as the sole (or primary) source of morality. Certainly, proportionality is a central concept in the Catholic tradition. However, what is crucial to a proper understanding of double effect and Catholic morality is that all four conditions must be met or the action is impermissible. Proportionality does not trump the other conditions. Double effect has also been misunderstood by ethicists outside the tradition, who have thought that either intentionality or direct causality was the sole or primary determinant of the principle.

Others have argued against double effect by saying that "the conditions of the principle itself have no necessary, a priori internal coherence."[33] It is difficult to understand this argument, since as I have shown, all parts of the principle are drawn from the natural law tradition—the existence of intrinsically evil acts, the emphasis on intentions for moral evaluation, the related but distinct concept of causation, and the prudential judgment concerning proportionate risks. Indeed, in many ways, the principle of double effect is an elegant distillation of the main components of natural law.

I turn now to a few specific examples of the use (and abuse) of double effect in health care.

Examples of Double Effect in Health Care

There are many examples of the usefulness of the principle of double effect in Catholic bioethics. In end-of-life care, we know that euthanasia, whether active or passive, is never morally permissible and that "Catholic health care institutions may never condone or participate in euthanasia or assisted suicide in any way."[34] We also know, however, that it is morally permissible to address the suffering and pain of a dying patient with medication that will in all likelihood hasten death.[35] The principle of double effect explains the difference here. Since a high dose of pain medication is not intrinsically evil, the first condition is met. Condition 2 is also met, as relief of suffering is the intention behind the administration of the medicine, the hastening of death being foreseen only and not intended. Con-

---

[33] J. F. Keenan, S.J., "The Function of the Principle of Double Effect," *Theological Studies* 54.2 (1993), 298; quoted in Cataldo, "Principle of Double Effect," 81.

[34] ERDs, n. 60.

[35] Ibid., n. 61.

dition 3 is met because the hastening of death is an indirect effect of the pain medication, and the relief of pain is not obtained by the means of death (as it would be in euthanasia). Finally, the good to be achieved and the evil risked are surely proportionate (condition 4). Although there are those who would characterize this procedure as euthanasia because of its external similarity to passive euthanasia, the moral nature and hence evaluation of the act is completely different, as shown by application of the principle of double effect.

Directive 47 of the ERDs is a clear example of the principle of double effect as applied to reproductive issues:

> Operations, treatments, and medications that have as their direct purpose the cure [conditions 1 and 3] of the proportionately serious pathological condition of a pregnant woman [condition 4] are permitted when they cannot be safely postponed until the unborn child is viable, even if they will result in the death of the unborn child [condition 2].

The principle of double effect is often invoked and often misapplied in regard to protocols for sterilization in Catholic healthcare facilities. Recently, a Catholic hospital designed a protocol for surgical sterilization that contained the following language: "The request for sterilization will be granted only for patients with extremely serious medical conditions, i.e., that a pregnancy will significantly compromise the health of the patient or possibly cause death." The serious medical conditions for which the request could be granted included hypertension, heart disease, renal disease, insulin-dependent diabetes, chronic thrombophlebitis, and pulmonary embolism.[36] The thinking behind the protocol appeared to be that this guideline was justified under the principle of double effect, since the good effect (maintaining health) was the goal and the evil effect (sterilization) was tolerated in the service of the good.

While the protocol does respect the fourth condition, that of proportionality, it directly violates conditions 1, 2, and 3. The act is intrinsically evil, for the object of the procedure is to induce sterility or infertility, which is a direct violation of a basic human good. The surgery is neither morally neutral nor good in itself, since its moral object is evil. Directive 70 of the ERDs states that "Catholic health care organizations are not permitted to engage in immediate material cooperation in ac-

---

[36] This protocol was sent to The National Catholic Bioethics Center for review in 2004. All identifying information was removed from the document prior to my examination of it.

tions that are intrinsically immoral, such as abortion, euthanasia, assisted suicide, and direct sterilization."

The intention behind the surgery is to permanently render a woman incapable of pregnancy, so that her health will not be affected by a pregnancy; therefore, this protocol entails a direct violation of the second condition. Finally, while the long-range goal may be the good of protecting health and life, this good is to be obtained by means of the evil, which violates the third condition. It is crucial, too, that the precondition for invoking double effect—ensuring that there is no other course of action that does not entail the evil effect—also has not been met. In fact, it could easily be argued from tradition that the most good would be promoted not by the subjection of a woman (whose health in such cases is already somewhat compromised) to surgery (which may not be 100 percent effective), but rather by the exercise of free will by the couple to regulate sexual intercourse.[37]

In brief, the principle of double effect cannot be used to justify direct sterilizations. In some circumstances the principle may support operations, treatments, and medications that indirectly induce sterility if they are used for proportionately grave reasons, if the direct effect of their use is a cure or alleviation of a serious pathologic condition, and if no other treatment is available. A hysterectomy for uterine cancer or severe fibroid tumor disease that has not responded to other treatment may be justified by a proper application of the principle of double effect. A hysterectomy to remove a uterus that might not be able to carry a future pregnancy without medical risk, however, cannot be justified by the principle of double effect, because both the intention and the goal of the surgery are precisely to prevent pregnancy. and the procedure is, by definition, a direct sterilization.

What about the premenopausal removal of ovaries from a woman who has a strong family history of ovarian cancer? There is no disease now, so the issue concerns a risk of a disease

---

[37] Current statistics for success rates for avoiding pregnancy using natural family planning methods are comparable to those for the birth control pill. See Richard J. Fehring, "The Future of Professional Education in Natural Family Planning," *Journal of Obstetrics, Gynecology and Neonatal Nursing* 33.1 (January–February 2004): 34–43; M. Arevalo et al., "Efficacy of the New Two-Day Method of Family Planning,"*Fertility and Sterility* 82.4 (October 2004): 885–892; and N. Matis, "Natural Family Planning: A Birth Control Alternative," *Journal of Nurse Midwifery* 28.1 (January–February 1983): 7–16.

versus induced sterility. The difference between this case and the one above (concerning the removal of the uterus to avoid a risky pregnancy) is that this is an example of indirect sterilization. The first condition of double effect is fulfilled, since the moral object of the procedure is not contraceptive in nature. The second condition is also met, since the intention is to protect the woman from disease, with sterility foreseen but not intended. Furthermore, sterility is not the means of protecting the woman's health, so condition 3 is met. In regard to condition 4, some types of ovarian cancer have been shown to be genetic. Ovarian cancer is also one of the most deadly types of cancer, since the presentation of symptoms is long delayed, usually until the cancer is advanced and a cure unlikely. If it could be reasonably determined that a particular woman had such increased risk, in all probability the procedure could be morally justified according to the principle of double effect.

This particular case can also be evaluated by another essential moral principle, that of totality. I turn now to a brief discussion of the principles of totality and integrity.

The Principles of Totality and Integrity

> Only in reference to the human person in his "unified totality," that is, as "a soul which expresses itself in a body and a body informed by an immortal spirit," can the specifically human meaning of the body be grasped. Indeed, natural inclinations take on moral relevance only insofar as they refer to the human person and his authentic fulfillment, a fulfillment which for that matter can take place always and only in human nature. By rejecting all manipulations of corporeity which alter its human meaning, the Church serves man and shows him the path of true love, the only path on which he can find the true God. — JOHN PAUL II, *Veritatis splendor,* n. 50

Totality and integrity of the body are complementary principles founded upon the Christian anthropology of the human person that was discussed in the first section of this paper. The human person exists as a rational, embodied spiritual being made in the image of God. Respect for human dignity means respecting this "unified totality." In his comprehensive volume on Catholic health care, Rev. Msgr. Orville Griese provides a complete definition of these principles:

> "Integrity" refers to each individual's duty to "preserve a view of the whole human person ... in which the values of intellect, will, conscience, and fraternity are pre-eminent."
> ... "Totality" refers to the duty to preserve intact the physical

component of the integrated whole, whereby, in the words of St. Thomas Aquinas, every member of the human body "exists for the sake of the whole as the imperfect for the sake of the perfect. Hence a member of the human body is to be disposed of according as it may profit the whole ... if ... a member is healthy and continuing in its natural state, it cannot be cut off to the detriment of the whole."[38]

These principles reflect that humans must exercise responsible stewardship for all that we have received from God, including our very personhood and our bodies. The principle of integrity is "perhaps best understood as being respectful of the hierarchical ordering of the members of the body."[39] Totality refers to the obligation to preserve functional body wholeness.[40]

Both principles find expression in the ERDs. Directive 29 states,

> All persons served by Catholic health care have the right and duty to protect and preserve their bodily and functional integrity. The functional integrity of the person may be sacrificed to maintain the health or life of the person when no other morally permissible means is available.

The principle of integrity is supported by directive 33:

> The well-being of the whole person must be taken into account in deciding about any therapeutic intervention or use of technology. Therapeutic procedures that are likely to cause harm or undesirable side-effects can be justified only by a proportionate benefit to the patient.

The centrality of the "profound respect for the body" is ever present in Catholic morality. In the words of John Haas,

> The human body shares in the dignity of the "image of God"... and it is the whole human person that is intended to become, in the body of Christ, a temple of the Spirit (*Catechism of the Catholic Church*, n. 364). The principles of totality and integrity guide our actions in the care of this spiritual and bodily creature for whom God has such love.[41]

---

[38] Griese, *Catholic Identity in Health Care*, 204–205. Internal references are to *Gaudium et Spes*, n. 61, and to Aquinas's *Summa Theologiae*, II-II, Q. 65.1c.

[39] Germain Kopaczynski, "Totality and Integrity," in Cataldo and Moraczewski, *Catholic Health Care Ethics*, 3A/2.

[40] John Haas, "The Totality and Integrity of the Body," in Furton, *Ethical Principle in Catholic Health Care*, 87.

[41] Ibid., 88.

Examples of Totality and Integrity in Health Care

I return now to the example used at the end of the section on the principle of double effect. This woman had a strong family history of ovarian cancer and was considering having her ovaries removed. According to the principle of double effect, this was morally permissible. However, is such an operation a violation of the principle of totality?

In 1953, Pope Pius XII taught that three circumstances justify the removal of an otherwise healthy organ:

> 1) when the preservation of the organ would cause serious damage or even endanger the life of the entire organism; 2) when the damage could not be avoided in any other way than through surgery, and there is reasonable hope of success; and 3) when the surgery and removal of the organ or suppression of its function will lead to a diminution or elimination of the threat to the organism.[42]

This third circumstance appears to fit our case, so such an operation could be justified according to both double effect and totality.[43] The principles of totality and integrity do not, however, justify a tubal ligation, because that is not the treatment of a disease but an attempt to avoid a pregnancy that would be the result of freely chosen sexual intercourse. This matter is reflected in the *Catechism of the Catholic Church*: "Except when performed for strictly therapeutic medical reasons, directly intended *amputations, mutilations*, and *sterilizations* performed on innocent persons are against the moral law" (n. 2297).[44]

Organ donations after death do not violate totality, for there is no more functional wholeness, nor do they violate integrity, for the spirit of the person is no longer present with the body. (Directives 63 through 66 of the ERDs address organ donations.) What about donations from the living? Appar-

---

[42] Pius XII, "Address to 26th Congress of Italian Association of Urology," *AAS* 45 (1953), n. 14; quoted in Haas, "Totality and Integrity," 86.

[43] This conclusion is supported by Peter Cataldo in an unpublished analysis, "The Ethics of Mastectomy or Oophorectomy as Prophylactic Measures against Breast or Ovarian Cancer" (personal communication).

[44] *Catechism of the Catholic Church: Modifications from the Editio Typica*, second edition, trans. U.S. Catholic Conference (Vatican City: Libreria Editrice Vaticana, 1997).

ently, there is no problem with blood donation or even in some cases bone marrow or partial liver donation, for these are not detrimental to functional bodily wholeness. Donation of a paired organ, such as a kidney, may be licit if there is a grave reason for making the donation, free and informed consent has been given, and "the anticipated benefit to the recipient is proportionate to the harm done to the donor."[45]

Haas, however, has said that one could not donate a cornea, for example,

> because even though eyes come in pairs, the elimination of one of them would severely diminish the wholesome functioning of the body. A person loses considerable peripheral vision and depth perception with the loss of an eye.[46]

Corneal transplants from living sighted persons are not performed at the present time, because of the general understanding that one does need both eyes for optimal functioning (unlike kidneys).

However, directive 30 of the ERDs states, "The transplantation of organs from living donors is morally permissible when such a donation will not sacrifice or *seriously impair* any essential bodily function and the anticipated benefit to the recipient is proportionate to the harm done to the donor" (emphasis added). The issue of corneal transplants from living, normal, sighted donors hinges on the definition of "seriously impair" and on the proportionate good versus harm.

Although a person who loses an eye will lose depth perception, "there are monocular cues to depth that can be learned through experience."[47] In addition, most activities of daily living are not affected, and those that are may still be accomplished through adaptation and rehabitation. Most states allow persons with vision in only one eye to drive, since the visual field requirements can usually be met.[48]

While the loss of vision in one eye does entail risks and some degree of functional impairment, it is *possible* to imagine a case in which the impairment is not serious in a given person's

---

[45] ERDs, n. 30. See also Haas, "Totality and Integrity," 87–88.

[46] Haas, "Totality and Integrity," 88.

[47] Thomas Politzer, "Implications of Acquired Monocular Vision (Loss of One Eye)," Neuro-Optometric Rehabilitation Online, http://www.nora.cc/patient_area/monocular_vision.html.

[48] Ibid.

life,[49] no other option is available for the potential recipient, and proportionality is achieved between benefits and harms. An example of such a case might be a woman with young children who has a condition called keratoconus, in which even glasses and contacts cannot aid sight. Since the wait for a corneal transplant from a dead donor is currently years, would it be permissible for her sister—who is not a mother, is financially wealthy, and (let's say) engages in the hobbies of swimming and writing—to donate a cornea to her? I hold that an argument in principle could be made for this donation according to totality and integrity (although I do concede that in reality the likelihood of any such case is extremely remote, and that due to legitimate health concerns for donors, we should attempt first to increase corneal donations after death.)

These examples show the relevance of the principles of totality and integrity and also raise important questions about the kinds of treatments and procedures to which individuals may consent and the role of freedom in decision making. I now turn to the final principle, informed consent.

The Principle of Informed Consent

> The relationship between faith and morality shines forth with all its brilliance in the *unconditional respect due to the insistent demands of the personal dignity of every man,* demands protected by those moral norms which prohibit without exception actions which are intrinsically evil. — JOHN PAUL II, *Veritatis splendor,* n. 90

One of the most important principles in health-care ethics is informed consent.[50] This principle is founded on the respect due to human dignity and to the autonomy of man. Directive 26 of the ERDs states,

> The free and informed consent of the person or the person's surrogate is required for medical treatments and procedures, except in an emergency situation when consent cannot be obtained and there is no indication that the patient would refuse consent to the treatment.

---

[49] Many persons with only one eye lead successful and productive lives, including President Theodore Roosevelt, Edgar Degas (artist), Frank Brady (airplane pilot), and Sandy Duncan and Sammy Davis, Jr.(entertainers).

[50] Indeed, six of the seventy-two directives of the ERDs speak specifically about informed consent, and at least four others are relevant to the principle.

One of the most complete statements of the principle in the Catholic tradition is found in Griese:

> It is the right and duty of every competent individual to advance "his higher spiritual as well as his bodily welfare" by voluntarily consenting or by refusing consent (either implied or reasonably presumed)—free of all external pressures—to recommended and necessary medical or psychological procedures and/or spiritual ministrations, based on a sufficient knowledge of the benefits, burdens, and risks involved. For incompetent individuals, this right and duty is to be interpreted by the parents, spouse, or legitimate guardians in accordance (as far as possible) with that individual's known or reasonable wishes.[51]

I take in turn the central aspects of informed consent. Griese first addresses the principle in regard to competent individuals. Every conscious adult person (over the age of eighteen) is presumed to be competent to make health-care decisions on his own behalf unless proven otherwise. This is true even for individuals who have been deemed to be incompetent to handle their financial affairs, have diagnosed mental illnesses, or have known mental or physical disabilities. In health care, competency is considered in relation to specific decisions. This means that someone might be competent to make a particular health-care decision (regarding treatment options, for example) but simultaneously incompetent to make another, perhaps more weighty decision (say, regarding refusal of life-saving treatment). Competency is thus a threshold concept, with greater amounts of capacity required for decisions that have more grave risks to the individual or to others.

What precisely, though, are these capacities for competency, and who decides that a given individual possesses the requisite capacity for a particular health-care decision? The mental capacities necessary for competency are those that are central to the "consent" part of informed consent. First is an adequate understanding of the nature of the proposed treatment, its likely benefits and risks, and its purpose. Second is an adequate reasoning ability, to process the implications of each treatment or nontreatment option. Third is a level of deliberation sufficient to weigh the alternatives against one another, and fourth is the ability to communicate decisions in a clear and unambiguous manner. This last condition does not give any priority to oral communication, of course, but only stipulates effective communication.

---

[51] Griese, *Catholic Identity in Health Care*, 154.

If any member of a family or health-care team questions whether a patient possesses these necessary capacities for consent, then a formal competency determination ought to be sought. In the United States, competency is actually a legal concept that is usually determined by specific consultation with a psychiatrist.

Deciding that a conscious adult patient is incompetent to make a health-care decision is, therefore, a formal process. This is important to understand, as there is still much confusion about it in the United States, even among well-meaning health-care workers. I have known superbly caring and truly brilliant nurses and physicians who have told me that certain patients were not competent to consent because they had severe mental disability—this without benefit of a formal determination of the person's abilities concerning the specific decision at hand.

Informed consent is a crucial safeguard of the dignity of every individual, regardless of disability. This is reflected in directive 3 of the ERDs: "the person with mental or physical disabilities, regardless of the cause or severity, must be treated as a unique person of incomparable worth, with the same right to life and to adequate health care as all other persons."[52] At the same time, however, we need to appreciate that certain individuals, because of their conditions (e.g., comatose states, persistent vegetative states, psychotic episodes, paranoid delusions, or severe dementia), may not be competent to make any health-care decisions.

If it has been formally determined that an individual is incompetent to make a health-care decision or set of decisions, then his proxy must decide on his behalf, as Griese's definition stipulates. In the United States, an individual may execute a durable power of attorney for health care. This document allows someone, when competent, to choose a person to make health-care decisions for him when he is not competent to make them himself.[53] He may choose any person to be his surrogate. If a durable power of attorney for health care does not exist, however, then the usual course of action is to turn to family members in order of next of kin—spouse, adult children, parents, siblings, and other relatives. The justification

---

[52] To my knowledge, it is usually not the case in this country (except in California) that one is legally determined to be globally incompetent for health-care decisions.

[53] This is also addressed by directive 25 of the ERDs.

for turning to the family is that these are usually the people who know the individual best.[54]

The surrogate decision maker must use one of two standards when deciding for an incompetent patient. The preferred standard is called "substituted judgment," and it means that the surrogate must make a decision that the patient would have made if the patient were competent. If there is no way to know what the patient would have wanted, the "best interests" standard is used, which means that the surrogate makes the decision that she believes is in the patient's overall best interest, broadly construed.[55]

In addition to choosing a surrogate decision maker, an individual may also execute an advance directive for medical treatment. An advance directive allows him to express his wishes concerning certain types of care, in case he is deemed incompetent to do so in the future. In the United States, Catholic health-care facilities must comply with a federal law that requires all patients to be advised of their right to make advance directives.[56]

In all cases, the principle of informed consent cannot truly be met without the condition of freedom from coercion, or voluntariness. This usually refers to the patient's ability to make a decision without the controlling influence of another person. The crucial word is *controlling*. Certainly, as social beings, we live in close community with others and will be influenced by those we love. What is of concern for proper informed consent is the absence of any manipulative influence that would hinder free choice. This could be from family, friends, or physicians and could be in the form of emotional persuasion, rewards, offers, or encouragement.[57]

---

[54] In the United States, some states actually stipulate by statute the precise order of priority for a family member to become the surrogate decision maker, in the absence of a durable power of attorney for health care.

[55] For a full philosophical bioethical treatment of the standards of surrogate decision making, standards of disclosure, and informed consent in general, see Tom L. Beauchamp and James F. Childress, *Principles of Biomedical Ethics*, 5th ed. (Oxford, U.K.: Oxford University Press, 2001), 77–104.

[56] ERDs, n. 24.

[57] Beauchamp and Childress, *Principles of Biomedical Ethics*, 93–98.

The principle of informed consent also entails, for the health-care community, an obligation of disclosure. This means that institutions and health-care workers, especially physicians, have a responsibility to present "all reasonable information about the essential nature of the proposed treatment and its benefits; its risks, side-effects, consequences, and cost; and any reasonable and morally legitimate alternatives, including no treatment at all."[58] There are three common standards of disclosure: the professional practice standard, the reasonable person standard, and the subjective standard. The professional practice standard refers to a level of disclosure that is customary in the profession of medicine, which essentially leaves the decision of how much to disclose up to a physician. This standard is not based on adequate respect for the free choice of individuals and is no longer considered valid.

The reasonable person standard refers to a level of disclosure that any reasonable person would need or want in order to make his decision. The subjective standard refers to a level of disclosure that is specific to the actual needs of an individual person. The subjective standard is morally preferable to the other two, as it is based on the greatest degree of respect for individual human dignity; however, it is often not realistic in many health-care settings, and the reasonable person standard is also morally acceptable.[59]

It is incumbent on the health-care workers and system that standards of disclosure are met in reality, not in mere formality. This means that as much as possible, communication between physician and patient should be direct and in person (in addition to the written consent forms) and that the physician should use language that is understood by the patient.

Finally, and most importantly, whether or not informed consent is given by the patient herself, by a surrogate on her behalf, or in an advance directive, it ought never to be contrary to Catholic moral principles. This prohibition is conceptually grounded in the universal truths of natural law, the respect for human dignity, and the proper understanding of human freedom, all discussed elegantly by John Paul II in *Veritatis splendor* and referenced earlier in this article. Indeed, four directives of the ERDs specifically refer to the obligation of

---

[58] ERDs, n. 27.

[59] Beauchamp and Childress, *Principles of Biomedical Ethics,* 81–83.

individuals and institutions to act in concert with Catholic moral principles.[60]

I turn now to specific examples of informed consent which show its application in Catholic health-care settings.

Examples of Informed Consent in Health Care

Many examples may be provided of the role of informed consent. Consider the case of a man who presents at a Catholic hospital with an advance directive stipulating that, should he develop Alzheimer's disease to the extent that he no longer knows who he is, then he wishes no treatment at all, for he wishes to die sooner rather than later. Such a directive could not be honored in this hospital. Individuals are morally obligated to accept all treatment that has a reasonable hope of benefit and proportionate risks.

It is in cases like this that Catholic health systems, and sometime the tradition itself, are often accused of "imposing" values on others. Critics plead for a stance of moral "neutrality." But moral neutrality is anything but neutral. Those who espouse such an approach to health care and morality in general are really advancing something else, like the value of individual decision making or the value of tolerance, as the paramount ethical principle. The reply, then, to the "imposition of values" charge is that the Catholic tradition has a conception of the good (the dignity of the human person) just as the secular tradition has a conception of the good (toleration, individual relativism, etc.). The Catholic position, as a competing conception of the good, is seen as an attempt to "impose" values because it is not the culturally dominant conception of the good.[61]

---

[60] "The institution, however, will not honor an advance directive that is contrary to Catholic teaching. If the advance directive conflicts with Catholic teaching, an explanation should be provided as to why the directive cannot be honored" (n. 24). "Decisions by the designated surrogate should be faithful to Catholic moral principles and to the person's intentions and values..." (n. 25). "The free and informed health care decision of the person or the person's surrogate is to be followed so long as it does not contradict Catholic principles" (n. 28). "The free and informed judgment made by a competent adult patient concerning the use or withdrawal of life-sustaining procedures should always be respected and normally complied with, unless it is contrary to Catholic moral teaching" (n. 59).

[61] This point is not an original one; other scholars have drawn attention to the fiction of moral neutrality as well as to the idea of a

In another example of informed consent, a man with developmental disability evidences a high degree of functioning and lives in an institutional setting. He is verbal, has good mobility, and until recently built models. Mr. Y is capable of directed conversation and of stating his preferences and interests.

Recently, because of concerns about her brother's best interests (stemming in part, perhaps, from serious medical complications that Mr. Y had in the past, but we do not really know), his sister has refused consent for a diagnostic colonoscopy and bone marrow biopsy, both of which the physician believes are medically indicated. Furthermore, she has stipulated that Mr. Y not be informed of his medical diagnoses or treatment options.

This case initially appears to present an ethical dilemma centered on conflicting understandings of the best interests of the client, Mr. Y. His sister, by denying care for her brother and by asking for information to be withheld from him, appears to be operating out of a concern for her brother's best interests and well being. Ethically, she might be attempting to balance doing good for her brother with her perceived obligation to allow no harm to be done to him. The physician, however, also appears to be operating out of a framework of best interests. His judgment is that to deny or withhold any diagnostic or treatment plan is to fail the best interests of his patient. Furthermore, he is uncomfortable with the idea of not discussing with his patient the nature of his medical care and treatment.

Crucially absent from this discussion is the right of Mr. Y himself to make his own health-care decisions. The respect and dignity due to each person demands that we presume competence to consent to medical treatment unless we have reasons in a particular situation to doubt the person's capacities in this regard. If Mr. Y is capable of consent, the mere fact of his developmental disabilities should not preclude him from receiving information about his treatment options and having his choice respected, whether we agree with his choice or not. If Mr. Y on his own refuses the treatments offered, then in the absence of other relevant moral considerations, we must respect this. Alternatively, if he

Catholic worldview as a conception of the good that competes with more dominant, secular worldviews. The point, however, bears repetition.

waives his right to knowledge or decision making in this regard and leaves the decisions up to his sister, then we must respect his autonomy by acting according to the wishes of his appointed surrogate, his sister, unless her decisions conflict with Catholic principles and teachings.

Finally, consider the situation of a hospital in the United States that serves a significant population for whom a language other than English is the first language. The hospital is not promoting the principle of informed consent if, in some explicit and formal manner, translation services are not provided. Similarly, it is not promoting informed consent if members of the medical staff, especially the physician, do not speak the other language well enough that patients can comfortably understand them. This is because disclosure is central to informed consent. Without adequate communication with physicians, patients cannot understand, deliberate, and choose. Leaving translation to informal mechanisms (by family members or volunteers from the community, for example) does not give adequate respect to human dignity. Justice and human dignity require that institutional support be given to ensure adequate communication. For example, the health system may have to hire medical staff with different language competencies or pay for interpreters.

The complexity of issues that present in contemporary health-care settings demands careful analysis. The principles of double effect, totality and integrity, and informed consent are essential in Catholic health-care ethics, providing moral clarity and insight. This essay shows how these principles are grounded within the tradition of Catholic morality and how the work of John Paul II, especially in *The Splendor of Truth*, has so richly illuminated bioethical reflection.

STEM CELL RESEARCH AND CLONING

Rev. Tadeusz Pacholczyk

Certain misconceptions surrounding stem cell research and cloning have come to be routinely presented in the mass media. These are the ten great media myths in the debate over stem cell research:

Myth 1: Stem cells can come only from embryos.

In fact, stem cells can be taken from umbilical cords, the placenta, amniotic fluid, adult tissues and organs such as bone marrow, fat obtained by liposuction, and regions of the nose, and they can be taken from cadavers up to twenty hours after death.

Myth 2: The Catholic Church is against stem cell research.

There are four categories of stem cells: embryonic stem cells, embryonic germ cells, umbilical cord stem cells, and adult stem cells. Given that germ cells can come from miscarriages that involve no deliberate interruption of pregnancy,

---

Portions of this paper were published previously in the booklet *Stem Cell Research, Cloning & Human Embryos,* by Fr. Pacholczyk (Washington, DC: Family Research Council, 2004) and in *The Five Issues That Matter Most: Catholics and the Upcoming Election,* by Mark Brumley et al. (Carlsbad, CA: Catholic Outreach, 2004).

the Church really opposes the use of only one of these four categories, i.e., embryonic stem cells. In other words, the Catholic Church approves three of the four possible types of stem cell research.

Myth 3: Embryonic stem cell research has the greatest promise.

Up to now, no human being has ever been cured of a disease by the use of embryonic stem cells. Adult stem cells, on the other hand, have already cured thousands. An example is the use of bone marrow cells from the hip bone to repair scar tissue on the heart after a heart attack. Research using adult cells is twenty to thirty years ahead of research using embryonic stem cells, and holds greater promise. This is in part because stem cells are part of the natural repair mechanisms of an adult body, whereas embryonic stem cells do not belong in an adult body, where they are likely to form tumors and to be rejected as foreign tissue by the recipient. Embryonic stem cells really belong only in the specialized microenvironment of a rapidly growing embryo, which is a radically different setting from an adult body.

Myth 4: Embryonic stem cell research is against the law.

In reality, there is no federal law or regulation against destroying human embryos for research purposes. Although President Bush has banned the use of federal funding to support research on embryonic stem cell lines created after August 2001, such research is not illegal. Anyone using private funds is free to pursue it.

Myth 5: President Bush created new restrictions on federal funding of embryonic stem cell research.

The 1996 Dickey Amendment prohibited the use of federal funds for research that would involve the destruction of human embryos. Bush's decision to permit research on embryonic stem cell lines created before a certain date thus relaxed this restriction from the Clinton era.

Myth 6: Therapeutic cloning and reproductive cloning are fundamentally different from one another.

The creation of cloned embryos either to make a baby or to harvest cells occurs by the same series of technical steps. The only difference is what will be done with the cloned human embryo that is produced: Will it be given the protection of a woman's womb in order to be born, or will it be destroyed for its stem cells?

Myth 7: Somatic cell nuclear transfer is different from cloning.

In fact, somatic cell nuclear transfer is simply cloning by a different name. The end result is still a cloned embryo.

Myth 8: By doing somatic cell nuclear transfer, we can directly produce tissues or organs without having to clone an embryo.

At the present stage of research, scientists are unable to bypass the creation of an embryo in the production of tissues or organs. In the future, it may be possible to inject elements from the cytoplasm of a woman's ovum into a somatic cell (a nonreproductive cell, or body cell) to "reprogram" it into a stem cell. This is called "dedifferentiation." If so, there would be no moral objection to this approach to getting stem cells.

Myth 9: Every body cell, or somatic cell, is somehow an embryo and thus a human life.

People sometimes argue: "Every cell in the body has the potential to become an embryo. Does that mean that every time we wash our hands and are shedding thousands of cells, we are killing life?" The problem is that this overlooks the basic biological difference between a regular body cell and a cell whose nuclear material has been fused with an unfertilized egg cell, resulting in an embryo. A normal skin cell will give rise to more skin cells only when it divides, whereas an embryo will give rise to the entire adult organism. Skin cells are not potential adults. Skin cells are potentially only more skin cells. Only embryos are potential adults.

Myth 10: Because frozen embryos may one day end up being discarded by somebody, that makes it morally allowable, even laudable, to violate and destroy those embryos.

The moral analysis of what we may permissibly do with embryos does not depend on their otherwise "going to waste." In other words, the fact that somebody may commit an evil act (throwing away human embryos) does not permit us to jump ahead in line and do the evil act (destroying the embryo for its stem cells) first ourselves.

Common Questions

The following questions are frequently asked about stem cell research:

What are stem cells and why are they important?

A stem cell is essentially a nonspecialized or "blank" cell, which is capable of becoming another, more differentiated cell type in the body, such as a muscle cell, nerve cell, or skin cell. Stem cells can be used to replace or heal damaged tissues and cells in the body.

Where do embryonic-type stem cells come from?

Embryonic-type stem cells basically come from two sources: embryos and fetuses:

- *Embryonic stem cells* are extracted from living embryos that are three to five days old. The removal of embryonic stem cells invariably results in the destruction of the embryo.
- *Embryonic germ cells,* another kind of stem cell, can be obtained from aborted or miscarried fetuses.

Where do adult-type stem cells come from?

Adult-type stem cells come from three sources:

- *Umbilical cords, placentas, and amniotic fluid.* Adult-type stem cells can be derived from various pregnancy-related tissues.
- *Adult tissues.* In adults, stem cells are present in various tissues and organ systems. These include the bone marrow, liver, epidermis, retina, skeletal muscle, intestine, brain, and dental pulp. Even fat obtained by liposuction has been shown to contain significant numbers of adult-type stem cells.
- *Cadavers.* Neural stem cells have been removed from specific areas in postmortem human brains as late as twenty hours following death.

Which sources of stem cells are always morally objectionable?

The only intrinsically objectionable source for harvesting stem cells is the human embryo. This is because it is necessary to destroy the early embryo (sometimes referred to as a blastocyst) in order to procure the embryonic stem cells. On the other hand, there is no moral objection to using stem cells obtained from a fetus if the fetus died of natural causes (miscarriage) and the parents gave consent to use their child's stem cells. This would be analogous to an organ donation from their deceased child. It is not morally permissible to harvest stem cells from a fetus that was killed in an induced abortion.

In other words, of the five tissue sources listed previously (i.e., the two embryonic sources and the three adult sources), it can be permissible to make use of four of them to obtain stem cells. The Church therefore vigorously supports and encourages most types of stem cell research. Only stem cell research that depends on the direct killing of another human being is morally excluded.

To summarize:

- Research involving *embryonic stem cells is always morally objectionable,* because the human embryo must be destroyed in order to extract its stem cells.

- Research involving *embryonic germ cells* is morally objectionable when it uses fetal tissue derived from elective abortions, but it is morally acceptable when it uses material from spontaneous abortions (miscarriages) if the parents have given informed consent.

- Research involving *umbilical cord stem cells* is morally acceptable, since the umbilical cord is no longer required after delivery has been completed.

- Research involving *placentally derived stem cells* is morally acceptable, since the afterbirth is no longer required after delivery has been completed.

- Research involving *adult stem cells* is morally acceptable, if the adult donor has given informed consent.

Why are adult stem cells preferable to embryonic stem cells?

Adult stem cells are a "natural" solution. They naturally exist in our bodies, and they provide a natural repair mechanism for many tissues of our bodies. They belong in the microenvironment of an adult body, whereas embryonic stem cells belong in the microenvironment of the early embryo, not in an adult body. In an adult body, embryonic stem cells tend to cause tumors and immune-system reactions.

Adult stem cell research has been going on for decades, and many therapies in humans (such as bone marrow transplants) have been successfully developed using adult stem cells. In contrast, embryonic stem cell research in humans is a relatively new field; the first human embryonic stem cell lines were developed only in 1998. Thus, *adult stem cells have already been successfully used in human therapies for many years.* As of the date of this publication, *NO therapy in humans has ever been successfully carried out using embryonic stem cells.*

This point is an important one: Thousands of people have been cured of diseases using adult stem cells, but none has ever been cured using stem cells from embryos.

Why do many patient advocacy groups push so strongly for embryonic stem cell research if all the cures are coming from adult stem cells?

The bottom line is that promoters of embryonic stem cell research have sold a bill of goods to many of these patient advocacy groups. They have promised a cure for every ailment, as well as the betterment of mankind.

The trouble is that patients with debilitating diseases are a vulnerable group, and some will latch onto even the flimsiest hopes and most improbable solutions in their desperate desire for a cure. Those scientists and advocates of embryonic destruction who take advantage of the desperation and vulnerability of these patient groups are guilty of a grave injustice against them, not only by offering them a medically ineffective approach but also by encouraging them in their vulnerability to support an inherently immoral and disordered approach to obtaining cures.

Have there been many real-life success stories and cures using adult and umbilical cord stem cells?

Yes, there are many such success stories, which have taken place without the destruction of any embryonic human beings. People have been successfully treated for some very serious maladies, including spinal cord injuries, leukemia, sickle cell anemia, and Parkinson's disease, to name a few. Several of these stories are recounted later in this chapter, under "Success Stories from the Use of Adult and Umbilical Cord Stem Cells."

How long is the list of diseases that can be treated or cured today using stem cells from adults or umbilical cords?

The list is already very long, and growing longer all the time. A partial list of the diseases that can be treated using adult or umbilical cord stem cells appears at the end of this chapter.

But if it were possible one day in the future to find cures for sick people by using embryonic stem cells, would that not be worthwhile? Is it not always a good thing to cure people?

Curing people is generally a good thing, but not always. If we commit a grave evil in order to cure somebody's disease, the cure will end up being worse than the disease. Consider, for example, a woman who is dying of heart failure. One approach to curing her might be to do a heart transplant from her daughter. If it were necessary to end the life of her healthy daughter in order to procure the organ and save the mother, would that kind of cure be good?

Clearly, it is not *always* a good thing to cure disease. We must use only the proper and fitting means to do so. Good medicine has always been built on such an understanding, which includes the moral recognition that the powerful should not exploit the weak in order to obtain cures. Embryonic stem cell research is an example of exploitation of the innocent and defenseless by the powerful, and is always an unjust and disordered human activity.

*But are embryos not just a bunch of cells? They are not
really human beings yet, are they?*

This is one of the most commonly promoted misconceptions about embryos. Human embryos are very small but complete organisms of the species *Homo sapiens*. Embryos are not merely cellular life; they are *beings* who are human, and are distinct from cells, tissues, or organs which are human. Human embryos possess an internal code for self-actualization and have an independent and inherent teleology (goal-directedness) to develop into adults, and they are physiologically alive and genetically human. Human embryos possess forty-six chromosomes, and their genetic identity as male or female has been irrevocably determined.

Are embryos human? Are they really one of us?

Embryos are no different in their essential humanity from a fetus in the womb, a ten-year-old boy, or a forty-year-old woman. At every stage of development, a human being (whether zygote, blastocyst, embryo, fetus, infant, adolescent, or adult) retains his or her identity as an enduring being who grows toward each subsequent stage; embryos are integral beings structured for maturation along their proper time line. Despite their unfamiliar appearance, embryos are what very young humans look like.

*Embryos are so tiny that they can fit on the point of a sewing
pin, and they are smaller than the period at the end of this
sentence. How can anybody take seriously the suggestion
that we should be protecting something so small?*

In carrying out the moral analysis, size is not a determinative factor in deciding whether human beings should be protected from exploitation and destruction. In fact, small size typically implies that *extra* protections are necessary, since the smaller the individuals, the less likely they will be equipped to defend themselves. Thus, we make special child labor laws to protect children from exploitation by ruthless businessmen who would use them to work in factories. We seek to protect babies and children from parents who have shown themselves to be irresponsible in the way they raise them or who plan to harm them. Those who have no voice to speak in their own defense need special protection, and embryonic humans are the preeminent example of those who are unable to speak in their own defense.

Is it not a matter of religious belief as to when human life begins?

No, it is not. It is actually a matter of biology. A human embryo is a human being, a being who is clearly and unmistakably human. It is not a zebra-type of being, a plant-type of being, or some other kind of being. Each of us was once an embryo, and this affirmation does not depend on religion, belief system, or the imposition of anything on anyone. It depends only on a grasp of basic biology. It is a matter of empirical observation.

Why is the destruction of human embryos immoral?

The well-known moral principle that good ends do not justify immoral means applies directly here. Once you are constituted a *human* being, which always occurs at fertilization (or at an event that mimics fertilization, like cloning), you are a new member of the human species and must be protected unconditionally. Once you are a being who is *human*, you are the bearer of *human* rights, and you are inviolable. Our existence as human beings is a continuum that extends all the way back to our origins in that humble ball of cells we call an embryo. Each of us had our origins in such an embryo, and embryos should never be instrumentalized for research purposes, even if the ends that might be achieved through that research would be very good.

What about the hundreds of thousands of embryos that are frozen in fertility clinics? They are just going to be thrown away anyway, so should we not get some good out of them by harvesting their stem cells?

This is a seductive argument, because at first glance it might seem that if frozen embryos may one day end up being discarded by somebody, it should be morally allowable, even laudable, to violate and destroy those embryos. However, the moral analysis of what we may permissibly do with an embryo does not depend on its otherwise "going to waste" or on the incidental fact that an embryo is "trapped" in liquid nitrogen.

Moreover, the statement that "they are just going to be thrown away anyway" needs to be scrutinized. Who says they must be thrown away? In fact, is not discarding human embryos (and thereby causing their demise) an immoral action in itself? Is not one immoral action being used to justify another immoral action in this scenario? The argument can be recast in another manner that also reveals its fallacious character. Because these embryos are about to die, it is argued, it should be morally acceptable to harvest their stem cells and thereby cause their demise. But there are many people who are about to die in our world, such as terminally ill cancer patients and children with incurable diseases. These individuals do not lose their right to protection and respect for their bodily integrity simply because of their terminal conditions.

Can human embryonic stem cells be obtained from sources other than embryos from in vitro fertilization clinics?

Yes, they can be obtained by making and destroying *cloned* embryos. This procedure would involve making an identical twin of a person, and then utilizing that twin brother or twin sister in their embryonic state to serve as a source for stem cells. This kind of cloning is sometimes called therapeutic cloning.

Do you always make an embryo when you carry out cloning?

Yes, cloning is a technique to make an identical twin of somebody. In order to make a twin in this way, you must first make an embryo. That embryo is a cloned embryo. Once you have successfully made a cloned embryo, you have two options available. You can strip-mine the cloned embryo for its stem cells or spare parts ("therapeutic cloning" or "research cloning"), or you can offer it the safe harbor of a woman's womb and allow it grow into a fetus, newborn, adolescent, and adult ("reproductive cloning" or "cloning to produce children"). Once again, the crucial difference between these two types of cloning is what you do with the cloned embryos that you make: Do you implant them into a womb, or destructively harvest them for their stem cells?

But do not reproductive cloning and therapeutic cloning really differ from each other in a fundamental technical way?

No, because both types of cloning rely on making a cloned embryo by the same series of steps, which are referred to as *somatic cell nuclear transfer*. This involves taking the nucleus of a body (somatic) cell and transferring it into an egg cell (oocyte) that has had its own nucleus removed.

The body cell thus provides a full complement of DNA (instead of the half-complement that the egg originally had). The newly constituted embryo is prompted to divide and grow toward adulthood, following the same developmental trajectory that a regular embryo, produced by union of sperm and egg, does. This cloned embryo is an identical twin of the person who donated the starting somatic cell.

In sum, then, therapeutic cloning involves making a cloned embryo by the same series of technical steps as reproductive cloning, but instead of being implanted into a uterus to be born, the clone is destroyed to harvest its stem cells. Therapeutic cloning is therefore identical to reproductive cloning except for the final step, since the cloned embryo is never placed into a uterus to cause the live birth of an individual. Instead, the identical twin is destroyed in order to remove his or her stem cells at the stage where he or she is still a blastocyst.

Therapeutic cloning is sometimes referred to as the clone-and-kill technique. The aim of this type of cloning is to obtain rejection-proof stem cells for transplantation into the person from whom the clone was made. Because stem cells from the clone are actually from the identical twin of the person cloned, they should theoretically be a good immune match and should not be rejected, since identical twins can exchange organs without immune reactions.

Is it true that cloning makes a carbon copy of a person?

No, the clone is not a carbon copy, with every detail exactly the same. Instead, the cloned embryo is essentially an identical twin of the person who donated the starting DNA. Clones are not carbon copies any more than identical twins are carbon copies. No human being is truly "identical" to another; subtle differences will always exist.

Would a cloned human being have his or her own soul?

Cloning is simply another way to make identical twins. Naturally born identical twins, of course, have their own souls. A twin born by cloning would likewise have his or her own soul. Any child who is a clone would be an individual and unique human being, with his own personality and unique defining characteristics. You might say that God is "beholden" to the biology he has set into motion when he created all things, so if we generate a bona fide embryo by a technique that is different from the usual way of joining sperm and egg, He still respects the biology governing the developmental trajectory of that new embryonic human and will infuse it with an immortal, immaterial soul.

*Will human therapeutic cloning raise any concerns about
egg procurement?*

The use of therapeutic cloning in an attempt to cure just
the class of people who have diabetes (leaving aside for the
moment any other diseases) would involve the donation of
numerous eggs (oocytes), which would require that many
women be used as donors. In order to donate oocytes, however, women must be treated with harsh hyperovulatory drugs
that cause the release of multiple eggs. These drugs have a
strong impact on each woman's body and are associated with
their own potential risks, such as dizziness, fatigue, and the
development of tumors or cysts. Complications can arise, and
in a few instances fatalities have been reported.[1] Hence, if
eggs were to be harvested from large numbers of women, some
women would suffer serious side effects and even death. Some
women's groups have been opposed to therapeutic cloning
for these reasons. They realize that women could be treated
as egg farms in order to provide the starting materials for therapeutic cloning. They recognize and object to this serious exploitation of women's bodies, especially of women who are
financially constrained or otherwise vulnerable.

Why is human reproductive cloning immoral?

Cloning, like in vitro fertilization, participates in the basic
evil of moving human procreation out of the setting of committed marital intimacy and into the laboratory. Human procreation
is not meant to occur in that setting, because it is inherently
dehumanizing to bring a new human being into the world through
means that replace the marital act. Each of us has a right to be
brought into the world as the fruit of marital love, rather than as
the product of technical domination and manufacturing protocols. Each of us is meant to be treated as a *subject* of inestimable
and unrepeatable value, rather than as an *object* for manipulation. Procreation is not meant to be replaced by production.

Cloning also represents a very radical sort of genetic engineering. Instead of choosing just a few of the features you
would like your offspring to have—like greater height or greater
intelligence—cloning allows you to choose *all* the features, so
it represents an extremely serious form of domination and
manipulation by parents over their own children. It represents

---

[1] Comment on Reproductive Ethics (CORE), "Death from Egg
Harvesting," press release, April 13, 2005, http://www.corethics.org/
document.asp?id=cpr130505.txt&se=2&st=4.

a type of parental power that parents are not intended to have. Ultimately, cloning is a type of human breeding, a despotic attempt by some individuals to dominate and predetermine the make-up of others. This is a power that does not properly belong to parents, who are called to accept the God-given designs of sexuality. These assure a natural variability in their offspring, which is partly reflective of each parent. The God-given designs of human sexuality also assure that parents stand in a properly "receptive" mode to their children, receiving them in their uniqueness and unanticipated originality.

This notion that children are always a gift, rather than a product to be manipulated or designed according to our own fancy, stands at the heart of what is objectionable about human reproductive cloning. With cloning you also distort the relationships between generations. If a woman were to clone herself, using her own egg cell and her own somatic cell, and bear the child in her own womb, she would not need to have sperm or any involvement of a man at all. Oddly, she would end up giving birth to her own identical twin—a twin sister who would also be her daughter.

Why is human therapeutic cloning immoral?

If human reproductive cloning (i.e., the bringing to birth of a new child who is an identical twin to somebody else) is wrong, then therapeutic cloning is worse—it is the creation of that same identical twin for the premeditated purpose of ending his life to harvest his tissues. In sum, a grave evil is involved in therapeutic cloning, where life is created for the explicit purpose of its destruction. With reproductive cloning, at least we would end up with a living baby. Human therapeutic cloning—the artificial creation of a human being for the sole purpose of his exploitation and destruction—will always be gravely unethical, even if the desired end is a very good one, namely, the curing of diseases. Therapeutic cloning sanctions the direct and unvarnished exploitation of one human being by another—in this case, the exploitation of the weak by the powerful. The danger of therapeutic cloning lies in the intentional creation of a subclass of human beings, who are still in their embryonic or fetal stages and who can be freely exploited by those fortunate enough to have already passed beyond those early stages of life.

Therapeutic cloning also raises serious "slippery-slope" concerns. The temptation to make embryos that can be exploited for their stem cells offers the further temptation to grow those cloned embryos within a uterus to the point where they become fetuses. Such a fetus can then be aborted and conveniently harvested for needed organs, so that the trouble of having to start from scratch with undifferentiated stem cells is avoided.

This line of slippery-slope analysis has been shrewdly analyzed by nationally syndicated columnist Charles Krauthammer:

> We would never countenance such work in humans, they say. Cows, yes, but we would never implant a cloned human embryo in the uterus of a woman and grow it to the stage of a fetus. We solemnly promise to grow human clones only to the blastocyst stage, a tiny eight-day-old cell mass no larger than the period at the end of this sentence, so that we can extract stem cells and cure diseases that way. Nothing more. No fetuses. No implantation. No brave new world of fetal farming.

> This is all very nice. But curing with stem cells is extremely complicated. First, you have to tease out the stem cells from the blastocyst. Then you have to keep the stem cells alive, growing one generation after another while retaining their pluripotentiality (their ability to develop into all different kinds of cells). Then you have to take those stem cells and chemically tweak them in complex ways to make them grow into specialized tissue cells— say, neurons for a spinal-cord injury. Then you inject the neurons into the patient and get your cure.

> The Advanced Cell Technology cow experiment suggests the obvious short circuit that circumvents this entire Rube Goldberg process: let the cloned embryo grow into a fetus. Nature will then create within the fetus the needed neurons, kidney cells, liver cells, etc., in far more usable, more perfect, and more easily available form.

> Tempting? No way, the cloning advocates assure us. We will never break that moral barrier. It is one thing to grow a cloned embryo, a tiny mass of cells not yet implanted. It is another thing to grow a cloned human fetus, with recognizable human features and carried in the womb of a woman.

> I am skeptical of these assurances. Why? Because just a year or two ago, research advocates were assuring us that they only wanted to do stem cell research on discarded embryos from fertility clinics but would not create a human embryo in the laboratory just for the purpose of taking it apart for its stem cells.

> Well, that was then. Today these very same advocates are campaigning hard to permit research cloning—that is, the

creation of human embryos for the purpose of taking them apart for their stem cells. They justify this reversal of position by invoking the suffering of millions. And they heap scorn on opponents for letting old promises and arbitrary moral barriers stand in the way of human betterment.[2]

Success Stories from the Use of Adult and Umbilical Cord Stem Cells

Spinal Cord Injury. Laura Dominguez broke her neck and was paralyzed from the chest down after a car accident in 2001. She was treated with a mix of adult stem cells and other cells obtained from olfactory tissue inside her nose. The cells were transplanted across the injury site in her damaged spinal cord. Several months after the surgery, she began to recover sensation in previously unresponsive parts of her body, and was able to move her foot. Her remarkable progress is continuing, and she is now able to walk short distances with the aid of braces. Several other patients with spinal cord injuries like hers are also showing remarkable benefits from the transplant surgery. The surgery on Laura Dominguez was carried out in Portugal, and neurologists in the United States are seeking FDA approval to begin offering the therapy here.

Leukemia. Patricia Durante was diagnosed with an aggressive form of leukemia six months into her pregnancy. Her daughter, Victoria Angel, was delivered early by cesarean section, so that Patricia could be treated with chemotherapy. Patricia was given only about six months to live. Fortunately, stem cells from her daughter's umbilical cord were saved after the delivery. After chemotherapy failed to halt the progress of the leukemia, her daughter's stem cells were used for a transplant. Several years later now, Durante is in full remission. "[Victoria] saved her mommy," Durante told reporters. "She's a little miracle. That's why we named her Victoria Angel. She's my little angel."

Sickle Cell Anemia. Keone Penn was born with sickle cell anemia, which means that his red blood cells were sickle shaped instead of round. The effect of the disease is that the sickle-shaped cells get caught in the small blood vessels of the body (the capillaries) and clog the vessels. Joint pain and

---

[2] Charles Krauthammer, "The Fatal Promise of Cloning," *Time* magazine (June 24, 2002).

swelling are one set of symptoms. The typical treatment is to carry out multiple blood transfusions as a child grows. Keone received many such transfusions, but eventually could not tolerate any more.

Doctors decided to destroy Keone's own immune system and perfuse in umbilical cord stem cells. These umbilical cord cells came from the New York Public Blood Bank, where Keone was fortunate enough to have found a match. After the transplant, Keone's blood type changed from one type to another. He is now considered cured of the disease, and is able to play basketball and participate in a range of other demanding physical activities for the first time in his life.

Parkinson's Disease. Dennis Turner was diagnosed with Parkinson's disease and, by early 1991, suffered extreme shaking of the right side of his body and stiffness in his gait and movements. Putting in his contact lenses became difficult or nearly impossible. He became unable to use his right arm.

Neurosurgeon Dr. Michel Lévesque removed a small tissue sample from Mr. Turner's brain, and isolated adult neural stem cells from it. Dr. Lévesque multiplied and matured these cells into dopamine neurons, and injected these cells back into the left side of Mr. Turner's brain, which controls the right side of the body. Soon after, the Parkinson's symptoms began to improve in Mr. Turner's right side. Mr. Turner's trembling decreased until to all appearances it was gone, reappearing only slightly when he became upset or nervous. Neurological evaluation indicated a marked improvement, which lasted for about five years.

Because Parkinson's is a progressive ailment, Mr. Turner's condition is deteriorating again, but as he recently testified at a U.S. Senate Committee hearing, "I have no doubt that because of this treatment I've enjoyed five years of quality life that I feared had passed me by." He enthusiastically expressed a willingness to undergo a repeat surgery of this sort to further slow the progression of his symptoms.

Krabbe's Leukodystrophy. Gina Rugari was born with Krabbe's leukodystrophy. This is a rare, degenerative enzyme disorder of the nervous system, in which a baby shows initial signs of irritability and developmental delay or regression. Seizures and fevers often follow, then blindness and deafness, until the baby dies, usually before age two. Gina was tested for Krabbe's leukodystrophy shortly after she was born, because she had a brother who had died from the disease. Doctors treated Gina with chemotherapy to destroy her immune system, and introduced new umbilical cord blood stem cells from a closely matched donor. The transplanted cells produced the missing enzyme. Her body accepted the cells, and she is thriving several years after the transplant.

Human Diseases That Currently Can Be Treated or Cured by the Use of Adult or Umbilical Cord Stem Cells

What follows is a partial list of human diseases that can be treated or cured today using stem cells from adults or umbilical cords. None of these diseases has ever been cured in humans using stem cells from embryos.

Acute biphenotypic leukemia
Acute lymphoblastic leukemia
Acute myelofibrosis
Acute myelogenous leukemia
Acute undifferentiated leukemia
Adrenoleukodystrophy
Advanced chronic lymphocytic leukemia
Agnogenic myeloid metaplasia (myelofibrosis)
Aplastic anemia (severe)
Ataxia-telangiectasia
Bare lymphocyte syndrome
Beta thalassemia major
Chediak-Higashi syndrome
Chronic granulomatous disease
Chronic myelogenous leukemia
Chronic myelomonocytic leukemia
DiGeorge syndrome
Essential thrombocythemia
Ewing sarcoma
Familial erythrophagocytic lymphohistiocytosis
Fanconi anemia
Gaucher's disease
Hemophagocytosis
Histiocytosis-X
Hodgkin's disease
Hunter's syndrome (MPS-II)
Hurler's syndrome (MPS-IH)
Juvenile chronic myelogenous leukemia
Juvenile myelomonocytic leukemia
Kostmann syndrome
Krabbe disease
Leukocyte adhesion deficiency

Maroteaux-Lamy syndrome (MPS-VI)
Metachromatic leukodystrophy
Morquio syndrome (MPS-IV)
Mucolipidosis II (I-cell disease)
Mucopolysaccharidoses (MPS)
Multiple myeloma
Neuroblastoma
Neutrophil actin deficiency
Niemann-Pick disease
Non-Hodgkin's lymphoma
Omenn's syndrome
Paroxysmal nocturnal hemoglobinuria
Plasma cell leukemia
Polycythemia vera
Prolymphocytic leukemia
Pure red cell aplasia
Refractory anemia
Refractory anemia with excess blasts
Refractory anemia with excess blasts in transformation
Refractory anemia with ringed sideroblasts)
Renal cell carcinoma
Reticular dysgenesis
Sanfilippo syndrome (MPS-III)
Scheie syndrome (MPS-IS)
Severe combined immunodeficiency
Sickle cell disease
Sly syndrome, beta-glucuronidase deficiency (MPS-VII)
Waldenstrom's macroglobulinemia
Wolman's disease

Bishops, Bioethics, and Sound Bites

Using the Mass Media

Rev. Raymond J. de Souza

For many years I have used an analogy about the relationship between the mass media and the life of the Church. After the tragic tsunami in Indonesia of December 26, 2004, it is even more powerful. Theology and philosophy are like the deep, deep waters. If you go down deep in the ocean, it is so still it is almost as if there is no motion and nothing happens. But whatever does happen down there, whatever slight deviation occurs down deep, has by the time it gets to the surface a huge effect. In like manner, the tsunami took place on the seabed and then came up to the surface.

The media, where I do much of my work, is the surface. On the surface of the water everything is in motion. The tides and the moon, the wind, the current, the fish that come to the top—all create a disturbance, but it is transitory, it disappears, and it is gone almost as soon as it takes place.

It is tempting to say that what happens on the surface does not matter, because the really important things occur

---

This text was prepared from an audio recording of the talk given by Fr. de Souza at the Bishop's Workshop.

down deep; everything on the surface is just transitory. The mass media, therefore, does not require a lot of attention; it is just a passing phenomenon. This would be true if we did not live on the surface. If you want to sail somewhere, it makes a great difference whether there are white caps or not, whether the wind is blowing or not. We live on the surface, so although things come and go and it seems to have a transitory nature, that is where we live, on the surface of the waves, on the surface of the ocean.

All the froth from the mass media is very important. It is where we live, and it is also, unfortunately, where most of our people live all the time. Very few of our people—and all too few of our clergy, too—ever venture down into the deep waters. We live on the surface. The consequence is that the mass media becomes a bishop's principal teaching tool. Not the only teaching tool, but the principal teaching tool. Indeed, it is likely to be the most powerful tool you have for preaching the gospel and teaching the faith.

Consider the large amount of work a bishop devotes to his homilies. Those homilies are heard probably by a few hundred people; of those who hear them, perhaps a small proportion, less than 10 percent, remember much of what was said the next day. Preaching is important, but sometimes the effort put into it does not bear much fruit among our people. The diocesan paper, where the bishop might have a regular column, is read by only a very small proportion of practicing Catholics. Many dioceses have to subsidize the diocesan papers because the number of readers is not sufficient to generate subscription revenue or attract advertisers; many parishes end up of throwing out many copies of their subscription to the diocesan paper. And these Catholic channels of communication reach only practicing Catholics, not non-practicing Catholics, who are the majority of our Catholic population, to say nothing of the non-Catholics in the diocese.

While we experience these limitations on Catholic channels of communication, our people are voraciously consuming information and news from other sources: newspapers, television, cable, and the Internet. That is where they spend their time, and our Catholic channels of communication do not reach them there. In my own home archdiocese of Kingston, Ontario, I would guess that the daily circulation of the main newspaper in a city of about 120,000 is about 25,000 people. There are other newspapers that are read in addition. That is every day. That would be roughly comparable to the total number of Catholics in our diocese who attend Mass on Sunday. So every day our local secular newspaper reaches as many people as we have coming to Mass in every parish on Sunday. That is a big difference in reach. As a result of all this, most of our Catholics, practicing as well an non-practicing, get the bulk of their news about the Church, including what the local bishop has to say, from the secular media, not from Catholic channels of communication. Consider some examples of the power of the mass media. These should be encouraging examples, because they are, for the most part, recent successes.

Cardinals Luciani, Pell, and O'Connor

Remember Albino Luciani, who was the patriarch of Venice before he became Pope John Paul I? When he first went to Venice, he would preach most Sundays at St. Mark's and work very hard on his homilies. One of his friends came to him and said, "Why are you spending so much time on your homilies for a few hundred people at St. Mark's? Half of those in attendance are not even Italians. They don't even understand what you're saying—they're tourists." That encouraged him to start writing for the secular press. A column he wrote in the paper reached so many people with such an endearing style that eventually he published a book, *Illustrissimi*, which contained his much-noted letters to famous historical figures.

At the current moment, in the archdiocese of Sydney, Australian cardinal George Pell writes a weekly column in the *Sunday Telegraph*, which is the largest-circulation Sunday newspaper in Sydney. Now Cardinal Pell, for those of you who know him, represents the worst possible enemy of the secular, liberal mindset; he speaks robustly, without apology, and does not trim on the claims of the Catholic faith. The paper is not a friend of the Catholic Church, but they run his column because it is prestigious for them to do so. Two years ago, when Anthony Fisher, a Dominican moralist, was ordained as his auxiliary bishop, one of the competing papers came to Fr. Fisher and asked him if he would write a column. Why? Because it adds to the prestige of the paper to have the leaders of the community writing in its pages.

Another example, closer to home, is a powerful one. In 1998, the New York Yankees held their home opener at Yankee Stadium on Good Friday. It was scheduled for one o'clock in the afternoon, and Cardinal O'Connor was incensed that baseball would be played on Good Friday, let alone during the sacred hours of noon to three. He said he would not go

115

to any baseball game that whole year, in protest against games played on Good Friday. He made the point that he had decided this because the Yankees played during those sacred hours. For several days, his comments and his protest were on the front page of every newspaper in New York. Most of the newspapers across the country also covered the story in their front section, not just the sports section. You may remember that episode. It is a marvelous example! He taught the whole country that there was something important about Good Friday. It turned out to be a real sacrifice, too, because that year the Yankees won the World Series, beating the San Diego Padres. Some say that the 1998 Yankees were even better than the Yankees of 1927, which are considered by many to be the best team in the history of baseball. So he made a sacrifice for this teaching!

So it is possible, even in a hostile media environment, to have great successes. Let me hasten to add that it is also possible to have failures. It is possible to say something that comes back to haunt you and cause you a lot of grief and worry. But just as it is possible for a priest or bishop to give a bad homily, so it is possible to make a mistake when talking to the media. If you do enough interviews, you will give one that goes badly.

We should not let the danger of failure make us reluctant to engage the media. I know that dioceses often have policies about speaking to the media, authorizing only certain people in the chancery office to do so. Whatever the rules are, they should not encourage the mentality that talking to the media is a risk to be avoided, or that it is actively discouraged by one's superiors. Mistakes are to be expected, to be tolerated, to be corrected; but they are worth risking because the media is a means of evangelization. We would never stop preaching just because we deliver a bad homily. Indeed, there are far fewer mistakes made in media relations than there are bad homilies preached!

Specific Media Challenges Relating to Bioethics

There are particular media challenges in the field of bioethics. The first is that we are seen as not willing to celebrate medical advances. Typically, what happens is that some medical advance is reported in the news, and then the cameras cut to some Catholic figure saying why we cannot do it. We have a real "church lady" problem on medical ethics, because it often appears that we are just there clucking about why something cannot be done. This is a real challenge, because sometimes we do have to say that something cannot be done. To do so without sounding like a church lady is a real challenge.

Second, there is the problem of suffering. You cannot practice Catholic medical ethics without speaking about the potential expiatory and redemptive value of suffering. However, unresolved suffering runs directly contrary to one of the deepest biases in the media—a bias that is neither liberal nor conservative but might be called "solutionism." Every problem must have a solution. Almost every media report about anything, whether it is violence in the inner city or low grain prices, will always end with some appeal to a solution—by the government, by a new policy, by a new initiative. When a bioethical question concerns the nature of suffering, and we must admit that suffering will continue rather than be "solved," we run into a very deep bias. This is a challenge that cannot be avoided, but of which we have to be aware.

The third challenge is the moral law. To speak about the moral law runs contrary to another deep bias of the modern media, namely, that progress, especially technological progress, is always good. So to say that a new possibility should not be pursued runs against a very strong bias in favor of "technological progress."

Let me illustrate with a case study: This goes back once again to Cardinal Luciani. The first IVF baby was born on July 25, 1978. In the ways of Providence, she was born ten years to the day after the promulgation of *Humanae vitae*. There were a lot of comments about this, and the most famous remark made from a Catholic perspective was that of Cardinal Luciani, who was then still the patriarch of Venice. He congratulated the parents on the birth of this child and shared in their joy before noting that there were also moral considerations that had to be taken into account. Now, to understand how difficult these cases can be, his statement was interpreted by some as being permissive toward the idea of IVF because he congratulated the parents, which is a natural thing to do. I do not find fault with Cardinal Luciani's statement; this just shows how difficult it can be. At the same time, those prelates who highlighted the moral difficulties were thought to be a little heartless, because they did not even acknowledge the obvious joy of the parents at the birth of this child. There are situations in which, one way or the other, you are not going to be successful. Things you say will be misinterpreted. But it does not mean you should stop trying.

The final media challenge in bioethics is the game of expectations. One of the biases of the media is that it loves novelty. "We're in the news business." The bias is in favor of what is new. Therefore, the expectation of novelty and change always trumps the expectation of continuity. So if you leave something uncertain, the expectation will be that it is going to change. The release of *Humanae vitae* fell victim to this problem. If you read the history of that time, the expectations of a change in the Church's teaching caused part of the turmoil when the teaching, in fact, did not change.

Consider a practical example of managing expectations. Say you are doing a hospital merger between a Catholic and a non-Catholic institution, and you say at the press conference something like, "Well, because there are difficult issues here with sterilizations and abortions, we're going to have a committee look this over and work it out." The expectations are going to be in favor of some kind of change. And when you announce that there will not be a change in the Catholic hospital's policy, it is going to be more difficult. It is better to say that because a Catholic hospital will never do sterilizations or abortions, we are going to have this committee formed to determine how the non-Catholic hospital is going to respect that. That way people know in advance what to expect from the committee.

John Paul II's Moral Vision: *Veritatis splendor* in Fifteen Seconds

When *Veritatis splendor* came out, it was criticized on literary grounds as an encyclical about moral theories to which had been attached two pious meditations, one at the beginning and the other at the end, about the rich young man and the cross of Christ. But in fact *Veritatis splendor* has a unity, because its three parts highlight what John Paul II wished us to remember about the moral life. The first part, about the rich young man, concerns the necessity of the commandments and the possibility of moral heroism. More generally, John Paul II tells us that moral excellence is possible. The middle part concerns moral theory and affirms the reality of universal, moral, negative prohibitions. There are some things that may never be done. The third part, titled *Lest the Cross of Christ Be Emptied of Its Power*, is about the role of sacrifice, suffering, and martyrdom in the moral life. These are the three pillars of John Paul's moral vision.

When we speak about bioethical issues, the challenge is to keep all three of those points in play. We may have only a paragraph, or a few sentences, or even just fifteen seconds, to say it. So let me just give you some examples of how I think that might be done.

Say the question is about euthanasia or physician-assisted suicide. You might say something like this in general about the topic. "The Christian life is not immune from suffering, as Christ Himself suffered. But with God's grace it is possible to live that suffering heroically and with peace and joy. It is never necessary to do what may never be done, namely, to take a human life." We talk about suffering. We talk about the possibility of moral excellence, God's grace, and what may never be done. All three elements are there in one short statement.

Let me give you another example. How does one talk about new reproductive technologies? Something like this: "The greatness of man is not in what he can do, but in what he chooses to do. We can always refuse to do what is wrong even if it means sacrifices. The suffering of infertile couples is real. Christ knows that suffering and provides the necessary grace, as well as opening up other doors, such as adoption."

Say you are talking to young people about sexuality: "The Church must teach the reality of the moral law, which is the same today as when God gave the commandments on Sinai. We teach it because Christ Himself taught it and died on the Cross for it. It is not easy to follow the moral law, but it is possible with God's grace to do so. Is chastity hard today? It has always been hard, but Christ invites the young to live it because young people are capable of doing great things."

Words to Avoid

We have to be very disciplined in our interventions with the mass media because our time to speak is so very short. There are also key phrases to avoid when speaking about bioethics. The first is the word *ban*. Catholic News Service (CNS), which is owned by the American episcopal conference, frequently uses the word *ban*. I worked in the Vatican press corps for five years, and never could persuade my friends at CNS not to use the word *ban*, as in the "Church's ban on artificial contraception." They use it all the time, so it appears in all your diocesan papers because CNS is in all your diocesan newspapers. "The Church's ban on such and such" is how they put it. It is not a *ban*. The Catholic Church cannot ban anything. It can only declare that certain actions are immoral.

A ban suggests a prohibition that can be reversed; if you can ban something, then you can permit it. When it comes to bioethics, the Church is not a creative author of morality; she is only a witness to natural law.

Another word we can avoid saying is *policy*. We do not have policies on moral issues. There is no Catholic Church policy on stem cells. There is the reality of the moral law. When we use words like *policy* and *ban*, they put us in the category of politics.

Other words to avoid are *now* and *today*, in the sense of "Well, today the Church teaches this" or "Now the Church teaches that." As soon as you say *now* or *today*, the suggestion is that maybe tomorrow will be different. Other things to avoid saying are "Rome says" or "the bishop says." I was on an ethics committee at one of our Catholic hospitals, and the question of vasectomies came up. A religious sister on the panel said, "Well, we can't do them here because the archbishop said we can't." Which is true, but it really does not matter what the archbishop of Kingston thinks about vasectomies. What matters is whether he is teaching the truth about whether they are morally licit and, therefore, whether you can do them in a Catholic hospital. But when you say, "The archbishop says we can't do it," it gives completely the wrong idea. The sense becomes that perhaps the archbishop would allow this if we only asked him more nicely, or if we managed to ask him when he was not paying attention.

Another thing to avoid, although it may seem a bit odd, are phrases like "Catholics believe" and "I believe" when you are talking about things that are not specifically Catholic. We err when we say things like "Catholics believe in the sanctity of life." Given the environment, if you are speaking to the whole of your city, you might prefer to say something like, "The sanctity of life is valued by every culture." This is true, and it avoids a very big problem. If we speak about what "Catholics believe" or what "I believe," issues that are not specifically Catholic become defined as Catholic, and in a pluralistic environment, the media immediately thinks there must options, then, for non-Catholics.

Another issue word to use with great delicacy is *conscience*. This is very difficult, because of the central role conscience plays in the moral life. My advice is not to speak about conscience except in a very controlled way, when you have sufficient time to talk about what it really means. Otherwise, we end up having to say something like, "Well, we always respect the conscience of individuals" or "A man must follow his own conscience," and as soon as we say that, which is true, we are in a whole heap of trouble. In the United States, Senator Kerry spent the election year of 2004 confusing people about what conscience is. In my country, Canada, the prime minister, who is Catholic, does the same thing almost every time he speaks on moral issues. Both speak about conscience not as a judge of the moral quality of acts, but as having the power to *determine* the moral quality of acts. That is what most people understand by conscience. So if you are on a long interview program, fine, you can get into it and make all the necessary definitions and distinctions. But otherwise, I think it is advisable to avoid the word *conscience* entirely, given the widespread confusion on the subject.

Practical Suggestions on What to Say

What are some things that might be helpful to say? I am a university chaplain, and I do a lot of work with Catholic school teachers. Whenever I talk about a moral subject, I spend the first hour hammering away against the point that something is wrong *because* the Church teaches that it is wrong. To the contrary, the Church teaches that something is wrong because it is, in fact, wrong. You could say that from now until the day you die, and you would not be saying it too often, such is the confusion on this subject. We need to repeat it over and over again: "It is not wrong because the Church says so. The Church says so because of what it is." When we elaborate, we can use words like *nature* and *contrary to nature* or *reason* and *contrary to reason*. We can use the language of human rights. That language should not be used solely by those who favor abortion "rights" or the "right" to same-sex marriages. Human-rights language belongs to Christians, too, and we can use it and should use it.

Finally, we should use the name of Jesus Christ. In the three examples I gave you earlier, all included the name of Jesus Christ. When I was in the seminary, Monsignor (now Archbishop) Timothy Dolan was very fond of telling us that just saying the name of Jesus Christ has its own power. (He credited that advice to Billy Graham.) This is the only Name under heaven by which we might be saved. And we should use that Name. I work with university students. Other than during Mass, most of them hear the name of Jesus Christ only in violation of the second commandment. We should not be afraid to use it.

A handy rule of thumb is to look at a quotation you have given or at something you have written, whether a paragraph, a sentence, or the key passage of a homily, and if you realize it could have been said by someone other than a Catholic bishop or Catholic priest, then you need to rework the statement. It is a very good rule of thumb. There are many people who can speak in our media; you are the only ones who can speak as bishop. The same thing goes for priests. Our people have no shortage of voices. They hear them all the time, especially the younger generation, who live in the cable television and Internet environment. There are no shortages of voices. *Your* voice should be distinctive. Usually, the name of Jesus Christ, aside from being good in and of itself, also makes it clear that the one who is speaking is a Christian believer and a Christian disciple.

Here are a few other practical suggestions about what you might say. When we talk about sterilization, we should not be afraid of using the word *mutilation*. That is the proper word for removing a healthy organ from the body. Now, if you are confronting a woman who has been sterilized, you probably will not use that word. But we should not be afraid of these harsh-sounding words, because they immediately change the terrain of the debate. The use of the word *mutilation* immediately makes it clear that something healthy is being damaged. It frames the issue immediately.

When talking about euthanasia, you could say something like: "Life is not disposable. It always remains a gift. It requires care, not killing." These are words that are hard to use but that quickly change the tone of the debate.

When it comes to contraception, many people talk about pregnancy as if it were a disease. You might say, "At St. Elizabeth's Hospital we do not consider pregnancy to be a disease." That is probably three seconds, or six seconds, and it changes the terrain of the debate. That might be the only thing you get to say on the news, but you convey a Catholic perspective in just a few words.

Practical Steps to a Better Media Presence

Here are some practical steps to increase the effectiveness of your media presence. We have a bishop in Canada, Bishop Frederick Henry of Calgary, who appears more than any other bishop in our national media. He is very out-spoken. He has a very colorful way of expressing himself, so he gets a lot of coverage. When I went to see him, I asked him about his media strategies, and he said, "Well, I do not have a press secretary, I do not have a communications office." I said, "Well, how do you handle it?" And he said, "I have a rule. I return all journalists' phone calls, usually the same day." Bishop Henry knows that if you call the next day, it is too late. So he returns all media phone calls right away, and as a result he is probably the most quoted Catholic bishop in our country. Now, it is also a matter of how he expresses himself, but it begins with returning the phone calls. If you cannot do it yourself, someone in your office should. A good rule: If a journalist calls in the morning, he gets a callback by lunch. If he calls after lunch, he gets a callback before the end of the day. It's great if you can return the call yourself, but it does not have to be you. It has to be somebody, though, and soon!

A second suggestion is to hold regular meetings with the local media. Invite them in. In most cities there are probably no more than a dozen people in television, radio, and the newspapers who would actually be involved in covering the Church or potentially assigned to do a story. Invite them in. Have dinner or lunch with them. Invite them twice a year. If you do that, they will know that when something comes up there is already a rapport and relationship there. You are not meeting for the first time when there is a scandal.

Third, know your market. If you are in a large market, like Chicago, New York, Miami, or Philadelphia, then you might have to have professional help in terms of a media relations firm. Media coverage gets pretty complicated. But if you do, be careful. When they start telling you what you should say, rather than how you should say what you have already decided you want to say, that is when you fire them. Because media experts who tell you what to say are not helping you preach what you want to say. For the most part, they work for corporations and political candidates who are looking for something to say; that is their bias. This is not a criticism of that profession. Their job is to tell a corporation that is doing an advertising campaign what would be a good thing to say, but being a bishop is different from being a corporation. You already know what you want to say, and you want help in saying it. So they have to know that if they are working for you, an adjustment is required.

The vast majority of bishops will not need professional firms, because their diocese can be considered a small market. Even a place like Dallas, which is a big city, has one principal newspaper and probably a couple of major television stations. St. Louis is similar. Even in Toronto there are only two principal newspapers, maybe three, so it still possible to know all the parties involved. And if you know all the parties, you can give them a heads-up on local events.

If you have a diocesan communications officer, his job is not just to do press releases and take reporters to lunch. That is part of his job, but not all of his job. He should also have strong relationships with your parish priests because that is how what goes on in the parishes, whether it is a new school opening, a bake sale, or a fund-raising drive, gets into the local media. We have a right as Catholics to be represented in the media of our communities. We belong to those communities. But how does the newspaper or the television station know what is going on at St. Bonaventure Parish unless they are told? Who is going to tell them unless the diocesan communications officer knows what is going on there himself? He should know what is going on in the parishes.

Whether or not you have an communications officer, one of the things that your chancery offices can do is provide experts, both priests and laity, who can respond when people call them. Sometimes they want a priest, especially if it is television, because it looks more authoritative. If they want a collar, give them a collar. But also be able to refer them to lay experts and spokesmen. The U.S. bishops' conference has been very savvy about their pro-life secretariat, by often having a woman speak on camera. You have to have a lay person on your list of referees, because bishops and priests should always speak as bishops and priests, that is, they should speak in explicitly Christian ways. You also need some people in the diocese who speak in the way of natural reason, appealing to natural law. If the bishop or the priests are always going to speak from the Christian point of view—and they should— and use the name of Christ Jesus, you also need some who do not. You need those who are going to make the natural law or natural reason argument. And the lay faithful are the experts at that.

It is important to get the good news out. Probably every week in the bishop's schedule there is an anniversary, a launch, or a blessing—something that would be of interest to the local media. Everybody wants local stories. We are part of the community and therefore a source of good local stories. Probably every week in a bishop's schedule there is something the media might cover if they were informed about it in advance.

Finally, you have pastoral letters, special homilies, and such, which amplify your voice when you are speaking in your most authoritative way. But these need to be widely disseminated, and only the secular media can do that. Therefore, when you issue a pastoral letter, have a launch. For example, if you have a pastoral letter on health care, release it at a hospital. Put on a press conference at a hospital and have the archbishop move around the wards. It seems exploitative, because we think we are doing it just for the cameras, but the cameras are the only way our people find out about this. If you are writing a pastoral letter about gambling, go to a casino parking lot, set up your podium there, and say, "Isn't it sad what's going on in this diocese?" If you release it just at the chancery office or send it out to the parishes, the story will probably not get out. If you go to the casino parking lot and do the launch there, I guarantee that you will be at least the third story in the news. We have to create media opportunities, not because we are looking for vainglory, but because it is the only way our people will learn about what is going on.

A comment about attire: If you go to bless a school in your clerical suit and invite the media, they will probably cover it. If you do it in your choir cassock, you will get a photo in the paper. If you do it in a cope and miter, you will be on the front page, because they love pictures. Now there is always a balance between the ascetical life and dressing up just to call attention to ourselves, but the media loves pictures, and Catholic bishops have the coolest outfits of anybody in the public square. So if you wear all the regalia, you will get pictures. If you get pictures, the story gets higher play. That is just how newspapers and, especially, television work. Therefore, if you want to call attention to something, consider how you are dressed.

The last point I want to make is about your "*urbi et non orbi*" addresses. I say "to the city but not to the world" because you address your local pastoral flock. Five years ago, I was in Rome working for the National Catholic Register while studying. Perhaps the least interesting and newsworthy events were the Holy Father's *Urbi et Orbi* addresses. These addresses are a beautiful tradition, but if you read the text of what he says, they are similar to speeches he gives all the time. In any given week, he probably has two or three addresses that are more interesting than the *Urbi et Orbi* address, which is very pro forma and usually involves a call for peace. But the *Urbi et Orbi* addresses are the most covered of all the papal speeches. Everybody covers them because that is part of the tradition. Christmas and Easter, that is what the Pope does.

It is possible in your local diocese to develop that tradition every Christmas and every Easter. In short order, "The Bishop's Christmas Message" could become an annual chance for you to speak to your diocese, Catholic and non-Catholic, as a whole. If you do it every year, it will become part of the local scene, and every December there will be a press conference to release the Christmas message. It will be covered, and the press will pick up the themes you want, especially because Christmas and Easter are slow news days.

There are many other such initiatives that can amplify your voice. It is good pastoral strategy to amplify that voice in the media. For if the flock never hears the voice of the shepherd, how will it know whom to follow?

Application

SURGICAL STERILIZATION

THE SEDUCTIVE LIE

Very Rev. Russell E. Smith

Tennessee Williams's play, *Cat on a Hot Tin Roof*, is about sex and mendacity. Much of Pope John Paul II's pontificate was about the language of human sexuality and truth. The characters of the play and the Holy Father would probably agree that much of the misery that occurs in marriage occurs because mendacity is allowed to permeate the language of love. In Act One, Big Mama has it out with Maggie, points to the bed the latter no longer shares with her husband, Brick, and says, "Something's not right. You're childless and my son drinks.... When a marriage goes on the rocks, the rocks are *there*, right *there*!"[1]

Aristotle taught that "a small error in the beginning becomes greater in the end" [*error minor in principio fit maior in fine*].[2] Theological reflection in our times has become increasingly inarticulate and vague, not only because of open and ac-

---

[1] Tennessee Williams, *Cat on a Hot Tin Roof* (1954; New York: Signet Books, 1985), 37.

[2] Aristotle, *De caelo et mundo*, I, 5, 271b13.

knowledged dissent, but also because of the natural desire not to give offense to those who do not share our doctrinal perspectives and truths. This vagueness haunts not only contemporary ecclesiastical documents[3] but also interfaith dialogues. The late Fr. Carl Peter, Dean of Religious Studies at the Catholic University of America and a participant in the Catholic-Lutheran dialogue, made this same point with his students, saying that the Catholic-Lutheran dialogue was among the most contentious, but was also the most substantial, because each group held clear doctrinal positions that could be articulated and examined, whereas the Catholic-Anglican dialogue was undoubtedly the most pleasant but least productive, because of the wide latitude of Anglican doctrine.

The Theological Horizon: It Is All about Sex

One of the areas that leads to easy confusion is an overly vague articulation of the Church's doctrine on matrimony. As Edward Schillebeeckx said a generation ago, marriage is both a human reality and a saving mystery.[4] As such, marriage is moored in both philosophy *and* theology. Often in the seminary, this sacrament is treated only as a spiritual reality, when in essence it is integral to human nature as well. Marriage is a covenant involving bodies as well as souls. Overemphasis on the spiritual aspects of matrimony bypasses the logically fundamental anthropological aspects of matrimony's "material cause." The contract of marriage consists of an exchange of consent between a man and a woman involving "rights" over each others' bodies, to engage in acts apt for the procreation of offspring.

---

[3] See the turgid explanation of directions for the reception of Holy Communion by the U.S. Conference of Catholic Bishops, a stultifying adventure to comprehend. See, for example, *Daily Roman Missal* (Chicago: Midwest Theological Forum, 2003), 2186. Michael Davies, in *Liturgical Time Bombs in Vatican II* (Chicago: TAN Books, 2003), chronicles the exploitation of the vagueness of liturgical documents for "auto-destructive" purposes, to use the language of Pope Paul VI. See also Paul Mandowski, S.J., "Atheistic Catholics," *Faith, Moral Reasoning, and Contemporary American Life*, ed. Sr. Madonna Murphy, C.S.C. (Boston: Cambridge Center for the Study of Faith and Culture, 1995), 89–103.

[4] E. Schillebeeckx, *Marriage: Secular Reality and Saving Mystery* (New York: Sheed & Ward, 1965).

Far from a romantic notion of holy wedlock, this articulation of the material cause of matrimony (which is clearly not an exhaustive understanding of it), if stated clearly at the beginning of a dialogue, say, about alternative domestic partnerships involving same-sex couples or groupings, would answer many questions before they are asked. This articulation clearly states the heterosexual essence of marriage, marriage's primary purpose of procreation, the distinction made between the *ius ad corpus* and the *ius in corpore*, and that the *ius in corpore* in no way implies a "right" to have a child, but rather the right to engage in acts apt for a child's procreation. This determines the Church's teaching regarding the remedies of infertility. The further implication of the articulation of material cause of matrimony is the moral imperative to respect the very nature of the conjugal act. It has been the patrimony of humanity's moral sense that the procreative and unitive aspects of the conjugal act must be respected and never treated as a pathology.

It has been a universal sense of humanity that there are two fundamental "sacred" moments for a person: one's arrival and one's departure from life. Among other respected sacred moments, these have been surrounded with rituals and taboos, chronicled through every corridor of humanity's expression, from basic anthropology to the most sublime theology. Among Christianity's most constant moral doctrines is the inseparability of the procreative and unitive aspects of the conjugal act. Since 1930, however, this doctrine has all but disappeared from Christian teaching, with the exception of the teachings of the Catholic Church.[5] In 1930, the Lambeth Conference of the Anglican Communion became the first Christian body to claim that contraception could be a good.[6] This drew, for us, a lightening quick response from the Vatican in the form of the thunderous encyclical *Casti connubii* of Pope Pius XI.[7]

---

[5] A very interesting exception is *The Bible and Birth Control*, by Protestant writer Charles D. Provan (Monongahela, PA: Zimmer Printing, 1989).

[6] Lambeth Conference of Catholic Bishops, 1930, Resolution 15, at http://www.anglicancommunion.org/acns/archive/1930/1930-15.htm.

[7] Pius XI, *Casti connubii* (December 31, 1930), AAS 22 (1930): 565. See n. 6, regarding the contract of marriage, and n. 24 regarding the chief reason for marriage being the mutual perfection of spouses

Prior to the challenges to marriage that developed in the twentieth century, however, there was a trend in philosophy—most notably in the thought of Catholic René Descartes, but certainly the other idealists as well—which reintroduced dualism into philosophical anthropology and into the quickly evaporating metaphysics that remained. The rational, or spiritual, aspect of the human person and, therefore, intentionality were determinative of ethical propriety. The body was sub-personal and merely functional and vehicular. Immanuel Kant would give this philosophical legitimacy, and his dualism of phenomenal-noumenal realms would later be imported into Catholic theology, most notably in the articulation of theology by Karl Rahner, S.J.[8]

Many have criticized some of the twentieth century theologians of the *nouvelle theologie* for destroying the gratuity of grace by misunderstanding the "natural desire" to see God.[9] However, I think an equally strong case can be made for their destruction of nature, denigrating it to the realm of mere functionality.[10] Material nature becomes a circumstance of the subject's action. Of itself, material reality harbors no inherent moral significance. This, of course, is the fundamental and primary mistake of proportionalism that has so plagued moral

---

as the wider meaning of marriage, "provided matrimony be looked at not in the restricted sense as instituted for the proper conception and education of the child, but more widely as the blending of life as a whole and the mutual interchange and sharing thereof." This teaching would become confused after the Second Vatican Council, inasmuch as the late council was sometimes described as changing the primary purpose of matrimony from procreation to unity of spouses. See Richard A. McCormick, *The Critical Calling: Reflections on Moral Dilemmas since Vatican II* (Washington, DC: Georgetown University Press, 1989), 277.

[8] For example, see Karl Rahner, "The Theological Concept of Concupiscentia," in *Theological Investigations*, vol. 1, *God, Christ, Mary, and Grace*, trans C. Ernst (London: Darton, Longman & Todd, 1974), 347–382.

[9] Joseph Cardinal Siri, *Gethsemene* (Chicago: Franciscan Herald Press, 1981).

[10] See Brian Mullady, *Man's Desire for God* (Bloomington, IL: First Books Library, 2003). Taken to its extreme, this dualism crescendos into Manichaeism, which despises materiality. This has taken many forms in the history of the Church. See also John Saward, *Cradle of Redeeming Love: The Theology of the Christmas Mystery* (San Francisco: Ignatius Press, 2002): "The evil spirit in his pride loathes everything

theology since the mid-twentieth century.[11] However, proportionalism is the consistent metastasis of modernism into the tissues of moral theology.

Only a proper metaphysics can bring one to a theological appreciation of the material cause, and this leads, regarding our topic, to the appreciation of the conjugal act and its dual procreative and unitive aspects. The matrimonial vow is, among other things, about sex. We turn to the lusty English for perhaps the highest expression of the vow. The Sarum Use of the rite of marriage is contained in the first prayerbook of Edward VI:

> With thys ring I thee wed: Thys golde and siluer I thee geue: with my body I thee worship: and withal my worldly Goodes I thee indowe. In the name of the father, and of the sonne, and of the holy goste. Amen.[12]

So, to summarize, the marriage contract involves the exchange of consent, which includes the imparting one to the other of

---

bodily and therefore tempts men into despising or doubting the bodily truths of Divine Revelation (the Virgin Birth, the Resurrection, the miracles, the Real Presence) as well as all the spatial and temporal circumstances of our Savior's earthly life and works. [A footnote here references Marie Dominique Phillipe, *Wherever He Goes: A Retreat on the Gospel of John*. (Laredo, TX: Congregation of St. John, 1998), 95.] In his fury, the devil 'sweeps down a third of the stars of heaven, and casts them to the earth' with sovereign scorn, finding them meaningless. *The fact that the devil holds matter in scorn explains many things. He did not accept that God be Creator of a world which includes matter. He wants a God who is only Light. He wants only justice. Being only 'intellectual' he pleads justice above all else. He is 'cerebral,' with a cold, purely metallic intellect, for he has lost love and contemplation*" (325), original emphasis.

[11] For a full examination of this and how it developed historically through the modern period, see Russell E. Smith, "*Veritatis splendor* Teaches the Truth," *Faith and Reason* 21.1–2 (1995): 62–69. "The aspect of nature is understood to include all that is given prior to free decision. Nature is the material about which the personal aspect 'decides.' It is that which is determined, while the personal aspect is that which determines. Nature is the chaotic, inertial matter given meaning or purpose by our creative intellects. Matter is purely instrumental, not inherently meaningful. The operative 'virtue' becomes 'efficiency'" (67). For a fuller—and magisterial—treatment of an even longer history, see Servais Pinckaers, *The Sources of Christian Ethics* (Washington, DC: Catholic University of America Press, 1995), 191–323.

[12] *The First and Second Prayerbooks of Edward VI* (New York: J. M. Dent & Sons, 1927), 254.

rights over the other's body to perform the conjugal act, and this is the only morally licit forum for genital sexuality. Only the unhindered conjugal act speaks the language of human sexuality truthfully.

The Integrity of the Conjugal Act

While contraception has been practiced since the fall of man, and accepting the fact that the Catholic Church from its beginning has taught that contraception is wrong, the integrity of the conjugal act has been challenged even from friendly quarters. Biological science, for example, allows us to separate aspects of naturally integral body functions. Today, every aspect of motherhood can be abstracted and assigned to different agents. A child can have a legal mother, a genetic mother, a gestational mother, and a rearing mother, none of whom have to be the same person.

The first challenge to the integrity of the act came in the nineteenth century from the application of artificial insemination, used in animal husbandry, to the human model. After all, since it worked for breeding good cattle (a little bit of eugenics), could it help an infertile couple? At the time, a husband's semen was obtained by masturbation. This would occupy the moralists' reflection to begin with. Eschbach and Lehmukuhl held that an intrinsically immoral means (masturbation) was placed to obtain a good end; therefore, it was not permitted. Berardi and Palmieri disagreed, maintaining that masturbation in this instance (that is, the artificial insemination of a wife by her husband's semen when conception would not occur in the usual way) was not masturbation in the immoral sense, as the act retained its fundamental direction toward procreation.[13]

---

[13] Russell E. Smith, "Artificial Insemination: Harmonizing Some Perspectives Consonant with the Magisterial Teaching," *International Review of Natural Family Planning* 5 (1981): 126. See also Gerald Kelly, "The Morality of Artificial Insemination," *Ecclesiastical Review* 39 (1939): 110; and Rodger Van Allen, "Artificial Insemination (AIH): A Contemporary Re-Analysis," *Homiletic and Pastoral Review* 70 [1969–1970]: 363–372. For a fuller history and discussion, see John C. Wakefield, *Artful Childmaking: Artificial Insemination in Catholic Teaching* (St. Louis: Pope John Center, 1978).

In 1897, the Holy Office of the Inquisition was asked, "Can artificial fecundation of a woman be used?" The answer: "It is not possible." To the moralists of the time, this decree meant that artificial insemination was immoral when the means of obtaining the semen was illicit, that is, involving either ipsation or onanism. This was reinforced again in 1929 when the Holy Office was asked if masturbation could be used to obtain sperm for diagnostic purposes in the cases of disease and possible cure. The response again was "in the negative." Prominent moralists, Gerald Kelly among them, thought that artificial insemination would be possible if the means of obtaining the husband's seed were not illicit. If that way could be found, artificial insemination would become a recourse to "extraordinary means" to achieve the purpose of procreation.

In 1949, in an allocution to Italian physicians, Pope Pius XII manifested his mind on this matter, and brought clarity to the theological debate.[14] First, he said, this is an issue involving more than just biological and medical competence: morality and law were necessary as well. Second, he condemned artificial insemination outside of marriage as immoral purely and simply, because it shattered the meaning of the marital union and shirked the morally required responsibility of care for the (illegitimate) child. Parallel to this was the principle that artificial insemination in marriage using the sperm of a third party was immoral since "only marriage partners have mutual rights over their bodies for the procreation of a new life, and these rights are exclusive, nontransferable and inalienable." The Holy Father concluded by saying that,

> although one may not exclude a priori the use of new methods simply on the grounds that they are new; nevertheless, with regard to artificial insemination, it is not only a case of being extremely reserved, but it must be rejected entirely.

However, he did qualify this statement by allowing for "assisted insemination," the facilitation of the natural act of intercourse by methods that would help it attain its end.

---

[14] Pius XII, "Discourse to Those Taking Part in the Fourth International Congress of Catholic Doctors" (September 29, 1949), AAS 41 (1949): 559–560, quoted in Smith, "Artificial Insemination," 127.

It is all about the integrity of the conjugal act. In the same allocution to Catholic physicians, the Holy Father was most explicit: "The marital contract has as its object *not* a child but the natural *acts* apt and destined for the generation of new life."[15]

These principles would again be invoked with the develop-ment of in vitro processes of insemination and their alternatives, such as the modified GIFT (gamete intrafallopian transfer) procedure of the 1980s—which were themselves developed in hopes of being forms of *assisted* rather than *artificial* insemination. The Congregation for the Doctrine of the Faith would articulate the application of the integrity of the conjugal act vis-à-vis forms of artificial insemination in its instruction on the dignity of human life and procreation, *Donum vitae*, in 1988.

The integrity of the conjugal act—the inseparability of its unitive and procreative aspects—has been defended as a consistent response to both questions of avoiding pregnancy and questions of seeking pregnancy. The Church's positions are perfectly coherent and logical, whether pursuing or suppressing conception.[16] We are all well aware of the stunning clarity with which Pope Paul VI stated this doctrine:

> The Church, which interprets natural law through its unchanging doctrine, reminds men and women that the teachings based on natural law must be obeyed and teaches that it is necessary that each conjugal act remain ordained in itself to the procreating of human life.[17]

The conjugal act must be allowed to speak its message, and to speak it truthfully.

---

[15] Ibid., 128, emphasis added.

[16] See the appendix to this article.

[17] Paul VI, *Humanae vitae*, n. 11, trans. Janet E. Smith, in *Why Humanae Vitae Was Right: A Reader*, ed. Janet E. Smith (San Francisco: Ignatius Press, 1993), 549. *Humanae vitae* was Pope Paul VI's seventh and last encyclical. See Ermenegildo Lio, *Humanae Vitae e Infallibilità: Il Concilio Paolo VI e Giovanni Paolo II* (Vatican City: Libreria Editrice Vaticana, 1986).

The Rise of Contraceptive Culture and Its Expression in the Church

The contraceptive mentality has many roots.[18] The immediate causes are several: a mentality of eugenics;[19] the technological imperative; (originally) atheistic feminism;[20] the sexual revolution (theoretical and hedonistic);[21] and theological,

---

[18] Although not precisely about contraception and the integrity of the conjugal act, an intimately related question (one that assumes a shared perspective of atheism) is abortion. A must-read is the page-turner by Germain Kopaczynski, *No Higher Court: Contemporary Feminism and the Right to Abortion* (Scranton, PA: University of Scranton Press, 1995). The preface opens with these haunting words: "How did the practice of human abortion go from its atheistic root in the existentialist philosophy of Jean-Paul Sartre and Simone de Beauvoir to the classrooms of Christians?" (xvii). Again, John Saward, in *Cradle of Redeeming Love*, states poignantly: "With regard to birth control, Chesterton argued that it is always and in all circumstances, objectively and in practice, an act of hostility towards the child. The very name was dishonest, concealing as it did, behind words of clinical cleanness, the squalid alliance of hatred and lust. 'They insist on talking about Birth Control when they mean less birth and no control.' The man and the woman must have their pleasure, but the child, at all costs, *must not be.* Chesterton realized that the contracepting couple no longer see the child as a beautiful person, the fruit of love and gift of God, but as a horrible thing to be avoided, a disaster to be averted. This is the outlook of Herod in the heat of his passion and of Lucifer in the cold of his pride ... 'cruel Herod has immolated [you Holy Innocents], not for any evil you have done, but *solely out of hatred for the God of whom you are the image.*' And one of his comrades says, 'There is nothing the devil abominates so much as a little child ... Human wickedness is seen at its most diabolical in crimes against the child" (358–359). The reference within this quotation is to G. K. Chesterton, "The Thing," in *The Collected Works of G. K. Chesterton*, vol. 3 (San Francisco: Ignatius Press, 1990), 170.

[19] See the works of Margaret Sanger and Planned Parenthood.

[20] See Kopaczynski, *No Higher Court*; and Donna Steichen, *Ungodly Rage: The Hidden Face of Catholic Feminism* (San Francisco: Ignatius Press, 1991).

[21] The urtext of the sexual revolution is, perhaps, Joseph Fletcher's *Situation Ethics* (Philadelphia: Westminster Press, 1966), and its chronicle his *Moral Responsibility: Situation Ethics at Work* (Westminster, 1988), which was published the same year *Humanae vitae* was promulgated.

pastoral, institutional, and religious dissent.[22] The limits of time and topic forbid a detailed account of each of these roots. Suffice it to say a few generalities. Eugenics is as old as the Fall of man. Caste systems, genocide, wars, intrigue, and arranged marriages all have an element of asserting some aspect of genetic prominence. But serious proposals for societal cleansing have been openly proposed in soi-disant civilized cultures, like England, for over a century. Margaret Sanger's project was originally explicitly eugenic. Hitler's projects were overwhelmingly eugenic. In the early twentieth century, forced sterilization of poor and black women in aptly named Lynchburg, Virginia, was explicitly eugenic. Planned Parenthood is tacitly eugenic. We could go on.

(Feminism is not innately atheistic. Pope John Paul II's impressive articulation of theological anthropology gave exquisite voice to this. His expansive magisterium of this anthropology is the subject of an emerging specialty in moral theology.[23] Also, it is unnecessary to address the reader of this volume about the sexual revolution that underwent societal expression from 1955 to 1975. The infamous Kinsey report became something of its playbook. This twenty-year period witnessed some of the most dramatic revolutions in public mores in western history—from a professedly Christian moral stability [at least by law and overt culture] to virtual antinomianism, say, with the promotion of the "right to privacy" and the abolition of American anti-abortion laws with *Roe v. Wade*.)

The technological imperative can be described as the moral obligation to pursue any action that becomes technologically feasible: "If we can do it, we should do it." It is the first principle of utilitarian ethics. This goes hand in glove with the dualism mentioned earlier. In a paper for an earlier volume in this series, titled "'Medicalizing' Moral Decisions in Repro-

---

[22] See also John T. Noonan, Jr., *Contraception: A History of Its Treatment by the Catholic Theologians and Canonists* (Cambridge, MA: Harvard University Press, 1986); and Steven Phillip Rohlfs, *The Notion of Public Dissent in the Thought of Charles Curran, and the Response of the Holy See* [dissertation] (Rome: Pontifical University of St. Thomas de Urbe, 1988).

[23] In English language circles, this has become known as the "theology of the body," a phrase that John Paul II himself does not use, with good reason.

138

ductive Medicine," Dr. Thomas Murphy Goodwin described the draining of ethical appreciation of a patient's condition by recasting it only in terms of the model of the medical condition that presents itself or the legal strictures on the medicine practiced.[24] One example he gives is that of a pregnancy accompanied by fetal anomalies. A physician is obligated to discuss this with the mother as part of the process of obtaining informed consent for treatment proposals. One option these days is abortion, and not to present this possibility may result in a lawsuit for "wrongful birth." (There is no such thing as wrongful abortion, so long as the mother freely chooses the abortion.) The choice to abort is thus wrenched from its moorings in the moral order, and is assessed solely from the medical facts of pathology and the legal parameters (or their lack) for termination of pregnancy.[25] This creates a great bias in favor of abortion.

This is applicable also to surgical sterilization, which is routinely presented as an option to women who have had multiple deliveries by cesarean section, resulting in the infamous "weakened uterus," which Dr. Goodwin has showed to be a completely unstudied reality. Dr. Goodwin continues:

> With regard to fetal abnormalities, the burden is equally one-sided and even more clearly delineated in law. Physicians have legal and, some would say, ethical duties to inform pregnant women of prenatal tests that would affect their willingness to continue the pregnancy. The concept of "wrongful birth" in law establishes that failure to inform of tests that are widely accepted in the medical community as part of the standard of care could lead to legal liability. The related concept of "wrongful life," although less commonly invoked legally, is instructive for distilling the idea behind the law. In such cases, the child sues, claiming that it would be better not to have been born than to have been born with defects.[26]

The decision to undergo surgical sterilization is far less dramatic than of the decision to abort—and, therefore, it is far

---

[24] Thomas Murphy Goodwin, "'Medicalizing' Moral Decisions in Reproductive Medicine," in *Faith and Challenges to the Family—Proceedings of the Thirteenth Workshop for Bishops*, ed. Russell E. Smith (Braintree, MA: Pope John Center, 1994), 79–99.

[25] Ibid., 86.

[26] Ibid.

easier to make. After all, now we are led to reinterpret human dilemmas not as situated in the larger drama of life and the meaning of suffering, but as problems awaiting a medical or legal "fix."

In the sultry summer of 1968, amid widespread social unrest throughout the world—but especially in the United States and Europe—Pope Paul VI promulgated the long-awaited encyclical *Humanae vitae*, to the shock and dismay of many (and their ultimate rejection), beginning with significant figures in the theological community.[27] Catholic physicians and the large cadre of Catholic hospitals, along with the many religious who sponsored and staffed them, would not be unaffected.

Before we recount how the thermals from the torrid societal landscape below created turbulence for Catholic hospitals, however, let us examine surgical sterilization in Catholic theology prior to the period of dissent. Earlier, we discussed the conjugal act in the context of attempts to achieve pregnancy, and the damage done to the unitive aspect of the act by artificial insemination. From the other direction come questions of the treatment of diseases of women's reproductive organs, of risky pregnancies, and of interventions that render pregnancy impossible. We know that a hysterectomy, for example, can be justified by the principle of double effect when the uterus is pathological. From a purely clinical perspective, however, this procedure has the effect of rendering the woman sterile.

For years, too, there was discussion about the removal of the uterus after a number of deliveries by cesarean section which, it was asserted, rendered the uterine wall weak. Fr. Gerald Kelly, S.J., stated that

> when competent physicians judge that, by reason of repeated cesareans (or some similar cause) a uterus is so badly damaged that it will very likely not function safely in another pregnancy, he may, with the consent of the patient, remove the uterus as a seriously pathological organ.[28]

Reflection on this problem (which Dr. Murphy had shown to be an undocumented "pathology"[29]) led even non-dissenting

---

[27] For an excellent history of this period, see Rohlfs, *The Notion of Public Dissent*, 2–42.

[28] Gerald Kelly, *Medico-Moral Problems* (St. Louis: Catholic Health Association, 1957).

[29] Ibid., 89.

theologians to theorize "uterine isolation" by tubal ligation, which is less surgically invasive. Fr. Thomas O'Donnell, S.J., is given the credit for developing this concept.[30] It was based on an understanding of the medical ethical principle of totality, which enjoyed widespread acceptance among non-dissenting theologians. "Uterine isolation," assisted by Fr. O'Donnell's good name, almost became permitted by inclusion in the 1971 *Ethical and Religious Directives for Catholic Health Facilities.* However, on the advice of Fr. John Connery, S.J., Fr. O'Donnell quietly withdrew this consideration, because it was thought its inclusion in the *Ethical and Religious Directives* would further theological dissent, which was reaching fever pitch at the time.[31]

Only much later would the Congregation for the Doctrine of the Faith deem "uterine isolation" to be wrongly justified because it was based on a false understanding of "pathology," and the practice was eventually rejected definitively as a theory and a practice in Catholic health-care facilities.[32] The congregation determined that a uterus with a weakened wall would be pathological *only* during pregnancy. Therefore, the "moral object" of uterine isolation is the prevention of pregnancy— that is, it is contraceptive. The point here is that surgical sterilization was a question for Catholic health-care providers even before the rise of theological dissent.

Returning to dissent, now, we return to the dreaded year 1968. At 5:00 p.m. on July 29, 1968, the day *Humanae vitae* was promulgated in Rome, a conference was held to "read, analyze, discuss and evaluate the Papal Letter" (and ultimately reject it) at the Catholic University of America in Washington, D.C.[33] At a press conference the next morning, a statement titled *Statement by Theologians* was issued, declaring the right

---

[30] Thomas O'Donnell, *Medicine and Christian Morality* (New York: Alba House, 1976), 134.

[31] Orville N. Griese, *Catholic Identity in Health Care: Principles and Practice.* (Braintree, MA: Pope John Center, 1987), 224–225. For an interesting history of directives for Catholic hospitals in the United States, see pp. 1–19.

[32] Congregation for the Doctrine of the Faith, *Responsa ad proposita dubia circa "interclusionem uteri" et alias quaestiones* (July 31, 1993), AAS 86 (1994): 820–821.

[33] Charles Curran, *Faithful Dissent* (Kansas City, MO: Sheed & Ward, 1987), 5; cited in Rohlfs, *The Notion of Public Dissent,* 4.

of Catholics to dissent from non-infallible doctrine. It had eighty-seven signatories that day, and was sent to one thousand two hundred Catholic theologians, half of whom subscribed to it as well. It stated in part:

> As Roman Catholic theologians, ... we conclude that spouses may responsibly decide according to their conscience that artificial contraception in some circumstances is permissible and indeed necessary to preserve and foster the values and sacredness of marriage.[34]

This was the shot heard around the world. We were off to the races.[35]

The rest of the theological arena of dissent need no longer detain us. Attention turns to Catholic hospitals. Religious life was in the midst of radical changes after the Second Vatican Council. The religious who staffed Catholic hospitals were still present in significant, if waning, numbers in the early 1970s. Many were young enough to return to graduate school and study theology. The dissent of the academy soon entered chanceries, motherhouses, and Catholic hospitals.

To counter the tsunami of confusion and dissent, the Congregation for the Doctrine of the Faith issued its "Response to Questions of the Bishops of North America about Sterilization in Catholic Hospitals."[36] The document made the following points:

- Sterilization which, of its nature or intention, has as its purpose or immediate effect to render the sexual faculty incapable of procreation is "direct sterilization" and is absolutely forbidden. [*Quaecumque sterilizatio quae ex seipsa, seu ex natura et conditione propria, immediate hoc solummodo efficit ut facultas generativa incapax reddatur ad consequendam procreationem, habenda est pro sterilizatione directa, prout haec intelligitur in declarationibus Magisterii Pontificii, speciatim Pii XII.*]

---

[34] Charles Curran et al., *Dissent In and For the Church* (New York: Sheed & Ward, 1969), 24-26, quoted in Rohlfs, *The Notion of Public Dissent*, 4f.

[35] See Charles E. Curran and Richard A. McCormick, *Readings in Moral Theology, No. 6: Dissent in the Church* (New York: Paulist Press, 1988).

[36] Congregation for the Doctrine of the Faith, "Response to Questions of the North American Bishops' Conference" (March 13, 1975), AAS 68 (1976): 738–740.

- Also absolutely forbidden is the performance of sterilization with the purpose of relieving some physical condition (unrelated to the sexual organs themselves) or mental condition. [*Absolute, ergo interdicta manet iuxta doctrinam Ecclesiae, non obstante quacumque recta intenione subiectiva agentium consulendi curae vel praeventioni mali sive physici sive psychici, quod ex praegnatione praevidetur vel timetur eventurum.*]

- Neither a civil mandate nor the principle of totality can justify direct sterilization in Catholic hospitals. [*Neque invocari potest ullum mandatum publicae auctoritatis, quae ex titulo necessarii boni comderet [sic!] dignitatem et inviolabilitatem personae humanae. Pariter invocari non potest in casu principium totalitatis, quo iustificantur interventus in organa propter maius bonum personae.*]

- This is the meaning of the National Conference of Catholic Bishops' *Ethical and Religious Directives*, no. 20, issued in 1971. [*Hinc articulus 20 Codicis ethicae medicalis a Conferentia a. 1971 promulgati reddit fideliter doctrinam tenendam, eiusque observantia urgeri debet.*] [37]

- The congregation acknowledges the existence of dissent but denies the validity of this dissent and disavows the opinion of dissenting theologians, saying that the opinions of such theologians do not constitute a genuine theological *locus* and so should not be followed by the faithful. [*Congregatio ... non ignorat factum dissensus ex parte plurium theologorum adversus eam (traditionalem doctrinam) existens. Negat, tamen, significationem doctrinalem huic facto, ut tali attribui posse ad constituendum "locum theologicum" quem invocare valeant fideles...*]

- Institutional cooperation permitting direct sterilization in Catholic hospitals is absolutely forbidden. [*...cooperatio institutionaliter adprobata vel admissa...est absolute interdicta.*]

---

[37] Directive 20 of the 1971 ERDs reads: "Procedures that induce sterility, whether permanent or temporary, are permitted when: (a) they are immediately directed to the cure, diminution, or prevention of a serious pathological condition and are not directly contraceptive (that is, contraception is not the purpose); and (b) a simpler treatment is not reasonably available." U.S. Conference of Catholic Bishops, *Ethical and Religious Directives for Catholic Health Facilities* (Washington, DC: USCCB, 1971).

- The traditional principles of material cooperation may be applied with the utmost prudence, avoiding at all costs scandal and confusion of the faithful. [*Traditionalis doctrina de cooperatione materiali, cum opportunis distinctionibus inter cooperationem necessariam et liberam, proximam et remotam, in vigore manet, prudentissime applicanda, si casus ferat...omnino scandalum et periculum cuiusvis confusionis mentium caveatur per opportunam explicationem realitatis.*]

The President of the National Conference of Catholic Bishops, then Archbishop Joseph Bernardin, made the teaching of the congregation quite clear. His letter accompanies the presentation of the congregation's response and states:

> direct sterilization is not to be considered as justified by the common good, the principle of totality, the existence of contrary opinion, *or any other argument.* This means that Catholic hospitals, as a matter of institutional policy, may not authorize sterilization procedures for reasons other than those contained in the guidelines.[38]

Much later, in 1993, the Congregation for the Doctrine of the Faith would again address the issue of surgical sterilization in its *Responsa ad dubia*, applying this directly to tubal ligation and in the presence of the so-called weakened uterus.[39]

Despite the clarity and specificity of the magisterial teaching on contraceptive sterilization through the 1970s, things

---

[38] Archbishop Joseph Bernardin, quoted in Benedict M. Ashley and Kevin D. O'Rourke in *Health Care Ethics: A Theological Analysis* (St. Louis: Catholic Health Association, 1977), 283 (emphasis added). This phrase in the archbishop's letter was roundly criticized by many theologians at the time.

[39] Congregation for the Doctrine of the Faith, "Responses to Questions Proposed Concerning Uterine Isolation and Related Matters" [*Responsa ad proposita dubia circa "interclusionem uteri" et alias quaestiones*], July 31, 1993, AAS 86 (1994):820-821. The congregation responded to three questions: (1) Can the uterus be removed during a delivery or cesarean section "in order to counter an immediate serious threat to the life or health of the mother? A: Yes. (2) It is permissible to remove the uterus when it does not pose a present risk to the life or health or the woman, but which is foreseeably incapable of carrying a future pregnancy to term without danger to the mother? A: No. (3) In the same situation as (2), can a tubal ligation be performed in place of the more invasive hysterectomy? A: No. The latter two dubia clearly reveal the intent, purpose, and effect of the tubal ligation—to prevent pregnancy. Therefore, it is directly contraceptive.

came to, at least, a symbolic head in what theologians call "the Mercy Affair." Fr. Richard McCormick summarizes the problem thus:

> In 1978 the Sisters of Mercy of the Union, sponsors of the [then] largest group of nonprofit hospitals in the country, began a study of the theological and ethical aspects of tubal ligation. The study resulted in a recommendation to the General Administration of the Sisters of Mercy that tubal ligations be allowed when they are determined by patient and physician to be essential to the overall good of the patient. The General Administrative Team accepted this recommendation in principle. In a November 12, 1980, letter to their hospital administrators the General Administrative Team reported the results of the study and indicated a desire to draw concerned persons into dialogue on the issue. They did not, as was inaccurately reported to the bishops of this country, mandate a policy.[40]

This led to a lengthy investigation by the Congregation for Religious and Secular Institutes. This dicastery formed a Committee of Verification, headed by an American Bishop (James Malone of Youngstown Diocese). Two years of wrangling created a very heated and at times somewhat hostile environment. Eventually, in 1982, the administrative team of the Sisters of Mercy of the Union responded: "We receive the teaching of the Church on tubal ligation with respectful fidelity in accord with *Lumen gentium* 25 (*obsequium religiosum*.)"[41] This was deemed by the Roman congregation as too little.

In July 1983, Sr. M. Theresa Kane wrote to hospital administrators, with a copy to Cardinal Pironio in Rome. Her letter reads in part:

> As requested by [the congregation] to reevaluate, we, the Mercy Administrative Team, have spent additional time in study and consultation on tubal ligation. In obedience to the magisterium we will take no public position on this matter contrary to Church teaching. As you face pastoral problems regarding tubal ligation, we ask that you continue to work in close collaboration with your local ordinary in implementing Church teaching.[42]

---

[40] Richard A. McCormick, *Notes on Moral Theology 1981–1984* (Lanham, MD: University Press of America, 1984), 187. See also McCormick, *Critical Calling*, 273–287.

[41] McCormick, *Notes*, 190.

[42] McCormick, *Critical Calling*, 284.

Nor was this enough. The congregation insisted on the following wording:

> In obedience to the magisterium we will continue to study and reflect on Church teaching with a view to accepting it. We, therefore, direct that the performance of tubal ligations be prohibited in all hospitals owned and/or operated by the Sisters of Mercy of the Union.

This wording was a "formal precept." Fr. McCormick notes that

> the sisters recognized both the rock and the hard place. Failure to comply might, indeed assuredly would, lead to consequences that would compromise or nullify their important work in many other areas. Accordingly, on October 26, 1983, Sister M. Theresa Kane sent the required letter to the Mercy Hospital administrators.[43]

The issue was over . . . for them.

Surgical Sterilization Today and the Catholic Hospital

As it was eleven years ago when Dr. Goodwin addressed this assembly, so today surgical sterilization by tubal ligation is the most commonly used method of contraception for women in the United States.[44] The number of tubal ligations has remained largely unchanged since the 1970s,[45] and about 700,000 are performed annually in America.[46] Twenty-seven percent of women who contracept choose surgical sterilization. Women are three times more likely than men to undergo surgical sterilization because of its effectiveness.[47] Not surprisingly, the majority of women who choose this method

---

[43] Ibid.

[44] See Goodwin, " 'Medicalizing' Moral Decisions," 89. See also I. Cori Baill et al., "Counseling Issues in Tubal Sterilization," *American Family Physician* 67.6 (March 15, 2003): 1287, http://www.aafp.org/afp/20030315/1287.html.

[45] "History and Epidemiology of Tubal Sterilization in the United States," *Clinical Proceedings of the Association of Reproductive Health Professionals* [ARHP], May 2002, http://www.arhp.org/healthcareproviders/cme/onlinecme/sterilizationcp/history.cfm?ID=47.

[46] "Tubal Sterilization Overview," *eMedicine Consumer Health* (July 22, 2004), http://www.emedicinehealth.com/articles/29895-1.asp.

[47] Baill et al., "Counseling Issues." "Tubal Sterilization Overview," *eMedicine Consumer Health* (July 22, 2004), at http://www.emedici nehealth.com/articles/29895-1.asp.

(around 50 percent) are over forty years old, because the procedure is considered irreversible.[48]

Between 1987 and 1995, a significant shift occurred in the locations where these procedures are performed. While half remained in in-patient hospital settings, because they were performed immediately after deliveries, there was a significant increase in procedures performed in out-patient hospital settings, as the technique was becoming less invasive—and is even less so now in the 2000s. Except when performed after cesarean deliveries, tubal sterilizations are now performed laparoscopically, and are no longer surgically invasive.[49]

The Recurrent Effort to Provide Surgical Sterilization in Catholic Hospitals

The reasons adduced today for providing surgical sterilizations in Catholic hospitals (as well as clinics and medical office buildings) are essentially the same reasons as always: pressure from physicians to provide all medically standard and safe procedures; the "business" side of the physicians' concern, namely, the continued provision of the obstetrical and gynecological services essential for the survival of the hospital; and the cultural acceptability of contraception. It would not be uncharitable to say that there is residual dissent from the Church's moral doctrine in some influential quarters (most concentrated in the arena of academic and university theology). The professional pressure on physicians and the first line of action for hospital administrators—appeasing trouble—combine to make this a concern, whether the Catholic facility is the sole provider in a given area or is set in a larger metropolitan area with many non-Catholic hospitals. The "sole provider" scenario carries with it the added argument of "we should not impose Catholic morality on non-Catholics. Ours is a pluralistic society." (This implies that the Church's institutions should not assert the Church's moral doctrine in a pluralistic society. Such submission on the part of religion would actually constitute a "secular society," not a pluralistic one.)

Add to this dynamic the evolution of the delivery of health care from the late 1980s to date. In this period, we have been

---

[48] "History and Epidemiology of Tubal Sterilization," ARHP Clinical Proceedings.

[49] Ibid.

witnesses to what is called the reconfiguration of health-care delivery. Although it was wrongly prophesied that the hospital would be displaced as the center of health care, much clinical care has moved to other forums, notably ambulatory surgical centers, physicians' offices, and the home itself. This has led to a "rationalizing" of health care, bringing together formerly rival and "stand-alone" institutions. These "reconfigurations" of health-care delivery have produced a variety of variously named partnerships, generally bringing together Catholic and non-Catholic providers: integrated delivery networks (IDNs), management corporations, PPOs (preferred provider organizations), IPOs (independent provider organizations), traditional mergers, and joint ventures of every type.

"Rules of engagement" had to be developed to chart the course for the Catholic mission to continue, for the stable patrimony to remain Church property and to remain faithful to Catholic moral doctrine. Book V of the *Code of Canon Law* is concerned with the "temporal goods of the Church." Early on, it was strongly proposed (and time has proved the wisdom of the proposal) that religious orders civilly incorporate their apostolates as corporations sole, with certain defining powers reserved to the members of the corporation, who represent and ideally are members of the sponsoring order.[50] Particularly important would be the powers over the philosophy and mission of the corporation, the ownership of the assets and patrimony of the apostolate, the naming of the board of directors of the corporation, and the hiring and dismissal of the CEO of the incorporated apostolate.

As the presence of religious women and men, and even whole congregations, diminished, the public juridic persons endowing Catholic hospitals with Catholic identity have frequently become civil corporations. These corporations have the approval of the competent dicasteries of the Holy See, but it seems that they are a pro tempore solution for holding onto the mission. In the long term, it seems that there will need to be some development in light of the Church's understanding of her *munus Communionis*. This is essentially a concern *ad intra*. This has been a fairly recent development in terms of actually creating these public juridic persons inasmuch as only now is the near total absence of non-retired religious manifest.

---

[50] Adam J. Maida and Nicholas P. Cafardi, *Church Property, Church Finances, and Church-Related Corporations* (St. Louis: Catholic Health Association of America, 1984), 271–272.

The concern *ad extra* arose earlier, when the myriad partnerships were first being proposed, generally in the latter half of the 1980s. How could Catholic institutions work with non-Catholic institutions that provide services at odds with the Church's moral doctrine and self-understanding? The "principles of cooperation" were given new life by theologians and ethicists in health-care systems, seminaries, and universities. These principles, first articulated in an orthodox manner by St. Alfonsus Liguori in the eighteenth century, suddenly became the radical chic of the late twentieth—and with the same cat fights that ensued between the moralists of that time. Until the mid 1980s, these principles generally received about fifteen minutes of one lecture in Moral Theology 101 (the first year of major seminary)! They were case specific and had dealt, up to that time, with individuals in difficult employment situations. Can a Catholic pharmacy clerk complete a sale for condoms? Can a nurse in the operating room assist in an abortion? Can a servant carry a ladder for a master about to commit a mortal sin? A far cry from boardroom headaches!

About all everyone could agree on was the fact that formal cooperation was not permitted, and certain types of material cooperation *could* be *permitted* as long as there was a sufficiently good reason to cooperate and scandal could be avoided. The National Catholic Bioethics Center developed principles of partnerships, which are well documented.[51] To my knowledge, no partnership crafted by these principles has failed because of these principles, or been disapproved by ecclesiastical authorities for reasons of ethical impropriety derived from action on them.

Pope John Paul II's Insistence on Resistance to Those Forces

It comes as no surprise that in the course of his long pontificate, Pope John Paul II was impressively articulate in forcefully asserting the Church's moral doctrine with regard to human sexuality and the intrinsic evil of contraception. The sheer volume of his pontifical magisterium is stunning. Perhaps

---

[51] See Russell E. Smith, "Ethical Quandary: Forming Hospital Partnerships," in *The Gospel of Life and the Vision of Health Care—Proceedings of the Fifteenth Workshop for Bishops*, ed. Russell E. Smith (Braintree, MA: Pope John Center, 1997), 113.

there is no better summation of the Church's doctrine on the immorality of contraception and contraceptive sterilization and affirmation of the witness to moral truth of the Catholic hospital than his allocution to the bishops of Texas, Oklahoma, and Arkansas on June 27, 1998:

> When the Church teaches, for example, that abortion, sterilization or euthanasia are always morally inadmissible, she is giving expression to the universal moral law inscribed on the human heart, and is therefore teaching something which is binding on everyone's conscience. Her absolute prohibition that such procedures be carried out in Catholic healthcare facilities is simply an act of fidelity to God's law. As bishops you must remind everyone involved—hospital administrations and medical personnel—that any failure to comply with this prohibition is both a grievous sin and a source of scandal....
>
> This and other such instances are not, it must be emphasized, the imposition of an external set of criteria in violation of human freedom. Rather, the Church's teaching of moral truth "brings to light the truths which [conscience] ought already to possess" ... and it is these truths which make us free in the deepest meaning of human freedom and give our humanity its genuine nobility.[52]

Little more can be added to this remarkably concise absolute prohibition of surgical sterilization in Catholic hospitals.

Our Relationship to God

Cat on a Hot Tin Roof climaxes with a wrenching and revelatory discussion between Big Daddy and his morally paralyzed son, Brick, whose marriage and other relationships have been shown to be thoroughly compromised by half-truths and lies. Brick, coming to a moment of clarity, admits, "[Big Daddy, m]endacity is a system that we live in. [I'm only] accidentally truthful—I don't know but—anyway—we've been friends ... — And being friends is telling each other the truth." [53]

There are many "reasons" given as to why surgical sterilizations should be provided in Catholic hospitals: the professional panoply of physicians' obstetrical and gynecological

---

[52] John Paul II, "*Ad limina* Address to the Bishops of Texas, Oklahoma, and Arkansas" (June 27, 1998), *L'Osservatore Romano*, English edition (July 1, 1998), 3.

[53] Williams, 94.

services, the administration's need to bring those services to the hospitals, the cultural acceptance of a contraceptive mentality, the reduction of sexuality to enjoyment, the technological imperative and its inherent utilitarianism, the denigration of the bodily aspects of the human person and anthropology, our focus on the product or results of our actions apart from moral considerations of the actions themselves. Each reason presents a "fact," but the "facts" make sense—that is, speak the truth—only in light of the fundamental, overarching truths about the human person and his relationship to God. Pope Paul VI wrote:

> The question of having children, like other questions regarding human life, cannot be addressed adequately by examining it in a piecemeal way, that is, by looking at it through the perspectives of biology, psychology, demography and sociology. Rather, [the question] must be addressed in such a way that the whole Man and the whole mission [*munus*] to which he has been called will be taken into account, for this [mission] pertains not only to his natural and earthly existence but also to his supernatural and eternal existence.[54]

Pope John Paul II concludes his encyclical *Veritatis splendor* by saying, "No absolution offered by beguiling doctrines, even in the areas of philosophy and theology, can make man truly happy: only the Cross and the glory of the Risen Christ can grant peace to his conscience and salvation to his life."[55] The Catholic hospital stands on the frontlines of the "culture wars" of our times. The witness of the Church to the truth of her Lord's teaching must be clear, strong, and articulate in the arena of health care. With the gentleness of Christ Himself, our hospitals must respect the right of everyone to the truth about themselves and the Lord who loves them.

The appendix appears on following page.

---

[54] Paul VI, *Humanae vitae*, trans. Smith, n. 7.

[55] John Paul II, *Veritatis splendor* (August 6, 1993), n. 120, http://www.vatican.va/edocs/ENG0222/__PA.HTM.

APPENDIX

The Two-fold Path of Doctrine regarding the Requisite Integrity of the Conjugal Act

Year	Artificial Insemination	Contraception
1897	Holy Office (infertility)[a]	
1929	Holy Office (masturbation for diagnosis)[b]	
1930		Holy Father, *Casti connubii*[c]
1949	Holy Father to physicians[d]	
1951	Holy Father to midwives[e]	
1968		Holy Father, *Humanae vitae*[f]
1971		NCCB, *Ethical and Religious Directives* (ERDs)[g]
1975		CDF, *Quaecumque sterilizatio*[h]
		Archbishop Bernardin's clarification[i]
		CDF, *Persona humana*[j]
1977		CTSA-commissioned study, *Human Sexuality*[k]
1978		CDF to Archbishop Quinn re CTSA study[l]
1988	CDF, *Donum vitae*[m]	
1993		CDF, *Responsa ad dubia*[n]
1994		ERDs revised[o]

NOTES: (a) "Response of the Holy Office" (March 17, 1897), *Acta Santæ Sedis* 29 (1896–1897), 704. (b) "Decree of the Holy Office" (August 2, 1929), *Acta Apostolicæ Sedis* (AAS) 21 (1929): 490. (c) Pius XI, *Casti connubii* (December 31, 1930), AAS 22 (1930): 546–547. (d) Pius XII, "Discourse to Those Taking Part in the Fourth International Congress of Catholic Doctors" (September 29, 1949), AAS 41 (1949): 559–560. (e) Pius XII, "Discourse to Those Taking Part in the Congress of the Italian Catholic Union of Midwives" (October 29, 1951), AAS 43 (1951): 850. (f) Paul VI, *Humanae vitae* (July 25, 1968), AAS 60 (1968): 483. (g) National Conference of Catholic Bishops, *Ethical and Religious Directives for Catholic Health Facilities* (Washington, DC: U.S. Catholic Conference, 1971). (h) Congregation for the Doctrine of the Faith (CDF), "Quaecumque sterilizatio" (March 13, 1975), AAS 68 (1976): 738–740. (i) Archbishop Joseph Bernardin, quoted in Benedict M. Ashley and Kevin D. O'Rourke, *Health Care Ethics: A Theological Analysis* (St. Louis: Catholic Health Association, 1977), 283. (j) CDF, *"Persona humana:* Declaration on Certain Questions concerning Sexual Ethics" (December 29, 1975), AAS 68 (1976): 77–96. (k) Anthony Kosnik et al., *Human Sexuality: New Directions in American Catholic Thought; A Study Commissioned by The Catholic Theological Society of America* (New York: Paulist Press, 1977). (l) CDF, "Lettura a Sua Ecc.za Mons. John R. Quinn, Presidente della Conferenza Episcopale Americana e osservazioni sul libro «La sessualità umana» a cura del Rev.do Anthony Kosnik" (July 13, 1979), *L'Osservatore Romano*, December 7, 1979, reprinted in *Documenta Inde a Concilio Vaticano Secondo Expleto Edita, 1966–1985* (Vatican City: Librera Editrice Vaticana, 1985), 148–154. (m) CDF, *Donum vitae* (February 22, 1987), AAS 80 (1988): 70–102. (n) CDF, "Responsa ad proposita dubia circa 'interclusionem uteri' et alias quaestiones" [responses to questions concerning uterine isolation and related matters] (July 31, 1993), AAS 86 (1994): 820–821. (o) National Conference of Catholic Bishops, *Ethical and Religious Directives for Catholic Health Care Services* (Washington, DC: U.S. Catholic Conference, 1995).

Rape Protocols and Emergency Contraception

Rev. Albert S. Moraczewski, O.P.

Gone are the halcyon days when there was a general public agreement on moral values, if that era ever existed. We know today there exist not only a wide divergence of values but also disagreement as to their relative importance. This situation makes it difficult to maintain reasonable public discourse on vital issues regarding life, sexual morality, war, and the like.

A case in point: What may a Catholic hospital do and not do for a female patient who is the survivor of a sexual assault? The protocols developed by secular hospitals generally are not morally acceptable for Catholic health-care facilities (or for Catholic health-care personnel). This is because the proposed treatments could result in the abortion of a newly conceived child. So what can a Catholic hospital do for such a survivor?

A Case Study

A fifteen-year-old rape survivor is brought to the emergency department of a local Catholic hospital by her mother, who vigorously demands that everything be done to make sure that her daughter does not get pregnant. What can the emergency personnel do while at the same time faithfully observing the requirement of directive 36 of the *Ethical and Religious Directives for Catholic Health Care Services,* that no abortifacient treatment be employed?[1] Directive 36 reads, in part:

> If, after appropriate testing, there is no evidence that conception has occurred already, she may be treated with medications that would prevent ovulation, sperm capacitation, or fertilization. It is not permissible, however, to initiate or recommend treatments that have as their purpose or direct effect the removal, destruction, or interference with the implantation of a fertilized ovum.

While the directive is clear, what is not clear—and, indeed, is controverted—is the certitude of the medical facts regarding the pharmacological action of the customary medications used in treating victims of rape. Are "morning-after" pills, such as Ovral, abortifacient or not? There are medical claims on both sides. In Peru, for example, the issue has drawn widespread public attention, because the Peruvian health minister, Pilar Mazzetti, has vigorously promoted the use of these medications in public health facilities, claiming that there is scientific evidence that these medications do not have an abortifacient effect.[2]

Others—apparently the majority of physicians—with equal vigor assert that these pills do have an abortifacient action.[3] In light of these conflicting assertions by the medical community, any ethical analysis rests on shaky grounds. Admitting this limitation, this presentation will be in two major parts: a brief review of the relevant reproductive biology and an ethical analysis of the case study briefly cited above.

---

[1] U.S. Conference of Catholic Bishops, *Ethical and Religious Directives for Catholic Health Services,* 4th ed. (Washington, DC: USCCB, 2001).

[2] See "Push for 'Morning-After' Pill," *Catholic World Report* (December 2004), 21.

[3] See, for example, D. C. Young et al., "Emergency Contraception Alters Progesterone-Associated Endometrial Protein in Serum and Uterine Luminal Fluid," *Obstetrics & Gynecology* 84.2 (August 1994): 266–271.

Review of the Relevant
Reproductive Biology

The relevant facts about the female reproductive tract prior to fertilization are, in brief, as follows:[4]

1. At puberty, the human female has about forty thousand oocytes (ova) in her ovaries.

2. The purpose of the menstrual cycle is to produce, each month, a single female gamete (the oocyte, or ovum) and a uterus in a condition to receive a fertilized embryo.

3. The hypothalamus of the brain secretes a hormone, gonadotropin-releasing hormone (GnRH) which stimulates the pituitary gland to increase its secretion of two gonadotropic hormones: (1) luteinizing hormone (LH); and (2) follicle-stimulating hormone (FSH).

4. Together, these hormones initiate folliculogenesis in the ovary and the proliferative phase in the endometrium.

5. Ovulation occurs about thirty-eight hours after the beginning of the ovulatory surge of FSH and LH.

6. The oocyte is actively scraped off the ovary by the fimbriated mouth of the oviduct (fallopian tube) and is moved into the ampulla (the enlarged end of the fallopian tube) by the beating of cilia on the oviduct wall. The oocyte remains viable for about twenty-four hours, after which it loses its capacity to be fertilized.

7. Fertilization involves a complex interaction between the sperm and the oocyte. The sperm has to be capacitated by factors in the oviduct which enable it to release enzymes from the acrosome (the tip of the sperm). These factors allow it to penetrate the tough zona pellucida surrounding the oocyte.

8. The entry of one sperm into the oocyte causes release of substances in the oocyte which alter the zona pellucida so that additional sperm cannot enter the oocyte subsequently.

---

[4] William J. Larsen, *Human Embryology* (New York: Churchill Livingston, 1993), 11–21.

9. The chromosomes of the oocyte and sperm are enclosed in the female and male pronuclei, respectively.

10. The fusion of the two pronuclei leads to the formation of the one-celled zygote, the beginning of the new organism, which immediately begins to cleave into two daughter cells, both remaining in close contact and enclosed in the zona pellucida.

11. The new organism (the zygote, or embryo) now travels down the fallopian tube, all while cleaving but not increasing in size. Before implantation, it will have gone through several stages, becoming first a morula and then a blastocyst, which is composed of about one hundred and fifty cells (blastomeres). About five and a half days after fertilization, it will begin to implant in the receptive uterine wall (endometrium) after having shed the tough zona pellucida.

Since the concern of this paper is to determine what medical procedures are morally acceptable for pregnancy prevention in a woman who is the victim of a sexual assault, it will be helpful to consider what procedures are theoretically possible before considering their moral acceptability as points of intervention. The possible points of intervention are as follows:[5]

- Follicle maturation
- The ovulatory process
- Sperm migration into and through the fallopian tube, including adhesion of spermatozoa to the epithelium needed to acquire and maintain fertilizing capacity
- Fertilization
- Zygote development in the fallopian tube
- Zygote transport through the fallopian tube
- Preimplantation development within the uterus
- Uterine retentiveness of the free-laying morula or blastocyst
- Endometrial receptivity
- Blastocyst signaling, adhesion, and invasiveness
- Corpus luteum sufficiency and responsiveness to hCG

---

[5] Horatio B. Croxatto et al., "Mechanism of Action of Hormonal Preparations Used for Emergency Contraception: A Review of the Literature," *Contraception* 63.3 (March 2001): 111–121.

After sexual intercourse, sperm can be found within five minutes at the mouth of the cervix. While an oocyte remains fertilizable only for about twenty-four hours, the sperm remains capable of fertilization for about four days in a suitable environment such as the cervical crypts. It should noted that:

> Neither the minimum length of time from coitus to fertilization, when the oocyte is waiting for the sperm, nor the shortest interval from ovulation to fertilization, when the sperm is waiting for the oocyte, have been determined in the human. Therefore the exact theoretical amplitude of the window for acting before fertilization is undetermined, less so the actual window in real cases.[6]

One other significant piece of biological information has to do with the implantation phase. As noted above, even though the endometrium may be altered by the "emergency contraception," it is not certain that implantation is thereby necessarily prevented. In fact, some question to what degree endometrial receptivity is actually altered:

> The most difficult parameter to assess with certainty is endometrial receptivity. Endometrial markers of receptivity have been established so far with certainty only in rodents. Even if endometrial receptivity is shown to be altered by [emergency contraceptives], other steps that precede implantation may also be altered enough to interrupt the process at an earlier stage.[7]

Ethical Analysis of Case Study

A critical issue in considering the morally acceptable treatment of a rape survivor relates to implantation. While all grant that the contraceptive drug will bring about changes in the endometrium, there is divergence as to whether these endometrial changes are sufficient to prevent implantation as a rule.

The moral decision which must be made when the treatment of a rape survivor is considered is the focus of this analysis. The opening words of directive 36 set the stage:

> Compassionate and understanding care should be given to a person who is the victim of sexual assault. Health-care providers should cooperate with law enforcement officials and offer the person psychological and spiritual

---

[6] Ibid., 118.

[7] Ibid., 119.

support as well as accurate medical information. A female who has been raped should be able to defend herself against a potential conception from the sexual assault.[8]

As was noted above, there are several points in the reproductive process where, by human intervention, a pregnancy could be avoided. In general, one can say that at any point before the completion of fertilization, intervention can be morally acceptable. However, once the zygote, the new organism, has come into existence, one may not initiate any procedure which would end the life of the new human being. Hence, a procedure that merely prevents ovulation, for example, could be morally acceptable (presuming the right of the woman to prevent a pregnancy), since a new human being has not yet come into existence.

However, a real problem that arises in the use of the current oral contraceptives is that they apparently they have several modes of action, which may include modification of the endometrium so that, presumably, it could not support the implantation of an embryo or would terminate an already-implanted embryo. Commonly, this action of the contraceptive is referred to as its abortifacient action.

On this point, as already noted, the medical community is divided: some physicians (the majority) assert and some deny that these medications have such an action. Assertions like the following support the position of those who deny it:

> These findings do not support the hypothesis that emergency contraception with [levonorgestrel] prevents pregnancy by interfering with post-fertilization events.[9]

> The hormonal methods, particularly the low-dose progestin-only products and emergency contraceptive pills, have effects on the endometrium that, theoretically, could affect implantation. However, no scientific evidence indicates prevention of implantation actually results from the use of these methods. Once pregnancy begins, none of these methods have an abortifacient action.[10]

---

[8] U.S. Conference of Catholic Bishops, *Ethical and Religious Directives*.

[9] M. E. Ortiz et al., "Post-coital Administration of Levonorgestrel Does Not Interfere with Post-fertilization Events in the New-World Monkey *Cebus apella*," *Human Reproduction* 19.6 (June 2004): 1352–1356.

[10] R. Rivera, I. Yacobson, D. Grimes, "The Mechanism of Action of Hormonal Contraceptives and Intrauterine Contraceptive Devices," *American Journal of Obstetrics and Gynecology* 181.5 (November 1999): 1263–1269.

The findings indicate that the contraceptive effect of post-coital treatment with [ethinylesteradiol-levonorgestrel] and danazol is mainly due to an inhibition or delay of ovulation and insufficient corpus luteum function. The direct effect on the endometrium is limited, if any.[11]

What complicates the matter is that pharmaceutical firms, apparently not concerned about the destruction of a nascent human life and wanting to reassure those women who wish to avoid a pregnancy at any cost, point out that this action is a backup in the event that the anovulatory action was not effective.

Furthermore, by a sleight of hand, as it were, the medical profession appears to have accepted a new definition of conception, as occurring at implantation and not at the completion of fertilization, which was the earlier definition.[12] The change in meaning apparently happened in this way.[13] In 1964, apparently as a public relations ploy, Dr. Christopher Tietze, of Planned Parenthood and the Population Council, advised his council colleagues:

not to disturb those people for whom it is a question of major importance [whether a birth control measure causes an early abortion].... Theologians and jurists have always taken the prevailing biological and medical consensus of their times as factual, [and] if a medical consensus develops and is maintained that pregnancy, and therefore life, begins at implantation, eventually our brethren from the other faculties will listen.[14]

This followed an earlier observation, in 1959, by Swedish researcher Bent Boving, that:

---

[11] M. L. Swahn et al., "Effect of Post-coital Contraceptive Methods on the Endometrium and the Menstrual Cycle," *Acta Obstetricia et Gynecologica Scandinavica* 75.8 (September 1996): 738–744.

[12] Thus, *Dorland's Illustrated Medical Dictionary*, 26th ed. (Philadelphia: W. B. Saunders, 1981), defined *conception* as "the onset of pregnancy, marked by implantation of the blastocyst; the formation of a viable zygote." Note well the ambivalence of the definition, which included in the defining sentence the formation of a viable zygote (which occurs about five days before implantation!).

[13] See "A Declaration of Life by Pro-Life Physicians," American Life League, n.d., http://www.all.org/article.php?id=10678.

[14] Sheldon J. Segal, Anna L. Southam, and K. D. Schafer, eds., *Intra-uterine Contraception: Proceedings of the Second International Conference* (Amsterdam: Excerpta Medica Foundation, 1965), 212, quoted in "Declaration of Life."

whether eventual control of implantation can be reserved

the social advantage of being considered to prevent conception rather than to destroy an established pregnancy
could depend upon something so simple as a prudent habit
of speech.[15]

To make the change "official," the American College of
Obstetrics and Gynecology proclaimed a year later that
"conception is the implantation of the fertilized ovum."[16] If one
accepts that definitional alteration of pregnancy, then even
with a potential abortifacient action before the completion of
implantation, the medical community can refer—albeit
erroneously—to these agents as *contraceptives*.

However, the juggling of words does not change the reality.
So what can a conscientious Catholic hospital do? The Pennsylvania bishops' conference proposed some guidelines in
1993.[17] More recently, a Catholic hospital has proposed a
medical protocol which appears to achieve the desired goal:
the prevention of a pregnancy in a female survivor of sexual
assault without the destruction of a nascent human life. The
protocol requires that the medical personnel ascertain with
moral certitude that the woman's reproductive status is such
that no human being will be aborted or destroyed when she
receives treatment. An alternative proposal distinguishes
between what the authors term the ovulatory approach and
the pregnancy approach.[18] They advocate the pregnancy
approach, which requires that before administering
appropriate treatment it is morally sufficient to determine
whether the woman was already pregnant at the time the
sexual assault took place.

If so, then "emergency contraceptives" would be not only
pointless but also possibly abortifacient. But if the pregnancy
test results were negative and the woman then became

---

[15] Bent Boving, "Implantation Mechanisms," in *Mechanisms Concerned with Conception*, ed. C. G. Hartman (New York: Pergamon Press, 1963), 386, quoted in "Declaration of Life."

[16] "Terms Used in Reference to the Fetus," *ACOG Terminology Bulletin* 1 (September 1965), quoted in "Declaration of Life."

[17] Pennsylvania Catholic Conference, "Guidelines for Catholic Hospitals Treating Victims of Sexual Assault," *Origins* 22.47 (May 6, 1993): 810.

[18] Ronald P. Hamel and Ronald R. Panicola, "Emergency Contraception and Sexual Assault," *Health Progress* 83.5 (September–October 2002): 12–19, 51.

pregnant shortly after the rape, that pregnancy would remain undetected, and the contraceptive medication could have an abortifacient effect by preventing implantation.

The Peoria protocol, which also determines the ovulatory status of the rape survivor, consists of the following requirements:[19]

1. Determination of the woman's pregnancy status as ascertained by suitable blood test and by urine dipstick test.

2. Determination of the woman's ovulatory phase in light of the woman's menstrual history and results of clinical tests:

   a. Preovulatory phase—Ovral[20] may be given

   b. Midcycle LH surge phase—Ovral may not be given

   c. Early postovulatory phase—Ovral may not be given

Even with careful assessment of the woman's ovulatory status, there remains the issue of a possible abortifacient action since we do not have clear certitude of the drug's mode of action in any particular case. May a conscientious medical professional act in the face of this doubt?

It is good to recall that in moral matters *absolute* certitude is generally not obtainable. Morality deals with contingent matters where only *moral* certitude can be attained. Absolute certitude, such as is found in mathematics, in metaphysics, and matters of faith, cannot be expected.

A few examples will illustrate the difference. From Euclidean geometry: if I have understood the proofs, I can know with absolute certitude that the square of the hypotenuse in a right triangle is equal to the sum of the squares of the other two sides. From philosophy: A being cannot both be and not be in the same sense at the same time. (The truth of that statement is self-evident once I have understood the meaning of the terms.) From theology: Jesus Christ is truly God and

---

[19] St. Francis Medical Center Interim Protocol for Sexual Assault (Peoria, IL). See discussion of this protocol by Gerald J. McShane, M.D., et al., "Pregnancy Prevention after Sexual Assault," in *Catholic Health Care Ethics: A Manual for Ethics Committees*, eds. Peter J. Cataldo and Albert S. Moraczewski, O.P. (Boston: National Catholic Bioethics Center, 2001), chapter 11.

[20] Ovral (Wyeth-Ayerst) is a commonly used "emergency contraceptive" composed of two compounds, norgestrel and ethinyl estradiol.

truly man. Of course, this is a truth of faith and not of reason; but reason can help to show that there is no intrinsic contradiction involved. Catholics accept (believe) this truth as revealed by God and taught as an article of faith by the Church.

It is true that the *principles* of moral science (e.g., "It is a grave moral evil to kill an innocent person"[21]) can have that kind of absolute certitude, but not in their application to specific cases, because of the contingent nature of the actual situation. This distinction is vital. In the issue being discussed here, only moral certitude can be attained. Hence, a prudential judgment has to be made, considering all the relevant facts of the rape survivor's situation. Then a decision must be made as to the treatment which with moral rectitude may be administered to this person.

Nonetheless, it is asserted by many that when a human life is at stake, one must be certain (but with what kind of certitude?) that our action does not endanger another person's life. Many of us will recall the old example of a deer hunter in the woods who is about to take a shot at a spot in the underbrush where he has detected some motion. He does not actually see a deer, but only the movement and sound of something— or someone—in the woods. He would be morally guilty of negligent homicide if he failed before shooting to make sure that it is not a man. (Of course, this example is not parallel, since the hunter knows there is something moving in the brush but does not know *what*, whereas with the rape survivor one does not know whether there *is* something in the first place.[22])

Yet, is it not true that human life in today's society is filled with actions which are potentially hazardous to human life? Any person driving on our streets has a finite chance of killing or injuring someone in an accident, and many jobs in industry are hazardous to the well-being of workers. All these situations involve a chance, albeit a small chance, that an individual will be seriously injured. Still, that incertitude does not prohibit acting with moral rectitude. In deciding, for example, to drive to a shopping mall or to Mass or visit a sick friend, we proceed without assessing the potential hazards.

---

[21] See Exod. 20:13 and 23:7; *Catechism of the Catholic Church*, n. 2258.

[22] See Peter J. Cataldo, "A Moral Analysis of Pregnancy Prevention after Sexual Assault," in *What is Man, O Lord?* ed. Edward J. Furton, (Boston: National Catholic Bioethics Center, 2002), esp. 254–259.

164

So with these medications. We need to take reasonable precautions to avoid an abortifacient action, if the medications have one. And that fact—that medical scientists disagree as to the reality of that action in connection with emergency contraceptives—makes the ethical analysis even more fuzzy. Experience has shown that people of good will and equal competence, exercising due diligence, can arrive at different, even opposite, prudential decisions.

Solution of the Case Study

In making the prudential decision whether "emergency contraception" may be employed in this particular case, two considerations are important: (1) Is the rape survivor at the safe stage of her cycle so that the administration of the medication will not cause an abortion? (2) Does the particular drug used have an abortifacient action in general, and will it have in this particular case? Absolute certitude is not possible as we have seen; but is moral certitude sufficient? It may not be emotionally satisfactory for some who like to be absolutely sure. Yet moral certitude is the best one can do in this matter.[23]

Consequently, the emergency department personnel may treat the fifteen-year-old rape survivor following diligently an approved protocol, such as the one described in this paper, without the *reasonable* fear of causing the death of a human being.

---

[23] For fuller discussion of this matter, see Hamel and Panicola, "Emergency Contraception and Sexual Assault."

Paying for Catholic Health Care for the Uninsured and Underinsured

Anthony R. Tersigni

My subject is paying for health care for the uninsured and underinsured and some of the challenges that Catholic health-care organizations face in working to resolve problems related to access in this country. I was asked to include in my considerations how Catholic health-care organizations are being pressured by various groups, institutions, and structures to perform or to support immoral procedures as a condition for payment. To be clear, these pressures are not the only challenge to our integrity that we face on a daily basis.

Underlying the practical problem of paying for health care for the uninsured and underinsured in this country is a grave moral injustice arising from our society's failure to acknowledge health care as the basic human right that it is. Although I do not propose to have any comprehensive answers to either challenge—that of resolving the tragedy of the under- and uninsured in this country or that of eliminating attacks against our freedom to serve in a manner consistent with our most fundamental beliefs and principles—I will share with you some of our experiences and the lessons I have learned during my tenure as a senior leader with Ascension Health. I am confident that you share my conviction that we must continue to strengthen our Catholic ministry of healing and health care in this country.

I believe we are called by Christ to be both a light on the hill and leaven in the bread. Certainly, prayer and discernment, asking for the guidance of the Holy Spirit and using Catholic moral principles and values, must guide our strategies. While routinely faced with external pressures to compromise our values and identity, Ascension Health has—through prayerful reflection and discernment—implemented a plan of action based on these very values, to address the problem of paying for health care for the uninsured and the underinsured. At Ascension Health, we have made resolving the plight of the uninsured and underinsured one of our top strategic priorities, so much so that we have made it one of the three pillars of our strategic plan's *Call to Action*: to create "Healthcare That Works, Healthcare That Is Safe, and Healthcare That Leaves No One Behind." Although these are admittedly ambitious goals, we are making progress every day.

Before I address our overall strategy, it will be helpful to examine the growing threat to our freedom to serve. The scope and danger of this hazard cannot be overestimated. The threats to our freedom to serve, from those who would see Catholic health care abandon its moral principles or see the Catholic Church leave health care altogether, impose on us a political and cultural environment that is wrought with strife. It is in this environment that all Catholic health care strives to carry out the healing ministry of Christ, and in this environment that Ascension Health has gladly taken up our *Call to Action*. After addressing the concern regarding our freedom to serve, I will share with you the approach that Ascension Health has taken in responding to one particular threat. Last, I will review for you our overall strategy for addressing the problem of the uninsured and underinsured.

Protecting Our Freedom to Serve

As we are all well aware, Pope John Paul II often spoke of the need to promote a *culture of life*, where human dignity and the sacredness of human life are promoted and protected, and where individuals flourish in a society governed by justice and the common good. Whether there is truly a "culture war," as some have suggested, is not clear, but there is a great struggle unfolding around us. I will refrain from engaging in my own theological reflection on the nature of this great spiritual and cultural struggle, but will focus instead on the practical realities of this struggle from a Catholic health-care *systems* perspective. The Catholic Health Association's research on the threats to our freedom to serve confirm that those opposed to Catholic health care are, with the backing of enormous resources, pursuing a goal of absolute "reproductive freedom."[1]

While some politicians claim to want only to "keep abortion safe, legal, and rare," this is not the more extreme strategy of many groups dedicated to keeping abortion widely available and well funded. These groups are actively opposed to Catholic health care's freedom to serve in a manner consistent with its core beliefs and fundamental principles. CHA's research indicates that the opponents of Catholic health care are indeed well funded and well organized. Under competent and experienced leadership, the opposition works through numerous organizations, pursuing a highly coordinated and aggressive advocacy agenda with a growing grassroots constituency. A list of these organizations can be found on the CHA Web site, in the *Freedom to Serve* section. What is remarkable is that these coalitions and organizations have a combined annual budget of nearly $81 million, funded for the most part by wealthy foundations supported by some of America's richest for-profit corporations and by the cultural elite. Many of these organizations and foundations share the same board members and use the same strategies and tactics in opposing Catholic health care.

Through legislatures, courts, and the media, at local, state, and national levels, these opposition groups are actively working to block the Catholic health ministry from serving people and communities in need, including the uninsured and underinsured. They first targeted mergers and acquisitions involving Catholic health-care organizations. More recently, some of these opposition groups have been making misleading claims that appear to be intended to discredit Catholic health care and to portray it as substandard.[2]

---

[1] The *Freedom to Serve* initiative's research and education materials are available to CHA members on the Catholic Health Association's Web site, at www.chausa.org.

[2] See, for example, Elena N. Cohen, *Truth or Consequences: Using Consumer Protection Law to Expose Institutional Restrictions on Reproductive and Other Health Care* (Washington, DC: National Women's Law Center, October 2003), http://www.nwlc.org/pdf/TruthOrConsequences2003.pdf.

Using flawed research, they are conducting a public relations campaign making false claims about the quality of care our Catholic hospitals provide to women who have been sexually assaulted. They misconstrue the *Ethical and Religious Directives*, claiming that we will not honor patients' advance directives; that we will let people endure agonizing deaths rather than provide appropriate pain management and relief from their suffering; that we would let a woman die in order to save her unborn baby; that we will not give patients the information they need to provide free and informed consent. They suggest that persons with AIDS will not receive the treatment or information they need in a Catholic hospital; that we will never allow a feeding tube to be removed; and that patients' close friends or loved ones will not be permitted to visit them in a Catholic hospital or nursing home or participate in treatment decisions as surrogates. In other words, they would have the public believe that Catholic hospitals are dangerous and uncaring places that routinely violate patients' rights.

Such strategies are being used to pursue state and federal legislation that would compel *all* hospitals to provide emergency contraception in *all* circumstances. So, too, state legislatures, state and federal courts, and state attorneys general have made significant inroads in making contraceptives a mandatory covered benefit in all employee prescription plans. The U.S. Supreme Court's refusal to consider the appeal of Catholic Charities of Sacramento in just such a case is no doubt empowering the opposition.

In many states and at the federal level, in collaboration with attorneys general, and with the favor of some courts, the opposition continues to challenge our religious exemption protections, our tax-exempt status, and our freedom to serve in accord with our beliefs—actions that threaten the survival and integrity of our vital ministry of healing. They go even further by claiming that our ministry of healing is secondary to our beliefs; that the "business of health care" is not "Church business" and therefore is not a constitutionally protected religious activity. Can you imagine what the Gospels would look like if they recorded only that Jesus forgave, taught, and preached? But that is *not* the whole truth. We believe as a matter of faith that comforting and healing the sick and infirm, and serving the poor and the vulnerable in accord with their human dignity, are *integral* to Christ's mission of restoring the reign of God, and to the Church's mission of carrying on the saving work of Christ in the world.

170

Although a culture war may, indeed, be sought by those who are opposed to our presence, purpose, and principles in health care, I believe that we ought to engage them not with the same misleading and demeaning tactics they employ against us, but with the gospel values and justice that animate our mission to be Jesus's healing presence in the world today. While as faithful Christians we know that God ultimately will win the day, this does not relieve us of our responsibility to seek an answer to the question, What is God asking of us now? I will now turn to recent developments that have presented a challenge for our Health Ministries (local health systems under Ascension Health) in New York State.

New York State Case Study

The Women's Health and Wellness Act of New York State, which mandates that employers who offer prescription coverage as an employee benefit include hormonal contraceptives in their benefits packages, took effect on January 1, 2003.

The New York State legislation is similar to California legislation in that its religious exemption clause is virtually impossible to meet for most Catholic service providers. In New York, however, there are options available to us that are not available with the California legislation. After talking through the issues thoroughly with both internal and external counsel, as well as internal and external ethicists, it became clear that we had three options for responding to the contraceptive coverage mandate in this legislation. Options one and two we consider to be morally licit. Option one entails complying with the legislation, but adopting disclaimer language that clearly explains why we, as a Catholic employer, are providing such coverage even though we do not promote or condone contraceptive acts. Option two entails taking advantage of ERISA plans available under federal law, which are not subject to the state's legislation. Option three, while creative, was not feasible. What follows is a detailed explanation of all three options and our moral reasoning behind each.

Option One: Compliance and Disclaimer

As mentioned, option one entails complying with the legislation but adopting disclaimer language. This disclaimer, which would be placed into the employee enrollment and benefits handbook where drug prescription coverage is discussed, reads as follows:

> Any benefits covered by this plan which are related to contraception are provided solely and exclusively by reason of legal requirements set forth by the "Women's Health and Wellness Act" enacted by the State of New York. Contraception is contrary to Catholic moral teaching and [the health ministry] does not endorse, approve, or intend contraception by complying with the aforementioned legal mandate.

Under this option, a local health ministry would continue to exclude coverage for any drug whose sole immediate effect is abortifacient, along with the usual beginning-of-life exclusions regarding in vitro fertilization and direct sterilizations. Health ministry leaders and human resources department heads who have the responsibility to explain this response, if this option is chosen, were instructed on five key points.

First, we must distinguish between contraceptive acts themselves and the coverage of contraceptive benefits within an overall drug plan that covers many other pharmacological services. In accord with Church teaching, directive 52 of the *Ethical and Religious Directives* makes it clear that, "Catholic health institutions may not promote or condone contraceptive practices."[3] Including contraceptive drugs as part of a prescription benefits package would be immoral and prohibited by the ERDs, if it is the organization's intention to promote or condone the actual practice of contraception.

There are, however, reasons other than promoting or condoning the actual practice of contraception that a Catholic health-care organization might include contraceptive drugs in a broader prescription benefits plan. For example, there are numerous medical reasons apart from contraception for which hormonal medication may licitly be prescribed, in accord with the principle of double effect. More to the point in this case, a Catholic health-care organization might include such coverage only with the intention of complying with the law.

The second point of concern follows immediately from the first, namely, that Ascension Health and its ministries may not approve, condone, or agree with contraception as a matter of our direct purpose or intention. Our purpose or intention for including contraceptive benefits in a plan falling under the

---

[3] U.S. Conference of Catholic Bishops, *Ethical and Religious Directives for Catholic Health Care Services,* 4th ed. (Washington, DC: USCCB, 2001).

state's mandate must be only to comply with the law, which is imposed on us externally. Done for this reason and with this intention only, we are able at the organizational level to avoid engaging in any formal cooperation with objectively immoral acts. Therefore, in those states where we are *not* under a legal mandate to include contraceptive drugs in our prescription benefit plans, we have made it clear that it remains inappropriate for us to do so.

Third, Ascension Health Ministries may not, according to directive 70, engage in immediate material cooperation in another agent's immoral act.[4] We understand this to mean that we may not deliberately contribute any circumstances that are essential to the occurrence of an immoral act. As a point of fact, including contraceptive drugs in our associates' prescription benefits package is *not* a necessary condition for them to obtain the contraceptives. They were able to obtain contraceptive drugs on their own even before the legislation was enacted. Moreover, the inclusion of contraceptive drugs as part of a larger prescription benefits package is not the same as writing a prescription for or dispensing contraceptives, which can be considered essential conditions of the immoral act. From a moral perspective, we believe that the inclusion of these drugs in a prescription benefits package is one step further removed from these more essential contributing circumstances.

Fourth, according to this line of thought, complying with the state's mandate would only entail our mediate material cooperation, which is permitted within the Catholic moral tradition if there is a proportionately serious reason for doing so, and if reasonable steps are taken to avoid scandal. According to our ethicists, "mediate material cooperation" means contributing circumstances that are *not* essential to the occurrence of another person's objectively immoral act, and that contribute to the immoral act only in a remote and indirect way. The disclaimer language included in this option is in part an attempt to address the issue of scandal and to clarify our intention.

While option one does involve us in mediate material cooperation, we believe there is a proportionately serious reason for our cooperation, namely, that we have a strong moral obligation in justice to provide our employees with prescrip-

[4] Ibid.

tion coverage as part of their overall benefits package. Failure to comply with the law would also entail legal and financial risks, some of which could potentially diminish our ability to maintain the level of uncompensated care for the uninsured and underinsured we currently provide. Likewise, if we were to fail to provide our associates with a prescription benefits plan as part of an adequate benefits package, we would probably lack the human resources needed to provide the hands-on services that are at the core of our mission. In the end, contraceptive coverage is only one small part of a much broader benefits package that we ought to provide to our associates as a matter of respect for human dignity, concern for the common good, and the promotion of justice.

Indeed, when it came time for the legislature of New York to vote on this particular piece of legislation, many pro-life legislators who voted in favor of it were in a very similar position politically: the larger legislation of which this piece was only one part mandated many items that are very good, and which no reasonable person concerned with justice would otherwise want to vote against. It was a moral-political dilemma not uncommonly faced by legislators.

Our fifth and final key moral consideration under option one was whether the disclaimer language could have been omitted from the actual contract with the insurance company without any change in the nature or conditions of the actual contract. As already stated, we concluded that the disclaimer language could help us avoid scandal and clarify our intentions to plan participants and others. But we also concluded that it would have to be included for us to proceed with integrity under this option. A contract, by its very nature, is a statement of agreement between two parties regarding a proposed course of action to be undertaken mutually.

With respect to avoiding scandal, not including the disclaimer statement in the contract could be taken to imply that we were agreeing with the state that our associates *ought* to have the contraceptive coverage, and therefore *ought* to have contraceptives. Putting the disclaimer language in the contract would make it clear that we are intending *only* to comply with the law, and not with contraception per se. It was our judgment, therefore, that this moral difference would impel us to include the disclaimer language in contracts with our insurance providers, if this option were chosen. Also, we reasoned that including the disclaimer language in the contract might better position us should we decide at a later time to pursue legal means for opposing the mandate.

Option Two: Adopt an ERISA Plan

Option two was to adopt an ERISA plan, if it would be financially and administratively feasible. This option does not seem to be available to the concerned parties in the California case. ERISA, the Employee Retirement Income Security Act, allows companies to self-insure under federal regulations, without meeting state insurance requirements. Therefore, Health Ministries that are self-insured under ERISA would not be required to provide contraceptive coverage in accord with the New York state mandate as part of their prescription benefits plan. This is what Lourdes Memorial Hospital in Binghamton, New York, chose to do by purchasing a turnkey, or prepackaged, ERISA option offered by Blue Cross. This option avoids cooperation, even remote mediate material cooperation, with contraception altogether. In the case of Lourdes, this option was sufficiently inexpensive that it did not interfere with the ability of the hospital to provide the same level of care for the underinsured and uninsured population in that community. This is not the case in every market, however.

Another possibility examined under this option was for all of our New York Health Ministries to consider asking Blue Cross for a competitive group bid for an ERISA plan that would be comparable to or cheaper than their current plans. Given the existing contractual agreements already in effect, this turned out not to be feasible. A significant disadvantage of this option is that, with an ERISA plan, the organization is limited in how far it can spread its risks. Thus, this option is accompanied by the risk that one devastating case could significantly impair the entire organization's ability to operate.

Option Three: Evoke "Religious Employer" Status

Option three would have been for our Health Ministries to communicate to their insurance company that they were religious organizations—and, therefore, exempt from the requirements of the law—and wanted to purchase insurance without this coverage. This was a complex option, similar to the New York archdiocesan proposal announced on December 9, 2002. External counsel with whom we consulted explained how this particular piece of legislation is open to interpretation, particularly in its definition of a "religious employer." Similar to the California legislation, the New York law states that a "religious employer" is an entity for which each and all of the following are true: (1) the inculcation of religious values is the purpose of the entity; (2) the entity primarily employs persons who share the religious tenets of the entity; and (3) the entity serves primarily persons who share the religious tenets of the entity.

It could be argued that the first criterion is satisfied by the fact that all Catholic health ministries are normally included in the *Official Catholic Directory* (New York: P. J. Kenedy and Sons, 2005) and by our 501(c)(3) status. In fact, most of our Health Ministries state explicitly in their articles of incorporation that the inculcation of religious values is one of their purposes. Regarding the second criterion, our internal counsel argued that this condition could be met by virtue of the fact that it does not say that employees must share *all* religious tenets of the entity—in fact, most of our associates do share many, if not most, of our religious tenets and values. Likewise, regarding the third criterion, the mere fact that most of the individuals we serve are Catholic, Protestant, Jewish, and Moslem means that those in the primary population we serve also share our most fundamental religious tenets—for example, belief in one God, love of God above all things, loving our neighbor as ourselves, and belief in the duty to serve all poor and vulnerable persons regardless of their creed. Insofar as these tenets sum up the divine law in the form of the Golden Rule, which is common to most religions, it could be argued that the third and final criterion is satisfied as well.

This approach, however, was considered a bit of a stretch, constituting a risky interpretation of the definition of a religious employer as defined under the law. Adopting option three would have exposed us to many possible consequences. First, the insurance companies available to us might simply say that they disagree with our interpretation of the law, and refuse to allow us to purchase a product without contraceptive coverage. In that case, we would have to fall back on option one or two. Or an insurance company might go along with us, but then an employee might object. We could then explain to the employee that we refuse to comply with the mandate on the basis that we are a religious employer. The employee could then choose to enlist the help of the ACLU, the National Women's Law Center, or another organization, and file a suit. This would then force us into court as a test case. We could then choose to comply at that time because of a need to avoid this risk.

In the end, what makes this new piece of legislation so distasteful—other than the fact that it compels us, against what we see as our right under the First Amendment, to do what we would not ordinarily do—is the manner in which the contraceptive coverage mandate was deliberately thrown in with a whole range of very positive and important women's health provisions, which few legislators would want to be caught voting against.

We ultimately recommended to our New York Health Ministries that they follow either option one or option two, depending on which was most feasible at the time. We also recommended that they wait and see how the California case panned out, how the New York Catholic Conference would respond, and how similar laws in other states are legally contested. Subsequently, we have supported the New York Catholic Conference through an amicus brief signed by the Catholic Health Association on our behalf.

I will now turn to the third part of my talk, explaining how Ascension Health hopes to achieve 100 percent access for the uninsured and underinsured in all the communities we serve.

How to Achieve
100 Percent Access to Health Care

While abortion is no doubt the gravest moral issue we face today, and it is clear that the agenda of most opponents of Catholic health care is not limited to contraceptive mandates, there is another grave issue that calls for our attention as we strive to be the healing presence of Jesus in the world today. It is the massive problem of the uninsured and underinsured. To rectify this problem, we need to collaborate with others who do not embrace the full scope of our values. Our ethicists advise me that licit forms of cooperation and even some toleration may be warranted when necessary to diminish the occurrence of evil or to preserve an important good in our society.[5]

If we exclude collaboration with others in our communities in our attempts to rectify the problem of access to health care for the uninsured, we risk the collapse of the entire health system in this country and even the eventual loss of our Catholic

---

[5] For a more detailed discussion of this point, see Benedict M. Ashley and Kevin D. O'Rourke, *Health Care Ethics: A Theological Analysis*, 4th ed. (Washington, DC: Georgetown University Press, 1997), 193–99.

health ministry altogether. The Catholic health ministry is one of the few remaining credible voices for the voiceless. We are a strong and substantial social institution, here to defend and promote the sacredness of human life, human dignity, the common good, and justice. If we lose this important good, then who will effectively stand and advocate against the further slide down the slippery slope toward the societal normalization of abortion, euthanasia, and assisted suicide? We believe that our country cannot afford to lose Catholic health care and that our Church cannot afford to lose its healing ministry. But Catholic health care is part of a much larger system, and we cannot resolve the problem in isolation from the rest of that system.

In 2004, there were more than 45 million people in the United States who did not have health-care insurance for an entire year.[6] There were also approximately 81.8 million people who lacked insurance for at least one month in 2002 and 2003, and 65.3 percent of these were uninsured for six months or more. Many of these people could qualify for help from existing safety net services and programs, but do not know how to access these services and programs.[7] Many of the uninsured and underinsured are particularly poor and vulnerable: immigrants, migrant workers, the frail elderly, the mentally ill, homeless adolescents, and the chronically ill who earn too much to make use of government programs but not enough to afford costly private health insurance premiums. Although many legislative reform efforts up to now have been designed to bolster the public hospitals and clinics that comprise a significant portion of the country's safety net, private providers continue to supply more than half of all uncompensated care, and among the largest providers of uncompensated care, 82 percent are

---

[6] Carmen DeNavas-Walt, Bernadette D. Proctor, and Cheryl Hill Lee, *Income, Poverty, and Health Insurance Coverage in the United States: 2004*, U.S. Census Bureau, Current Population Report P60-229 (Washington, DC: U.S. Government Printing Office, 2005), 16.

[7] Kathleen Stoll and Kim Jones, *One in Three: Non-elderly Americans without Health Insurance, 2003–2004*, Families USA publication 04-104 (Washington, DC: Families USA, June 2004). Data analysis was provided by the Lewin Group, Falls Church, Virginia.

[8] J. M. Mann et al., "A Profile of Hospital Uncompensated Care, 1983–1995." *Health Affairs* 16.4 (July-August 1997): 223–232.

[9] See Catholic Health Association, *A Commitment to Caring: The Role of Catholic Hospitals in the Healthcare Safety Net* (St. Louis: CHA, 2002), 1–20.

private.[8] In fact, 72 percent of Medicaid patient-days are delivered in private, not public, hospitals.[9]

Consistent with our mission of continuing the healing ministry of Jesus especially for the poor and vulnerable, we at Ascension Health not only believe that 100 percent access to health care in all our communities is achievable, but we have made it one of our highest priorities. That is why, as part of our *Call to Action,* we are trying to provide 100 percent access in those communities where we have a presence and to create a system of health care that leaves no one behind.

The first phase of our work toward this goal is well under way, and our Board of Directors has recently approved the strategic blueprint for the second phase. The first phase includes two parallel strategies: First, we seek federal support to strengthen the role of private providers in the health-care safety net for the uninsured. This requires collaboration and the building of friendships and relationships with public officials and community organizations that do not necessarily agree with all of our values. Second, through successful local access models, we are creating a new model of access leadership and are accelerating work to improve access to care in all the communities we serve.

The Ascension Health Access Strategy

We believe we have a strategy that will get us there. The hope is that we will create models of access that will work as well in other communities where Ascension Health does not have a presence.

National Legislative Leadership

The first component of our access strategy is national legislative leadership. Ascension Health has sought bipartisan support for a series of laws to help the private safety net meet the needs of the underserved. We began our journey by leading a successful effort for federal funding of the Healthy Communities Access Program (HCAP).[10] Over the last four years, nineteen communities partnering with Ascension Health Ministries have received significant federal grants to improve access. The members of each local coalition are addressing

---

[10] Healthy Communities Access Program grants are administered by the Bureau of Primary Health Care, U.S. Department of Health and Human Services, Rockville, Maryland.

the unique challenges presented by immigrant, homeless, minority, rural, and other populations who previously did not have reliable and steady access to health care.

Ascension Health provides staff resources to assist these coalitions in leadership development, strategic planning, and grant management, and we provide ongoing education through site visits, conferences, and the creation of networking opportunities. To further demonstrate our commitment, Ascension Health has provided a total of $7 million in matching funds to eight of these local access models. Their early results are impressive.

As we move forward, Ascension Health is also leading with a coalition that includes the nation's ten largest Catholic health systems, to advocate for federal support of critical access health centers. These are medical clinics and health centers operated by faith-based providers and located in places with the greatest need. In 2004, the U.S. Senate Republican Task Force on Health Care Costs and the Uninsured included a provision for new funding of religious-sponsored integrated health systems that provide primary care, specialty health care, and hospital services, along with other key provisions that the coalition supported.[11] Senate majority leader Bill Frist of Tennessee commended the work of the task force toward developing "the innovative ideas and real solutions we need to benefit Americans who do not have health insurance today and in the future."[12] The National Catholic Bioethics Center's clinical practice ethics guidelines, published in *Catholic Health Care Ethics: A Manual for Ethics Committees*, were of critical importance in obtaining the support of legislators who were in doubt as to whether Catholic-sponsored health centers would be able to meet the requirements of the federal regulations governing health centers.[13]

---

[11] See U.S. Senate Republican Task Force on Health Care Costs and the Uninsured, "Building on a Record of Creative Solutions," http://republican.senate.gov/costcoveragecare/SummaryPacket.pdf.

[12] Senator Bill Frist, M.D., "Frist Comments on IOM Report on the Uninsured and Increasing Health Care Costs," press release (January 14, 2004), http://frist.senate.gov/index.cfm?FuseAction= PressReleases.Detail&PressRelease_id=1558.

[13] National Catholic Bioethics Center ethicists, "Model Clinical Practice Ethics Guidelines for Affiliated Health Care Professionals with Respect to Prescription of Contraceptives," in Peter J. Cataldo and Albert S. Moraczewski, O.P., eds., *Catholic Health Care Ethics: A Manual for Ethics Committees* (Boston: National Catholic Bioethics Center, 2001), 8/12–8/14.

The Five-Step Model to 100 Percent Access

The second component of the Ascension Health access strategy is expressed in its five-step model to 100 percent access. Innovative ideas are flourishing locally, and Ascension Health seeks ways to catalyze these community breakthroughs and share them across the system. In Travis County, Texas, for example, voters approved the creation of a hospital district to address the increasing pressure health-care providers in the Austin area face, by better coordinating existing resources and targeting the use of local tax dollars to support of the district. It is expected that the hospital district funding will sustain important safety net initiatives in the Austin area, including those provided by Ascension Health's SETON Healthcare Network, to help serve people who are particularly poor and vulnerable. SETON's leadership played a key role in support of the hospital district proposal. We are deeply indebted to Bishop Gregory Aymond, who has been one of our greatest supporters.

With the establishment of the hospital district in Travis County, SETON has become the first Ascension health ministry to address all five of what we believe are the key steps in achieving 100 percent access to health care. Ascension Health's five steps include:

1. Enabling infrastructure, including the establishment of a formal coalition and the connection of information systems;
2. Filling service gaps, like dental, mental health, and others;
3. Redesigning the care model for the uninsured to provide a continuum of care, including preventive care;
4. Engaging private physicians to voluntarily accept a certain number of uninsured patients; and
5. Achieving sustainable funding.

Modeled through the lessons we have learned from our access-model sites over the last five years, all our Health Ministries are being challenged to achieve the five steps as we continue our efforts to deliver "Healthcare That Leaves No One Behind."

Raising Awareness and Serving as a Voice for the Voiceless

As mentioned earlier, there are more than 45 million uninsured in the United States at this time, and an estimated 81.8 million people, including millions of children, who lacked health insurance for all or part of the years 2002 and 2003.

This is a grave injustice, and until we can raise the consciousness and moral outrage of ordinary citizens throughout the
country, we will continue to falter in our attempts to fix the
problem. We have helped expand coverage for children through
our leadership in the national Children's Health Matters
initiative, and for the last two years we have raised public
awareness of the crisis through our system's 100 percent participation in Cover the Uninsured Week. The results of our
Cover the Uninsured Week efforts in 2004 indicate that our
Health Ministries made a strong impact system-wide. During
Cover the Uninsured Week:

- Our ministries enrolled individuals (including children)
  in existing health insurance programs, an increase of
  46 percent over last year.

- We organized more than 180 local Cover the Uninsured
  Week events or initiatives, which were attended by thousands of people. We provided health and wellness
  screenings, an increase of about 40 percent over the
  year before.

- We enhanced community-wide awareness and involvement in all of our Health Ministries by working in partnership with other community organizations on local
  Cover the Uninsured Week efforts.

Such attempts to motivate the grassroots movement and
create public outrage to support health-care reform have been
and will remain a priority for Ascension Health as we seek
100 percent access for all Americans. While many experts on
Capitol Hill tell us that now is not the time to engage in health-
care reform, we firmly believe that much can be achieved toward realizing the goal.

Responsiveness to Congressional Concerns about the Health-Care Industry

For over a year, congressional leaders have been studying how people without health insurance are treated in the
hospital billing and collection process. Ascension Health is
proud of its long-standing commitment to serve people who
lack the financial resources to pay for their care. In fiscal
year 2004, Ascension Health Ministries provided
$603,328,982 for the care of persons who are poor, commu-
nity benefit, and advocacy. For every dollar we earned from
our operations, we spent nearly four dollars on charity care
and community benefits.

As part of an effort begun in early 2003 to integrate a variety of management and information systems used by our Health Ministries, we reviewed the individual billing and collection policies of our hospitals. We determined that we needed more clarity and consistency in this important area, and identified several opportunities for improvement. A new system-wide policy was approved by our board of trustees in December 2003. It is based on several core values and principles, including our commitment to, and reverence for, human dignity and the common good; our special concern for, and solidarity with, persons who are poor and vulnerable; and our dedication to distributive justice and stewardship.

In June 2004, a congressional subcommittee hearing was held to investigate the issue of hospital billing and collection practices. Joined by the leaders of the nation's other large health systems, I had the opportunity to explain to the congressional subcommittee our commitment to all patients who seek our health services, regardless of their means to pay, while calling on congressional leaders to support universal health-care access for all Americans. While this was a difficult task, Ascension Health had the opportunity to get our message about the plight of the under- and uninsured in this country before Congress. My hope is that this issue and the congressional attention it is receiving now will call this tragic situation to the attention of the American public.

In the second phase of our work to create "Health Care That Leaves No One Behind," we will continue to build on our existing strategies while expanding our efforts to include three new strategies. The first of these new strategies is to become a critical partner and participant in national public policy. The goal of this strategy is to influence national health policy to create long-term health-care reform that eliminates the very need for a safety net.

The second new strategy is to engage in more proactive stewardship. Working in conjunction with the American Hospital Association and the Catholic Health Association (USA), we will address high-impact system-level reimbursement issues, such as Medicare disproportionate share calculations, that affect our financial ability to provide care for the uninsured and underinsured.

For our final new strategy under phase two, we have launched our Access Leadership Planning Program, which will contribute to developing a new model of Health Ministry leadership that accelerates achievement of our goal of 100 percent access to health-care services. We have selected CEOs from a dozen of our Health Ministries to participate with access leadership staff from our national headquarters to create and implement access plans for their Health Ministries. These plans will contain specific activities to improve access to health care for the uninsured, as well as specific measurements of the impact of these activites. Each CEO has committed to playing a pivotal and visible role in the implementation of his or her local plans.

Health Care Access for All

Ascension Health is convinced that 100 percent access is an attainable goal. To us, access is about more than the distribution of insurance cards or assignments to a medical home. We define 100 percent access to mean that "all persons, particularly those persons who are uninsured or underinsured, receive health care services that (1) create and support the best journey to improved health outcomes for each individual, and (2) are funded in an adequate and sustainable fashion." Improved access leads to improved outcomes. Ascension Health is beginning to deliver both as we make tangible our commitment to provide "Healthcare That Leaves No One Behind." Catholic health care must lead the charge for securing access to health care in America as a basic human right.

Twenty-five years ago, at the beginning of his pontificate, Pope John Paul II challenged us to lead the charge of reform:

> Social thinking and social practice inspired by the Gospel must always be marked by a special sensitivity toward those who are most in distress, those who are extremely poor, those suffering from all the physical, mental, and moral ills that afflict humanity ... But neither will you recoil before the reforms—even profound ones—of attitudes and structures that may prove necessary in order to re-create over and over again the conditions needed by the disadvantaged if they are to have a fresh chance in the hard struggle of life. The poor of the United States and of the world are your brothers and sisters in Christ. You must never be content to leave them just the crumbs from the feast.[14]

---

[14] John Paul II, homily at Yankee Stadium (October 2, 1979), nn. 3 and 4, quoted in National Conference of Catholic Bishops, *Health and Health Care: A Pastoral Letter of the American Catholic Bishops* (Washington, DC: U.S. Catholic Conference, 1981), part IV, section B, n. 3. The Italian text of the homily is available at http://www.vatican.va/holy_father/ john_paul_ii/homilies/1979/documents/hf_jp-ii_hom_19791002_usa-new-york-it.html.

The Catholic Church in America and its health ministries must give birth to a new cry of outrage through strong public advocacy on behalf of and through compassionate service to our most poor and vulnerable brothers and sisters—the sick, the elderly, the disabled, the chronically ill, the mentally ill, the dying, the suffering, the rejected, the despised, and the lonely.

Let me conclude by reiterating that, while no small feat to begin with, this task is further complicated by the well-organized and well-funded opposition to the Catholic institutional presence in health care, and growing pressures to abandon our principles and values. It is clear to me that we cannot simply close our eyes and hope that this opposition and pressure will go away.

At the same time, however, we should not allow those who oppose our ministry to succeed in their quest to pull us into an all-out war. To allow that would mean resorting to the very tactics that our opponents use against us, which benefit no one, especially not the poor and vulnerable, who remain our first and primary concern. Rather, guided by the gospel values and justice, we must seek to find a balance that will allow us to carry out our mission *with integrity*. To do this, we must rely on the very values that we seek to protect. We must rely on the guidance of the moral principles arising out of hundreds of years of tradition within the Church, in the hope of living out our mission to be Christ's healing presence in the world, while at the same time defending our freedom to do so.

Bioethical Challenges for the Catholic Church in Europe

Rev. Gonzalo Miranda, L.C.

A few years back, a group of Catholic doctors would visit parishes in Rome on Sundays, promoting organ donation. When they asked a certain pastor if they could promote organ transplantation in his parish, the priest responded very seriously, "That organ has been over there for three centuries, and it can't be moved anymore."

When I think about the current bioethical challenges of the Catholic Church in Europe, I remember this anecdote. Progress and practices in biological sciences and medicine currently present societal problems that are true challenges for the Catholic Church. And unfortunately, we clergy, priests and agents of pastoral care, are not always adequately prepared to confront them. For this reason, the periodic convocation of this workshop for the American bishops answers an important need of the Church, and deserves to be applauded.

This chapter is based on Fr. Miranda's original presentation in Spanish, which appears in Appendix A of this volume, on p. 305. The English translation is by Come Alive Communications Inc., West Grove, Pennsylvania, www.comealiveusa.com.

I have been asked to comment on the current bioethical challenges of the Catholic Church *in Europe*. On one hand, the problems faced in bioethics have a clear, universal character which applies to all countries and all churches everywhere: respect for developing life, respect for the patient as a person, and respect for the environment, for example, are values that affect all human beings, regardless of their geographical location. Moreover, increasing globalization quickly changes certain problems—problems that appear to be local at first— into problems that affect other parts of the planet. This occurs even where a specific practice does not appear to be a real possibility. Such is the case with cloning, for example. In many countries, the possibility of cloning is not yet foreseen, not by a long shot; nevertheless, in those very countries it has become a topic of heated debate, simply because it touches the heart of human understanding and respect for human life, and it evokes ethical concerns in the conscience of all human beings, regardless of their culture or religion.

In any case, every geographic and cultural region possesses a few specific characteristics that are worth keeping in mind as we consider the bioethical challenges facing the Catholic Church. Analyzing the situation of Europe in particular may help us better understand the challenges facing the Church in America. We must remember that the flow of ideas, ideologies, and lifestyles between these two continents is particularly significant. Therefore, we must keep in mind what happens on the other side of the Atlantic in order to better familiarize ourselves with our pastoral options.

Specific Bioethical Problems in Europe

During the meeting of the Council of European Bishops' Conferences celebrated in June 2001, Secretary General Aldo Giordano explained that the topic of bioethics had been included in the agenda to answer the concerns of bishops from many countries.[1] In reality, clergy members from many dioceses throughout Europe are seriously worried—and at times perplexed—about the increasingly complex cultural, legal, and practical circumstances arising at both the diocesan and the

[1] See Aldo Giordano, "Themes in the Agenda of the European Bishops' Conferences," annual meeting of general secretaries of the Concilium Conferentarium Episcoporum Europae (CCEE), Prague, Czechoslovakia, June 21–25, 2001, http://ccee.ch/english/press/segretarifinale.htm.

national levels. At times, these even involve legislative measures, resolutions or bills proposed within the European community itself (by one of its many authorities, such as the European Commission and the European Parliament), which have some influence on life in every region included in the mosaic of Europe.

In his report, Giordano recalled some of the most urgent problems in modern Europe. For example, he mentioned the European initiatives regarding genetic manipulation; the ambiguity and confusion of many legal codes on the judicial status of the human embryo; the legalization of euthanasia in a few European countries; the slavery of prostitution of women and children; and the concept of the family, which "in some countries has been broadened to the point of including two contradictory realities."[2] Giordano commented, "Conscious that these are issues which determine the future of Europe and humanity, the Bishops' Conferences feel the responsibility to safeguard life and act at cultural, pastoral, and legislative levels."[3]

It would be interesting for us to analyze some of the current, concrete challenges in the field of bioethics in terms of how they are being experienced in Europe. But it would also be too time consuming, and could easily become a mere chronicle of facts, which would not help us understand the core of the problems. I will limit myself instead to describing just a few aspects of the European situation. We can take into consideration, for example, the fact that the practice of abortion has already been legalized in the majority of European countries; in fact, only Ireland and Malta are off the list.

Practices of assisted reproduction have also been legalized in many countries on the Continent. Nevertheless, European laws in this area vary widely from country to country. England and Spain have very anarchistic laws, which permit almost everything. In contrast, assisted reproductive practices have been regulated in a more restrictive way in several countries of northern Europe. Germany also has quite a rigorous law, and in Italy a law curtailing many practices was approved in February 2004. Article 1 of the Italian law recognizes that the conceived embryo is a person with rights, and subsequent articles prohibit reckless, unsubstantiated practices. The production of more than three embryos is prohibited, and all em-

---

[2] Ibid.

[3] Ibid.

bryos must be transferred to the mother's uterus; the freezing of embryos is also prohibited, as is experimentation on them.

The equating of marriage and homosexual unions, extending even to adoption rights, has become a legal reality in Holland and Denmark, and the Spanish government has recently taken firm steps in the same direction, wishing to demonstrate to the world that Spain, under the leadership of a socialist government, is a modern nation.

Concerning bioethical problems at the end of life, Europe takes precedence in yet another sad way: euthanasia has been legalized on a national level in two countries, Holland and Belgium. And the pro-euthanasia movement continues to strive for legalization in several countries. In Spain, a cultural shift is currently being promoted by the government itself, which could lead to legalization.

These examples are sufficient for us to see that the European situation is very dramatic, and that it is accelerating at a powerful rate. It is more interesting now, as I was saying, to make an *in-depth* analysis of the challenges faced by the Church in Europe—an analysis of the *cultural substratum* in which these activities are nurtured and flourish.

Social and Cultural Characteristics of the European Situation

The emergence and growth of many current problems in bioethics are related to specific social, cultural, and religious aspects of our time, just as fruit is related to the root of a plant. For this very reason, it may be helpful if we stop for a moment to consider a few characteristics of modern Europe. At their root, the current bioethical challenges faced by the Catholic Church in Europe are played out on this level.

Progressive Secularization

Unfortunately, it does not take long to show that a serious and calculated process of secularization is under way in Europe. Numerous sociological studies clearly demonstrate the advance of this phenomenon.

In some countries (such as the Netherlands, England, and France), much of the general population can no longer be recognized within the realm of faith and Christian culture. In other countries (such as Ireland, Spain, and Italy), a deep substratum of Catholic identity persists, but along with it one notices the advance of a godless culture and lifestyle that are increasingly indifferent to the moral and evangelistic principles set forth by the Catholic Church. In other countries (such as Poland and Croatia), the winds of European secularization have been blowing strong since the fall of the Berlin Wall.

In reality, studies and attentive observation reveal very contradictory situations. At times it seems as if we are living in a spiritual desert. Methods used by the mass media, statements made by many politicians, the campaigns of many well-known and well-recognized cultural leaders (literary scholars, philosophers, and leaders in the entertainment industry, for example) give us the impression that faith and religion have almost completely disappeared.

Nevertheless, when one least expects them, surprises pop up to contradict this impression. This has happened, for example, in connection with the Holy Father whenever World Youth Day has taken place in Europe: six hundred thousand youth in Santiago de Compostela, a million youth in secular Paris, two million youth at the celebration of Jubilee 2000 in Rome. After each of these events, sociologists, political analysts, and critics of every stripe rack their brains for several weeks trying to interpret the surprising phenomenon, each observer in his own way and according to his own ideology or interests. Whatever the observers say, these youth are not mushrooms that suddenly sprouted because of a little humidity in the air. Few observers realize or want to recognize that these young people "were already there"—in the parish youth group or the little Christian community, enthusiastically motivated by the ideal of the laity movement, or being trained in that little school led by the nuns. These observers are also surprised when it is shown that a high percentage of families choose religion classes for their young children or that a large number of taxpayers check the box next to "Catholic Church" to designate where a fixed percentage of their income should go by law.

Having mentioned these contradictions, we should probably also acknowledge that the deep roots of Christianity are still alive in Europe, but they are continually devalued, especially among leaders, who have the greatest influence on culture, laws, politics, and public opinion. Evidently, a weak Christian identity at these levels provokes its gradual weakening on *all* social levels.

To my knowledge, a close relationship exists between secularization and the loss of a sense of what the universal

dignity of human beings means. This brings about, in consequence, the acceptance and promotion of practices that seriously contravene this dignity, such as abortion, the destruction of human embryos, and euthanasia.

In principle, the values and standards that help us understand the moral obligation to respect every human being—
regardless of condition, race, sex, religion, or age (and even if
he or she has not yet been born)—are rational concepts that
are deeply engrained in human nature. They should, therefore, be understood and accepted by all human beings, not
just by those who believe in God the Creator or in Jesus Christ.
But in fact, in many places it seems as if we who are Christians or Catholics have a sort of monopoly on respect for human life, a monopoly that we have neither sought nor desired.[4]

By being open to the current facts of embryology, anyone
can understand that the human embryo is a human individual
from the first moment of existence; and by purely natural reasoning, anyone can understand that every human being must
be respected in his or her right to life. Nevertheless, no sooner
does one acknowledge these rational scientific truths than one
is identified as a Catholic and accused of seeking to impose
one's religious ideology upon society.

This gives the impression that the Christian, who has not
found in Sacred Scripture specific details about the status of
the human embryo or about the moral condemnation of human cloning, has a tremendous natural tendency to comprehend certain scientific and natural truths and draw conclusions from them. It is not that the Christian can see more
truth because he or she possesses some special light; rather,
it is that the Christian *wants* to see, and looks at things as
they are.

This also gives the impression that, in contrast, those who
do not believe in God do not manage to see what science clearly
demonstrates, or perhaps they cannot understand truths
based on simple human reason. It may sometimes have to do
with an attitude that tends to justify certain practices already
in progress and to promote certain interests. And sometimes
the best way to justify one's own conscience is not to see, and
in order not to see, it is best not to even look.

But there is something deeper going on in this phenomenon, as John Paul II explains in *Evangelium vitae:*

---

[4] See John Paul II, *Evangelium vitae* (March 25, 1995), n. 21.

We have to go to the heart of the tragedy being experienced by modern man: the eclipse of the sense of God and of man, typical of a social and cultural climate dominated by secularism, which, with its ubiquitous tentacles, succeeds at times in putting Christian communities themselves to the test. Those who allow themselves to be influenced by this climate easily fall into a sad vicious circle: when the sense of God is lost, there is also a tendency to lose the sense of man, of his dignity and his life; in turn, the systematic violation of the moral law, especially in the serious matter of respect for human life and its dignity, produces a kind of progressive darkening of the capacity to discern God's living and saving presence.[5]

These considerations lead us to conclude that the best way the Church in Europe can promote human dignity and respect for life is by committing itself with renewed enthusiasm to the task of the new evangelization of the Continent. As the citizens and people of Europe rediscover the Gospel, they will also be able to discover the Gospel of life.

But the converse also occurs: as they discover the Gospel of life, they will be better prepared to receive the Gospel of salvation. This is mentioned by Pope John Paul II at the end of the text just cited: moral violations, especially in the area of respect for human life, bewilder the heart and mind, and make it difficult to perceive God's presence. Put in a positive way, if our patient work in the field of bioethics allows us to achieve the goal of making men and women in Europe better prepared to receive and respect human life, then they will be more willing to receive the Lord of life. In this sense, properly implemented bioethics proves to be a task of "pre-evangelization."[6]

Relativism and Libertarianism

Europe is not only losing faith; it is also losing reason. If faith was rejected by modern culture, the daughter of the Enlightenment, reason is dying in the postmodern culture. It would seem as if reason—placed on a pedestal that was not

---

[5] Ibid.

[6] A good illustration is the well-known case of Bernard Nathanson. A Jewish nonbeliever who was vigorously dedicated to the practice and legalization of abortion, he first "converted" to respecting and defending life. From there, he underwent a long, profound human and religious conversion, which brought him to the very doors of the Catholic Church, where he was eventually received in baptism.

her own and forced to play the counterfeit role of "goddess reason"—has become extremely weak and no longer believes in her own strength. This is what is referred to in Europe as "weak thinking."

To a great extent, the failure to trust reason comes from distancing oneself from God. As John Paul II says in his encyclical *Veritatis splendor:*

> Man is constantly tempted to turn his gaze away from the living and true God in order to direct it towards idols (cf. 1 Thess 1:9), exchanging "the truth about God for a lie" (Rom 1:25). Man's capacity to know the truth is also darkened, and his will to submit to it is weakened. Thus, giving himself over to relativism and skepticism (cf. Jn 18:38), he goes off in search of an illusory freedom apart from truth itself.[7]

Pope John Paul II clearly denounced the tendency toward absolute relativism in a speech delivered during his historic visit to the Italian parliament.[8] As if taking up the Holy Father's message, chairman of the Italian senate Marcello Pera, a philosopher and nonbeliever, recently devoted one of his speeches, delivered to the Pontifical Lateran University in Rome, to analyzing and denouncing the corrosive phenomenon of relativism.[9] He presented this phenomenon in its axiological dimension—"the idea that there are no solid proofs or arguments for establishing that something is better, or worth more, than something else."[10]

In his analysis, Pera identified two models of modern relativism: the contextual and the deconstructive.[11] The first holds that all concepts or values must necessarily be considered only within the cultural context in which they operate; thus, they cannot be compared with any concept or value that is part of some other cultural area. In this way, everything is relative—dependent on its reference point—so that we cannot say it has a value greater than the value of something else.

---

[7] John Paul II, *Veritatis splendor* (August 6, 1993), n. 1.

[8] John Paul II, "Address to the Italian Parliament (Palazzo Montecitorio)," (November 14, 2002), http://www.vatican.va/holy_father/john_paul_ii/speeches/2002/november/documents/hf_jp-ii_spe_20021114_italian-parliament_en.html.

[9] Marcello Pera, "Relativism, Christianity, and the West," address at the Pontifical Lateran University, Rome, Italy (May 12, 2004), http://www.chiesa.espressonline.it/dettaglio.jsp?id=7739.

[10] Ibid.

[11] Ibid.

The second, the deconstructive model, whose main proponent was Nietzsche, primarily references extreme cases in an attempt to show that supposedly absolute and universal concepts are intrinsically aporetic (or open to doubt) and contradictory. In this way, what some (or many) people think of as good in itself reveals itself as contrary to goodness; this thinking is used to conclude that good and evil are always relative.

Joseph Cardinal Ratzinger, now Pope Benedict XVI, wrote that relativism has in some ways become the religion of modern man[12] and represents the greatest problem of our age.[13] He and Pope John Paul II, as well as Marcello Pera, have verified the penetration of a relativist mentality even among believers—and into theology itself.

In bioethics, relativism has also spread like gangrene. The Italian philosopher Uberto Scarpelli, the master among Italy's so-called laics, has affirmed that it is not possible, not linguistically correct, to speak about truth in the field of ethics,[14] as he tried to demonstrate in a book titled *L'etica senza verità,* or *Ethics without Truth.*[15] Elsewhere he argues that those who think there is one true ethic, such that all others are false, should hold to that ethic and, from it, come up with a single bioethic. He asserts, however, that truth does not exist in ethics, and that the designations "true" and "false" apply appropriately to propositions of a descriptive discourse that is explanatory and predictive, not values-based.[16]

This mentality, widespread among devotees of bioethics but also very much present in ordinary society, leads to the justification of any type of behavior. Relativism thus leads to a libertarian mentality and practice: without the existence of an ethical truth, all that is left is the value of liberty itself, which becomes a kind of self-justification—my action is good because it is free. Self-determination thus becomes the only moral criterion used, for example, in relation to the practice and legalization of euthanasia.

---

[12] Joseph Ratzinger, *Fede, verità, tolleranza* [*Faith, Truth, and Tolerance*] (Siena, Italy: Cantagalli, 2003), 87.

[13] Ibid., 75.

[14] Uberto Scarpelli, "Giovanni Paolo e la Centesimus annus," in *Bioetica Laica* (Milan, Italy: Baldini & Castoldi, 1998), 58.

[15] Scarpelli, *L'etica senza verità* (Bologna, Italy: Il Mulino, 1982).

[16] Scarpelli, "La Bioetica: Alla ricerca dei principi," *Biblioteca della Libertà,* vol. 99 (1987), 227.

I am of the opinion that in many cases, this relativism is a convenient alibi, a covering, or shroud, that allows everyone to have whatever opinion he or she pleases, without having to pay any attention to reason itself. As a result, it is said that each person must independently decide, for example, when an embryo or fetus has developed enough that it is sufficiently valuable to merit respect.

During a debate at a medical congress, an Italian philosopher who is also a proponent of the so-called secular bioethics complained, saying: "For you Catholics, who believe in truth, everything is easier. You think that you have found the truth, and you rest assured; we on the other hand are always seeking, we live the tragedy of knowing that we will never find it." To this rather romantic reflection, I responded, "We Catholics, who believe in the possibility of finding some truth, feel obligated to search for it; you, on the contrary, do not have to look for something you feel cannot be found. We are afraid of making a mistake; you do not have to fear: if truth does not exist, neither does error. We have to strive to be coherent regarding known truths; you do not. Actually, your tragedy is this: you know that when you really get down to it, the assertion 'truth does not exist' is false."

The Church, spouse of the One who is "the Way, the Truth and the Life," must—with Him and like Him—give witness to the truth and serve every person in his or her dramatic search. This is perhaps one of the greatest contributions that we Catholics can currently offer the world regarding respect for human life: building ideas and considerations in bioethics that are not limited to justifying what is useful or agreeable or justifying only certain vested interests.

Exclusive and Intolerant Laicism

Secularization and relativism, so widespread in Europe, are also related to another movement on the continent: an exclusive and intolerant laicism that tends to dominate the whole public arena. The activity of the current Spanish government, which has come to be called "zapaterismo" [after José Luis Rodriguez Zapatero, Spain's newly elected prime minister], is a clear example of the virulence of certain groups in European society. The new ruling party had just barely taken power [in 2004] when they proposed a new social program, in which the following "conquests" are being considered: establishing an equal standing between homosexual unions and matrimony, which extends even to adoption rights; modifying the divorce law to allow for the so-called express divorce, which permits the dissolution of a marriage in just a few weeks; extending the legally permissible conditions for seeking an abortion; modifying the law with regard to assisted reproduction (which was just adjusted by the previous government in November 2003), to allow for experimentation using human embryos; and encouraging social debate regarding the legalization of euthanasia.

The attitude of such groups, which have now risen to power, is distinguished by an outward repulsion toward any type of religious expression—or, more precisely, any Christian or Catholic expression. In fact, while on one hand they seek to limit the teaching of religion in schools, on the other they have decided that the state should finance the teaching of the Islamic faith in the very same schools. The slogan used by Mr. Zapatero during his electoral campaign, "more exercise and less religion," helps us understand his solemn respect for the faith practiced by the majority of Spaniards.

We cannot deceive ourselves into thinking that this is a purely Spanish phenomenon. The European Union's refusal to mention Europe's Judeo-Christian roots in the preamble to the European Constitution was a clear sign of the stubbornness with which certain dominant groups seek to exclude the Christian faith from the public realm.

The recent Buttiglione case has also reverberated loudly at the very center of Europe. In October 2004, Rocco Buttiglione, Italy's European Affairs minister, was denied the post of European Union Commissioner for Justice because of his position on homosexuality. It was not that the Italian minister announced discriminatory measures with regard to homosexuals, or that he made any kind of pejorative remarks. It was simply that, during grueling confirmation hearings before members of the European Parliament, Buttiglione said, "I may think that homosexuality is a sin, but this has no effect on politics unless I say that homosexuality is a crime"—a statement he made after insisting that *personal moral belief* and *public policy* are very separate things and that the latter should never allow for discrimination against anyone.[17] In fact, as soon as he presented his name for candidacy to the European Commission, certain groups in Italy and other European countries protested the nomination of a person who was "too Catholic."

---

[17] Transcripts of the hearings are available at http://www.acton.org/press/special/buttiglione.php#3.

In 2004, Cardinal Ratzinger presented an interesting analysis of the phenomenon of fanatic and intolerant European laicism, comparing it to the situation in the United States. He observed that while secularization is progressing in America at an accelerated rate, there is still—much more than in Europe—an implicit recognition of moral and religious foundations that spring from Christianity and that surpass individual religion. In contrast, Europe is on a collision course with its own history, and often makes itself the spokesperson for an almost visceral rejection of Christian values in every possible public dimension.[18]

I find it enlightening to analyze the causes of this phenomenon. In the United States, the separation of church and state arose in response to the founding fathers' own religious experience, as they wanted to live their faith without being subjected to the dominant church of their European countries of origin. For that very reason, this separation seeks to allow religion to have its own nature; it respects and protects its vital role, distinct from the state and its regulations; it is separation envisioned in a positive way.

In Europe, on the contrary, Illuminism (which proclaimed autonomy of reason and liberation from traditional faith) and Catholicism (strongly anchored to its inheritance of the faith) were seen to be up against each other in an irresolvable conflict.[19] Since then, the separation between Catholics and laicists has become typical in the Latin European countries. As Cardinal Ratzinger describes it, being a "laicist" indicates that one belongs to the spiritual movement of Illuminism, and from there no bridge to the Catholic faith exists. The two worlds have become mutually impenetrable. And since "laicism" means free thought and freedom from any religious restriction, it also involves the exclusion of Christian content and values from public life. [20]

In light of these analyses, it is easier to comprehend the belligerent attitude of many European laicist groups. It is *not* an expression of "laicity," understood in the complementary

---

[18] Joseph Ratzinger, "Lettera a Marcello Pera," in *Senza radici, Europa, relativismo, cristianismo, islam* [*Without Roots: Europe, Relativism, Christianity, and Islam*], by Marcello Pera and Joseph Ratzinger (Milan, Italy: Mondadori, 2004), 99.

[19] Ibid., 104.

[20] Ibid., 105.

separation of the political and religious spheres, but *is* rather an expression of "laicism," understood as the intolerant exclusion of anything religious. Laicists thus seek to deny the Church the right to speak out on public issues, accusing it of seeking to impose its own morality and viewpoint on society. This has reached such a degree that, just recently, again in Spain, a bishop was denounced before a judge for having mentioned in a pastoral letter the doctrine of the *Catechism of the Catholic Church* on homosexuality.

In this situation, shepherds of the Catholic Church in Europe are under enormous public pressure that could tempt them to shut up and acquiesce—and to stop being the light of the world and salt of the earth. But it is interesting that the same people who cry out in protest when the Pope or a bishop makes some statement on moral or social issues are frequently the same ones who protest because, according to them, Pope Pius XII did not adequately denounce the outrages of the Nazi regime. So where do we stand? Were those not also moral and social issues?

In fact, although many people may deny it, European societies are still interested in knowing the Church's opinions about key moral issues and about the most debated topics on life and family. Recently, a well-known director of Italian films complained in a widely circulated newspaper that priests and religious show up too much in debates and on television shows. According to him, these people should not appear in situations where topics of public interest are discussed, because they represent only a minority of the population. But the fact is, the media assiduously seeks the presence of clergy members, because they know that a majority of the population is interested in knowing what the Church thinks and says on the most burning and critical topics.

This was demonstrated again very recently. A brief statement by the secretary and spokesperson of the Spanish Bishops' Conference regarding the use of condoms as protection against AIDS elicited a loud response. The news traveled around the world in just a few hours, and all kinds of commentaries quickly multiplied, coming from all types of people— from theologians of various leanings to representatives of homosexual groups. Why all the commotion? After all, are we not talking about the opinion of a religious person on a public topic, which the Church should not be commenting on anyway? Where do we stand?

Conclusions

We could continue analyzing other significant aspects of the European situation. Some of them are quite specific, such as the enormous complexity of the institutional network that represents the sociopolitical reality—still poorly defined—that we call Europe. Some problems in bioethics are addressed by the European Parliament, with resolutions that are not normative but may influence national legislation. Others are addressed by decisions of the European Commission or the Council of the European Union [or "Council of Ministers"], which in reality represents the various national ministries. And so on.

But I believe that the three characteristics of modern European culture that are analyzed here—progressive secularization, relativism and libertarianism, and exclusive and intolerant laicism—will help us understand the path that bioethical problems have traveled in recent times. They will also help us understand the challenges these problems and cultural characteristics represent to the Church in Europe.

For each characteristic I have presented a description, its repercussions in the field of bioethics, and finally, a very brief allusion to the possibilities and opportunities it presents to the Catholic Church in a difficult situation.

In fact, one of the first conclusions to be drawn from this analysis should be that the Church cannot hide, cannot escape into retirement, and cannot close itself up in silence. The Church in Europe (and on other continents) must question itself on the strength, clarity, and intelligence with which it has faced and continues to face these problems, which are so crucial to the good of humanity and so central to the acceptance of the Gospel.

At times it seems that a good portion of the clergy and agents of pastoral care do not sufficiently occupy themselves with these problems, that they are not sufficiently prepared and do not speak publicly about them. The earlier anecdote (about organ transplants) is an example of this situation. I believe that things are improving in this regard, as initiatives directed at formation and action are flourishing among bishops, priests, and Catholic laity.

As previously mentioned, it is important to be aware that present-day society—secularized, relativistic, and laicized as it is—continues to attribute great importance to the Church's viewpoint. For this very reason, some are attentive to what she says and others are worried when she speaks. At a recent

200

meeting with Church representatives, members of the Spanish Popular Party asked the clergy to speak out more loudly and clearly on these topics. And, truthfully, many Spanish bishops have done so in the last few months, eliciting anger from the most fanatic laicists. Nevertheless, Catholics who are active in politics still ask for a greater Church presence.

It is also important that we renew our confidence in how very effective the Church can be when it intervenes in such areas with intelligence, respect, and firmness. We may have the impression that society is not listening, and that speaking out on these topics in the public arena is nothing but a waste of time or, worse, a way of further distancing people from the Church and the Gospel. Nevertheless, numerous examples show that if the Church (her clergy, her agents of pastoral care, and her laity) mobilizes herself with intelligence, prudence, and at the same time clarity and firmness, important results can be obtained.

One example is the previously mentioned Law 40 in Italy, which has regulated assisted reproduction there since February 2004. It is a law which, despite a few defects, is a true "miracle" in a European society such as Italy. The groups that seek greater liberalization of assisted fertility practices have cried out in protest because, they say, the law was approved because of the influence of the Catholic Church. And they are correct: behind this law are years of intense effort on the part of many Catholic groups that are very active in society. And behind them was the support and at times the direct participation of a few clergy members, who were very conscious of the importance of the issues that were in play.

Pope John Paul II, well aware of the serious and urgent challenges facing the Church with regard to the defense of life in Europe and throughout the world, called bishops to enthusiastically confront these challenges. In *Evangelium vitae,* he says of bishops, "we are the first ones called to be untiring preachers of the Gospel of life." He continues:

> In the proclamation of this Gospel, we must not fear hostility or unpopularity, and we must refuse any compromise or ambiguity which might conform us to the world's way of thinking (cf. Rom 12:2). We must be in the world but not of the world (cf. Jn 15:19; 17:16), drawing our strength from Christ, who by his Death and Resurrection has overcome the world (cf. Jn 16:33). [21]

---

[21] John Paul II, *Evangelium vitae*, n. 82.

THE ETHICS OF INFERTILITY TREATMENT

AN UPBEAT UPDATE

Sr. Renée Mirkes, O.S.F.

All of us recognize the importance of finding moral solutions to infertility. We are acutely aware that we rise and fall collectively with the health of our social infrastructure. And since society's infrastructure rests squarely on the foundation of the family, the issue we take up here—appraising the moral character of the means by which infertile couples build their families—takes on critical importance.

The good news is that I have something genuinely innovative to report in the area of infertility treatment. Its moniker is NaProTechnology (an acronym for Natural Procreative Technology, or NPT for short). This comprehensive, versatile approach to women's health care has been developed and refined during twenty-eight years of clinical research conducted by Dr. Thomas W. Hilgers and his colleagues at the Pope Paul VI Institute. NPT protocols are aimed at the diagnosis and treatment of the diseases that cause infertility, so that infertile couples might achieve pregnancies naturally. You are about to discover why NPT and its disease-based approach to infertility is one-and-a-half to three-and-a-half times more effective than in vitro fertilization (IVF) in assisting infertile couples to achieve a pregnancy.[1]

As the phrase *"upbeat* update" suggests, I believe NPT is good news squared. It not only makes eminently good medical sense; it also makes elegant ethical sense.

My thesis, then, is this: When analyzed comparatively with homologous IVF/embryo transfer (hIVF/ET), only NaPro-Technology provides infertile couples with a good means to the good end of wanting to conceive their own biological baby. That is to say, its protocols assist infertile couples "to procreate in full respect for their own personal dignity and that of the child to be born."[2]

To prove my thesis, I will first contrast the medical regimen of hIVF/ET with that of NPT. Second, I will identify the moral dynamism that these respective infertility treatments evince when judged against the criteria of the dignity of human life and human procreation.

The Medical Facts

First, a medical textbook definition of infertility is a couple's inability to achieve a pregnancy after twelve months of unprotected sexual intercourse.[3] Primary infertility is the inability of the couple to achieve any pregnancy; secondary infertility is the inability to achieve further pregnancies after conceiving one or more times. The most current, nationally representative infertility statistics indicate that there are 6.2 million women of reproductive age in the United States who have impaired fecundity. This represents a significant increase, from 10.8 percent of married women in 1982, to 12.9 percent in 1995. Twenty-year projections suggest that by the year 2025, there could be as many as 7.7 million mar-

---

[1] Thomas W. Hilgers, *The Medical & Surgical Practice of NaPro-Technology* (Omaha, NE: Pope Paul VI Institute, 2004), 691.

[2] Congregation for the Doctrine of the Faith, *Donum vitae: The Gift of Life: Instruction on Respect for Human Life in Its Origin and on the Dignity of Procreation* (Boston: National Catholic Bioethics Center, n.d.), II. B. 8.

[3] Charles B. Clayman, MD, ed., *The American Medical Association Encyclopedia of Medicine* (New York: Random House, 1989), 586.

ried women in the United States who have compromised fertility.[4]

Second, the etiology of infertility[5] can be female factors, such as pelvic pathology (intrinsic tubal diseases, peritubal adhesive disease, or endometriosis), which may occur alone or in combination with other female factors (ovulatory dysfunction, hormonal deficiencies, diminished ovarian reserve, and immunological disorders); male factors (oligospermia or poor sperm motility or morphology); or both. The etiology of some infertility is simply unknown.

Third, the Centers for Disease Control,[6] in its 2001 report *Assisted Reproductive Technology Success Rates,* measured the risk of having multiple-infant births through ART cycles, including gamete intrafallopian transfer (GIFT), zygote intrafallopian transfer (ZIFT), and IVF cycles. In the year 2000 in the United States, 26,550 reported pregnancies resulted from ART cycles using fresh, non-donor eggs: 4,525 of these resulted in either miscarriage, stillbirth, or induced abortion, and 212 pregnancy outcomes were not reported. The remaining 21,813 pregnancies resulted in live births, with 32.0 percent twins and

---

[4] The 1995 National Survey of Family Growth (NSFG), in Stephen EH, Chandra A, "Updated Projections of Infertility in the U.S.: 1995–2025," *Fertility and Sterility* 70.1 (July 1998), 30–34, cited in Thomas W. Hilgers, *The Medical Applications of Natural Family Planning: A Contemporary Approach to Women's Health Care* (Omaha, NB: Pope Paul VI Institute, 1991), 477.

[5] Hilgers, *Applications of NPT*, 480.

[6] The CDC is very upfront in describing the increased risks of multiple births with ART: "Multiple-infant births are associated with greater problems for both mothers and infants, including higher rates of caesarean section, prematurity, low birth weight, and infant disability or death." It is less straightforward with the way it describes selective reduction, i.e., implying that induced abortion and miscarriage are morally indistinguishable: "Triplet (or more) pregnancies may be reduced to twins or singletons by the time of birth. This can happen naturally (e.g., fetal death), or a woman and her doctor may decide to reduce the number of fetuses using a procedure called multifetal pregnancy reduction." (Centers for Disease Control and Prevention and American Society for Reproductive Medicine, "ART Cycles Using Fresh Nondonor Eggs or Embryos," *2001 Assisted Reproductive Technology Success Rates: National Summary and Fertility Clinic Reports,* section 2 [Atlanta, GA: CDC, December 2003]: 20, http://www.cdc.gov/ART/ART01/PDF/ART2001.pdf.)

3.8 percent triplets or more. Comparing the 35.8 percent multiple-birth rate of ART with the 3 percent rate in the general U.S. population,[7] we begin to see why many in the IVF industry and many couples contemplating IVF are concerned.[8]

Fourth, the average cost of one cycle of IVF is between $10,000 and $14,200, including medications.[9] Currently, IVF treatment is not covered by insurance.

Fifth, I have singled out hIVF/ET for consideration because the majority of infertile couples who are advised to pursue IVF and subsequently present at the Center for NaProEthics are trying to discern the morality of this form of ART.[10] (Homologous IVF [hIVF] uses oocytes and sperm from the couple trying to conceive a child; heterologous IVF, which is not discussed here, uses gametes obtained outside the marriage—donor egg, donor sperm, or both). In my experience, many of the couples seeking hIVF/ET are blindsided by the ostensibly benign character of hIVF. "What possible objection," they wonder, "can the philoprogenitive Catholic Church have with a technology that, first, offers us a good chance to conceive a baby and, second, does so using our own, not donor, gametes?"

---

[7] Ibid.

[8] There is a movement within the U.S. IVF industry to reform certain of its practices. An amazingly candid article by Betsy Bates in *OB/GYN News* makes the following assertions about IVF's multiple birth rates: "Many couples do not seek infertility treatment out of fear of multiples, but many specialists continue to transfer three or more embryos. High order multiples are costly (triplets, on average, incur $140,000 in charges before they leave the hospital), and frighten people into believing that IVF will leave them with sick, low-birth-weight babies and unmanageably large families." Then the author approvingly quotes the chairman of Advanced Reproductive Care, Palo Alto, CA: "It's a major reason for bad press. It's a major reason the government is saying it wants to regulate us. It's a major reason for employers to say they're not going to cover it because, I guarantee you, they'd rather have a depressed, infertile patient than a woman with triplets.... It's no longer acceptable to have a 7 or 8 percent triplet rate. It is just not going to fly." (Betsy Bates, "Fear of Failure Deters Many from Infertility Tx," *OB/GYN News* 39.15 [August 1, 2004]: 20A.)

[9] Ibid.

[10] Of approximately 620 infertile couples who have consulted the Center for NaProEthics (the ethics division of the Pope Paul VI Institute) in the past eight years, more than 80 percent of them were considering hIVF.

Homologous IVF/Embryo Transfer

In hIVF, oocytes (obtained surgically from the wife's ovarian follicles in superovulated cycles) and prepared sperm (previously collected by the husband through masturbation) are brought together in a dish in the laboratory. Fertilization takes place in vitro (in glass) in a laboratory, that is, outside the body and outside an act of sexual union. For pregnancy to occur, cleavage-stage or blastocyst-stage embryos derived from the fertilized oocytes are placed in the uterus through a process called embryo transfer. Let us examine each step of the IVF/ET technique in turn.[11]

Semen Preparation. Sperm are capacitated by being centrifuged through a density gradient, with the healthiest sperm left at the bottom of the receptacle. This in vitro process mimics the sperm conditioning that occurs naturally in the female reproductive tract when sperm undergo the acrosome reaction. Sperm density is calculated to determine the amount of sperm needed for the fertilization medium (one million sperm per milliliter) and the incubation of oocytes and sperm.

Superovulation. The woman receives superovulation treatment with gonadotropins (such as follicle-stimulating hormone alone [Gonal-F and Follistim] or in combination with luteinizing hormone [Repronex]) usually preceded by pituitary suppression with a gonadotropin-releasing hormone (GnRH) analog (such as Lupron) or a GnRH antagonist (such as Ganirelix or Cetrotide). A careful balance of these drugs is needed to maximize safely the number of oocytes retrieved. Ideally, there should be enough eggs produced through superovulation to allow, after fertilization, a choice of embryos for the transfer process, as well as extra embryos for cryopreservation. The risk of ovarian hyperstimulation syndrome needs to be minimized, however. Ultrasonographic imaging of the ovaries and in some cases monitoring of the rise in plasma estradiol con-

---

[11] The description of each of the steps of IVF comes from summaries of several sources: Peter R. Brinsden, ed., *A Textbook of In Vitro Fertilization and Assisted Reproduction: The Bourn Hall Guide to Clinical and Laboratory Practice,* 2nd ed. (London: Parthenon, 1999); Peter Braude and Paula Rowell, "Assisted Conception, II: In Vitro Fertilisation and Intracytoplasmic Sperm Injection," *BMJ* 327.7419 (October 11, 2003): 852–855; and (3) personal communication with Dr. Jacques W. Ramey, MD, PhD, a reproductive endocrinologist from the Heartland Center for Reproductive Medicine, Omaha, Nebraska.

centration are both used to check the effects of superovulation. Human chorionic gonadotropin (hCG) is administered thirty-four to thirty-eight hours before planned egg retrieval, when the leading follicles are equal to or greater than 18 mm in diameter. About 10 percent of cycles are cancelled before the planned egg collection because the response to superovulation was either excessive—risking ovarian hyperstimulation syndrome—or, more often, inadequate.

Egg Collection. In the past, eggs were collected laparoscopically under general anesthesia, but now transvaginal follicle aspiration guided by ultrasonography is the method of choice. This procedure can be performed under intravenous sedation and allows access to ovaries that previously were not visible laparoscopically (e.g., in women with severe pelvic disease and adhesions). Most women are able to leave the clinic a few hours after transvaginal egg collection, and the procedure has minimal analgesic requirements.

Each follicle is aspirated in turn, usually through a single vaginal needle puncture for each ovary. The per-cycle number of eggs aspirated from both ovaries varies widely from clinic to clinic, with a conservative goal of five to ten eggs. The fluid collected from each follicle is examined immediately under a microscope for the presence of a cumulus mass that may contain an oocyte. Once the oocytes have been collected, they are placed immediately in a culture medium conducive to fertilization and maintenance of embryo growth.

Insemination. Each oocyte is inseminated with fifty thousand to one hundred thousand motile, morphologically normal sperm. The gametes are incubated in a culture medium for eighteen to twenty-four hours at 39 degrees Celsius in an atmosphere of 5 percent carbon dioxide. The culture medium contains the essential nutrients and electrolytes required for fertilization and maintenance of embryo growth.[12]

Fertilization can be detected twelve to twenty hours after insemination, by the presence of two pronuclei formed in the cytoplasm of the egg around the maternal and paternal chromatids, and by the presence of two polar bodies in the perivitelline

---

[12] The culture medium for in vitro fertilization of human oocyte and sperm includes: sodium chloride, potassium chloride, sodium bicarbonate, sodium phosphate, penicillin, pH indicator, sodium lactate, magnesium chloride, pyruvate salt solution, and bovine serum albumin.

space. More than 60 percent of the eggs collected are fertilized, although complete failure of fertilization can occur because of previously undetected sperm or oocyte abnormalities.

Around twenty-four hours after insemination, the pronuclear membranes dissolve, allowing combination of the maternal and paternal chromatids (syngamy). After syngamy, the single-cell zygote undergoes its first cleavage division to become a two-cell embryo. Further cleavages occur at around twenty-four-hour intervals.

Embryo Transfer. Generally, embryos are transferred to the uterus on the second or third day after fertilization, by which time they have usually divided into four or eight cells, respectively. Many IVF specialists today are allowing embryos to develop in the laboratory for a longer period of time, considering that this may be a better method for selecting the embryos most likely to implant. In theory, the pregnancy rate per transfer should be much higher when blastocyst embryos are transferred on days five to seven than when earlier-stage embryos are transferred on day two or three. The primary risk of attempting blastocyst transfer, however, is that some embryos will die in the laboratory, reducing the number of embryos available for transfer and freezing. Unfortunately, some couples who undergo IVF lose all their embryos in the laboratory and have no embryos available for transfer.

When excess blastocysts are available, they may be frozen. Some of these, however, will not survive the freeze-thaw process when they are utilized in a later attempt to achieve a pregnancy.

But of what does the transfer process itself consist? I will quote from what many consider the definitive text on IVF clinical practice, Brinsden's *Textbook of In Vitro Fertilization and Assisted Reproduction: The Bourn Hall Guide to Clinical and Laboratory Practice*:

> Embryo transfer is carried out in the operating theater under sterile conditions, scrubbing up and gloving, but not gowning up. Husbands are encouraged to attend, suitably gowned and with overshoes.

> On arrival in the theater, the identity of the patient is checked by the accompanying nurse, the surgeon and the embryologist attending to the case—all then sign the case records confirming that they have done so. The patient is placed in the lithotomy position and the surgeon places a perineal drape over her and inserts a Cuscoe vaginal speculum lubricated with warmed saline solution. The cervix is

exposed and any vaginal and cervical secretions are gently removed....

In the laboratory, the embryos are identified by the embryologist and scored, and their details are entered into the log. Those embryos that are to be transferred are placed into a drop of Earle's medium. At Bourn Hall, an Edwards-Wallace (Bourn) embryo transfer catheter ... is used for the majority of transfers. The catheter is fitted with a 1 ml tuberculin-type syringe and flushed through with medium. The embryo(s) are drawn up into the already charged catheter, so that a volume of 15–25 microliters is transferred. The catheter is taken through to the theater and passed to the surgeon. At this stage the lights in the theater are kept dimmed, but are switched up when the surgeon is ready to do the transfer. The catheter is gently maneuvered through the cervical canal and into the uterus.

... If difficulty is experienced in passing the catheter through the cervical canal, then the stiffer outer sheath can be introduced into the canal and the inner catheter "persuaded" through. If this fails, an Aliss single-tooth forceps may be applied to the anterior or posterior lip of the cervix and gentle traction applied to straighten the cervical canal. If it is still found to be impossible to pass the catheter after every reasonable means has been tried, and after a maximum of two minutes (because of the cooling effect on the embryos), then the embryos are returned to the laboratory and replaced in the culture dish.... The embryologist then returns with the embryo transfer catheter; it is threaded up the sheath and will usually enter the uterine cavity. When the operator is confident that the catheter is properly placed, the embryologist or the surgeon can slowly and gently inject the embryos into the uterus; the catheter is left in position for a few moments and then gently and slowly removed. The catheter is returned to the laboratory and checked to ensure that the embryos have not been retained. If they have, the embryologist will draw up the embryos again into the catheter and a further attempt will be made to transfer them to the uterus. On completion of the transfer, the speculum is withdrawn and the patient is made comfortable.[13]

Post-embryo Transfer Support. Most IVF centers administer progesterone supplementation via vaginal pessaries, suppositories, intramuscular injections, or oral micronized proges-

---

[13] Brinsden, *Textbook of IVF*, 181–183. (Bourn Hall Clinic was founded by Patrick C. Steptoe and Robert G. Edwards, who presided over the "conception" of the first IVF baby, Louise Brown, in 1978.)

terone tablets until menses occur or the woman has a positive pregnancy test. Alternatively, hCG may be given two to three times a week, but it can promote ovarian hyperstimulation syndrome in susceptible or heavily stimulated patients.

NaProTechnology

First, the NPT parameters for defining infertility are these:[14] If a couple have not achieved pregnancy within three cycles of fertility-focused intercourse, an infertility problem is likely. If pregnancy has not occurred by the sixth cycle, then testing for an organic or other underlying abnormality begins.

Second, NPT has one principal goal in reference to an infertile couple: to resolve the conditions causing their infertility so that they are empowered to achieve a pregnancy within their own act of intercourse.

Third, NPT takes a disease-based approach to infertility. In other words, infertility is viewed as a symptom of an underlying organic, hormonal, or ovulatory dysfunction. To date, NaProTechnology has been very successful in identifying and treating infertility precisely because it comprehensively evaluates and corrects the multiple causes of the "symptom" of infertility. Consequently, because the couple better understand *why* they are infertile and because they pursue only *reasonable* means to overcome the roots of their infertility, NPT couples are more apt to adjust to their situations with healthy acceptance and peace of mind.

Fourth, the reason that the diagnostic and treatment strategies of NPT manage infertility so well is that they are able to adequately (and therefore precisely) target the menstrual/fertility cycles of the particular infertile patient being evaluated.

To understand this nostrum, we need to examine the basics of the Creighton Model FertilityCare System of charting—the only prospective and standardized means of monitoring the various patterns of a woman's menstrual and fertility cycle for the natural regulation of fertility. Figure 1 (*next page*) shows a chart from an infertile woman who has normal vulvar mucus cycles of a regular length (i.e., between twenty-one and thirty-eight days). Her cycle begins with menses. The days of menses, marked on the chart with red stamps (which appear light gray in the figure), are followed by infertile days

---

[14] This entire section references Hilgers, *Applications of NPT*.

211

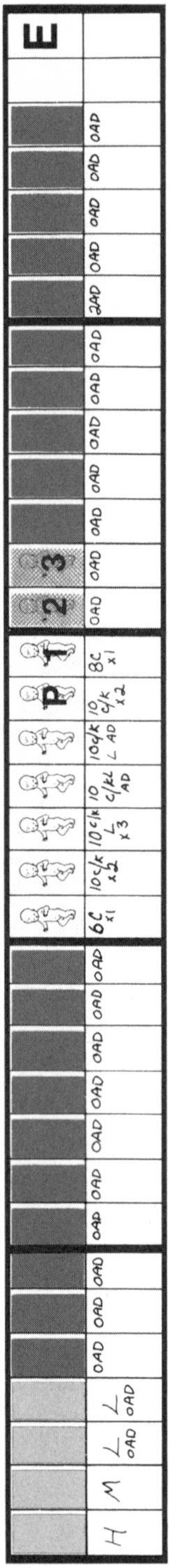

FIGURE 1. Chart from an infertile woman who has normal vulvar mucus cycles of a regular length.

marked with green stamps (dark gray in the figure), indicating that the patient does not observe either bleeding or cervical mucus. The infertile days are followed by fertile days, marked with white baby stamps, indicating that she observes cervical mucus at the vulva. These are followed by infertile days, marked with green (dark gray) stamps, when she no longer observes cervical mucus.

In the fertile or ovulatory phase of her cycle, the woman observes a cervical discharge at the vulva that begins as sticky/cloudy or tacky/cloudy mucus and eventually becomes clear, stretchy, or lubricative mucus. The presence of mucus tells the woman she is fertile and in the periovulatory phase of her cycle. She marks the last day of her discharge of mucus that is clear, stretchy, or lubricative with a "P" to indicate the peak day of cervical mucus and the peak day of her fertility.

With this chart, the woman and her husband know their window of fertile days, or the vulvar mucus cycle. They know that fertility-focused intercourse increases their chances of getting pregnant. More importantly, the infertile couple understand that if they direct their acts of intercourse to their days of peak-type mucus, they optimize their chances of achieving a pregnancy.

Because the infertile patient's charts tell an NPT physician where this patient is in her cycle, on any given day the physician is able to schedule phase-sensitive diagnostic protocols when they will yield maximum results. For example:

- A postcoital test can be timed to occur when the female patient observes good peak-type cervical mucus at the vulva, so that the infertile couple are assured a more accurate assessment of the husband's sperm.

- Diagnostic laparoscopy can be scheduled during the preovulatory phase of the woman's cycle, when it will not risk interruption of a pregnancy that could occur during the postovulatory phase. A selective hysterosalpingogram should be done during the proliferative phase of a woman's cycle—between day four and day eight or ten—when her endometrium is still thin and access to the internal os of the fallopian tube is relatively easy.

- The scheduling of follicular ultrasound studies for an infertile woman is directed by the timing of cyclic events recorded on her previous charts. For this infertile patient with a regular cycle, for example, the NPT physician would order a baseline pelvic ultrasound on day five, because he knows the preovulatory phase is the best time of her cycle to attempt an adequate structural assessment of her reproductive organs. He will order daily follicular ultrasound studies from the fifth day before her peak until follicular rupture, because he knows these periovulatory studies will adequately monitor ovarian folliculogenesis and development. Finally, he will order another pelvic ultrasound on the seventh day after her peak because he knows it will give him an adequate picture of endometrial pathology, should it be present, and the patient's postovulatory ovarian status.

- The way an NPT physician measures the ovarian hormones of an infertile patient illustrates how the patient's charts direct the timing of hormone profiles in such a way as to assure that they adequately assess or target estradiol and progesterone surges.[15]

---

[15] Contrast the NPT use of targeted hormone profiles with what a non-NPT physician does. The latter places a patient with a thirty-nine-day cycle (with a long preovulatory phase) into a twenty-eight-day-cycle schematic. Consequently, when the physician tests this woman's levels of periovulatory estradiol on day fifteen, the result is totally useless, since this woman is in her preovulatory, not periovulatory, phase on that day. When the same physician calls for a postovulatory progesterone and estradiol profile on day twenty-two, the finding is equally useless, since this woman, on day twenty-two, is in her periovulatory, not postovulatory, phase. As a result, the hormone profiles gleaned from non-targeted hormone profiles will be ineffective in diagnosing whether the infertile woman suffers from endocrinopathy, and will also result in less effective therapy design and delivery.

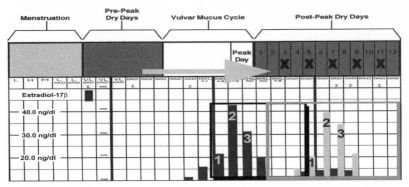

FIGURE 2. Targeted peri-ovulatory and post-ovulatory hormone profiles.

Figure 2 is a schematized drawing of the regular cycle chart that we have been examining. It helps clarify when the woman is in her periovulatory and postovulatory phases and can be used to adequately target the respective periovulatory and postovulatory hormone surges. With the woman's charts as reference, the physician will get an adequate periovulatory estradiol surge profile (at least three values, with the middle value being the peak estradiol level), if he orders a blood draw every other day from day six pre-peak through day two post-peak. Similarly, the physician will get an adequate post-ovulatory progesterone and estradiol surge profile (at least three values, with the middle value being the peak progesterone and estradiol levels), if the woman's blood is drawn at specified intervals (i.e., at peak plus three, five, seven, nine, and eleven).

The ultimate goal of these hormone assays is to compare the infertile woman's targeted profiles with normal profiles, to confidently determine whether abnormal levels of ovarian hormones are a part of the pathology underlying her infertility. If endocrinopathies are present, the NPT physician can initiate effective therapeutic regimens to correct the problem and thereby help the woman more easily conceive naturally.

Fifth, NPT surgical techniques effectively treat the various organic and structural abnormalities that underlie infertility, and they do so in a way that prevents postoperative pelvic adhesions.[16] This kind of prevention is significant, since pelvic adhesions could reduce the infertile patient's chances of conceiving on subsequent attempts.

---

[16] Hilgers discusses his accumulated wealth of surgical wisdom in Chapter 67 of *Applications of NPT*, 908–924. To prevent pelvic adhe-

FIGURE 3. Multiple-pregnancy rate in patients with infertility treated with NaProTechnology in the United States and Ireland (Pope Paul VI Institute research findings, Omaha, Nebraska, 2004). The twenty multiple births comprised seventeen sets of twins and three sets of triplets. There were no multiples beyond triplets.

Number of pregnancies	617
Number of multiple births	20
Incidence of pregnancies producing multiple births	U.S.: 3.2% Ireland: 3.4%

Sixth, NPT infertility protocols incur a low multiple pregnancy rate, illustrated in Figure 3 by a 3.2 percent rate at the Pope Paul VI Institute clinic and a 3.4 percent rate at a NaPro clinic in Ireland.[17] These rates compare *very* favorably with the previously cited 35.8 percent rate of multiple-infant births with ART cycles. Judged against these national statistics, the NPT approach to infertility evinces an 11.2-fold *decrease* in multiple births and all their adverse sequelae for baby and mother.

Seventh, the cumulative pregnancy rate for 1,054 infertile women who were treated at the Pope Paul VI Institute clinic with NPT for the full spectrum of infertility-causing diseases (Figure 4, *next page*) demonstrates that over 60 percent of these patients became pregnant within twenty-four months, and nearly 70 percent of them within thirty-six months.[18] Achieving a pregnancy may take longer with NPT than with with IVF, but the number of women who achieve a pregnancy with NPT is higher than the number of women who achieve a pregnancy with IVF. In addition, the already encouraging pregnancy rates cited from the recently published definitive textbook, *The Medical and Surgical Practice of NaProTechnology*, are expected to increase even more as surgical techniques and the ability to treat ovarian and target organ dysfunction (OTOD) improve.

---

sions following reconstructive pelvic surgery, the surgeon must pay attention to the details of skin incisions, intermittent irrigation, use of hydro-packs, choice of suture, the choice of cutting instruments, tissue closure, uterine suspension, adhesion barriers, the use of clear fluid for irrigation, and closure of the peritoneum.

[17] Ibid., 536.

[18] Ibid., 680–681.

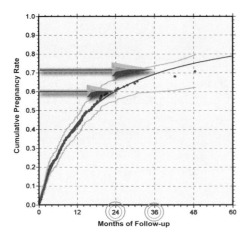

FIGURE 4. Cumulative pregnancy rate among infertile patients treated with NaPro Technology.

Eighth, the cost of NPT infertility protocols will vary from couple to couple depending on the more or less expensive medical or surgical interventions that are needed to successfully treat the pathology underlying the infertility. Increasingly, however, insurance providers are covering many of the NPT medical and surgical interventions because they categorize them (rightly, in our estimation) as treatments for disease.

NPT Treatment of Infertile Women with Regular Cycles

Since most of the infertile patients who have come to the Pope Paul VI Institute clinic have presented with regular cycles, that is, cycles lasting from twenty-one to thirty-eight days, I will only describe the evaluative, diagnostic, and treatment regimen for this category of patient.

First Visit. The NPT physician takes the infertile patient's history and determines her cycle category. In this case, the woman reports that she has "regular cycles," or cycles lasting somewhere between twenty-one and thirty-eight days. The physician directs the patient to a practitioner who will teach her and her husband how to chart their cycles using the Creighton Model System (CrMS).

Second Visit. The patient returns with at least two months of charts. The NPT physician accomplishes three goals during this second visit:

1. The physician conducts a physical examination.

2. The physician reviews the patient's charts with close attention to CrMS biomarkers. He or she categorizes the woman's chart according to mucus cycle type; determines the length and stability of its post-peak phase, the length (and

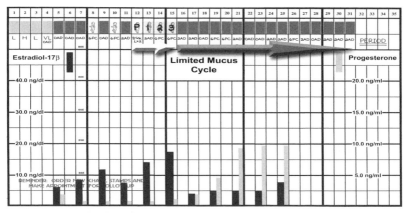

FIGURE 5. Chart showing very limited mucus cycles with a prolonged post-peak phase.

characteristics) of its pre-peak phase, and the length of the cycle as a whole; and notes whether there is premenstrual spotting or tail-end brown bleeding and their significance.

- If the infertile patient with regular cycles presents with charts like the one shown in Figure 5, the physician will categorize them as very limited mucus cycles with a prolonged post-peak phase. This kind of chart, the NPT physician knows, is suggestive of suboptimal preovulatory and postovulatory hormone profiles and a lutenized unruptured follicle.

- If the infertile patient presents with charts like those shown in Figure 6, the NPT physician categorizes them

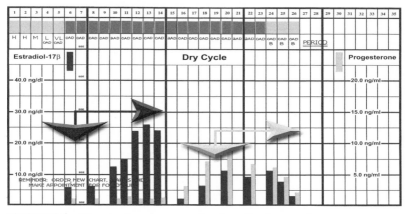

FIGURE 6. Chart showing regular-length dry cycles.

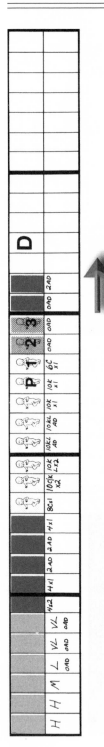

FIGURE 7. Chart showing a regular, short post-peak-phase cycle.

as regular-length, dry cycles. Regular, dry cycles suggest to the physician decreased hormone parameters associated with poor folliculogenesis and luteogenesis.

- When the infertile patient with regular cycles presents with charts like the one shown in Figure 7, the physician categorizes them as regular, short post-peak-phase cycles. A short phase after peak day suggests to the NPT physician an inadequate-length luteal phase, caused by suboptimal levels of progesterone due to an inadequate corpus luteum.

- If the infertile patient presents with charts of regular-length, normal mucus cycles, suggesting no major hormone abnormalities or ovarian dysfunction, the NPT physician knows that this sort of chart is often associated with male infertility factors, such as oligospermia or azospermia, or with female organic factors such as tubal anomalies, endometriosis, or polycystic ovarian disease (PCOD).

- If the patient's charts look like the chart shown in Figure 8, the physician classifies them as dry cycles with premenstrual spotting. Both premenstrual spotting (when blood is a pinkish color) and tail-end brown bleeding (when brown bleeding occurs at the end of the menstrual cycle) may indicate the possibility of low progesterone levels, which can be associated with endometritis (i.e., inflammation of the uterine lining).

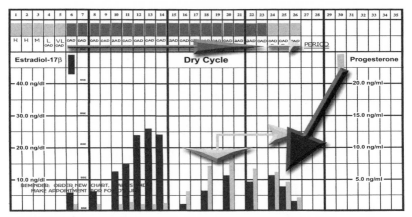

FIGURE 8. Chart showing a dry cycle with premenstrual bleeding.

The important point is that the characteristic biomarkers of these charts point the physician with consistent reliability to the underlying pathophysiology of the infertile patient.

3. The physician orders the following tests:

- *A seminal fluid analysis.* If the husband's sperm count is zero (azospermia), the count should be repeated to determine whether there is an obstruction of the vas deferens. If there is no obstruction and azospermia is the correct diagnosis, then the rest of the medical evaluation for this infertile patient is cancelled, unless the woman has gynecological anomalies that need to be addressed (e.g., chronic pelvic pain, severe dysmenorrhea, dyspareunia, or severe premenstrual symptoms). Even though there is no further NPT infertility treatment that could help this couple, the physician, drawing on the pro-family philosophy behind NPT, will discuss with them alternative means by which they can give life to other people's children.

  If the husband's sperm count is normal or only suboptimal, the remaining diagnostic tests are ordered:

- *A full-series menstrual cycle hormone profile*, which measures periovulatory estrogen levels, postovulatory progesterone and estradiol levels, male hormone levels, thyroid hormone levels, and gonadotropin and beta endorphin levels.

- *A follicular ultrasound series* (described on p. 213).

- *Surgical interventions*: diagnostic laparoscopy (to diagnose organic or structural anomalies of the pelvis associated with infertility), hysteroscopy (to diagnose uterine abnormalities associated with infertility), and a selective hysterosalpingogram (to diagnose and treat fallopian tube anomalies associated with infertility).

Third Visit. The physician shares the laparoscopy videotape with the couple, reviews all test results, and gives a comprehensive case management review with NPT medical and surgical solutions in mind.

Case Presentation[19]

Presentation of the case of a forty-two-year-old patient from California who was treated at the Pope Paul VI Institute for infertility is the best way to sum up NPT's characteristic management of infertility.

Evaluation. The patient presented to Dr. Hilgers with a history of regular-length cycles. Her responses on the "Female General Information Form" revealed that her previous diagnostic workup had been limited to annual gynecological checkups and that she failed two cycles of IVF with intracytoplasmic sperm injection (ICSI). Her husband's responses on the "Male General Information Form" indicated that he had undergone vericocele surgical repair after diagnoses of oligospermia and very low sperm motility. The woman reported that her obstetrician-gynecologist was convinced that she was ovulating normally, and her fertility specialist had suggested that, because of her age, the age of her eggs, and her husband's suboptimal sperm, IVF with ICSI represented her best shot at a pregnancy.

Diagnostic Protocols. Dr. Hilgers directed the patient to a CrM FertilityCare practitioner (FCP) in California so that she could learn to chart her cycles. Two months later, she returned to Omaha and presented Dr. Hilgers with two months of charting for his evaluation. The biomarkers of her charts revealed regular-length cycles (suggestive of endometriosis or PCOD) with borderline limited mucus (suggestive of hormonal abnormalities), no unusual bleeding, a normal post-peak phase length, and a normal menses. Dr. Hilgers ordered a full-series menstrual cycle hormone profile, a follicular ultrasound series, and a diagnostic laparoscopy and hysteroscopy. Results of the

---

[19] Ibid., 537–539.

hormone profile indicated suboptimal post-ovulatory progesterone and beta endorphin levels. The follicular ultrasound
series revealed normal ovulation with a single follicle showing
a complete rupture on day seventeen of the cycle, and normal
folliculogenesis. The diagnostic laparoscopy and hysteroscopy
showed endometriosis.

Treatment Protocols. The patient's husband was given low-
dose clomiphene citrate (Clomid), 5 mg. twice a day, to improve his sperm count. The patient's endometriosis was lasered
at the time of the diagnostic laparoscopy. The patient returned
to California and began a cycle-by-cycle treatment with Clomid
to induce ovulation and to help correct the underlying hormonal dysfunction. This segment of the treatment was moni-
tored long-distance by Pope Paul VI Institute clinicians.

Outcome. During the eighth cycle of treatment, the patient conceived. The pregnancy was supplemented with natural progesterone. At term, the patient delivered a healthy baby
girl.

Ethics Assessment

No couple has a right to a baby. Couples do, however,
have a right to marital acts and, with that right, the corresponding duty to collaborate *responsibly* with "the fruitful love
of God."[20] Here, I will compare and contrast the intrinsic morality of hIVF/ET with that of the NPT approach to infertility, in
hopes of resolving one central question. Do these respective
infertility treatments assist couples to collaborate responsibly
with God's life-giving love?

The (small-c) catholic norms that I will use to adjudicate
the morality of these respective treatments have certainly not
developed in a vacuum. They follow directly from the Church's
comprehensive vision of the human person, which is rooted
in reason and confirmed by faith. In turn, that vision and its
correlative norms shed light and meaning on an infertile
couple's lived experience of the personal nature of their procreative capacity. Thus, infertile couples who seek to realize
their good goal of wanting to conceive a baby of their own can
use these norms as guideposts directing them to a good
means—an infertility treatment that promotes the values of
life and procreation.

---

[20] *Donum vitae,* Introduction, n. 5.

The Catholic Vision of the Value of Human Life

The life of every human being is a gift from God, the way God shares with each human being "his breath of life," "his image and imprint."[21] *Shares* is the operative word here. God does not surrender his Lordship over life, but entrusts life to every human being as a proprietor would his household to a steward. Our ensuing responsibility, as human recipients of the gift of life, is to uphold and care for, rather than control and dominate, our own life and that of others.

Thus, God alone is the Lord of life from its beginning until its end: "no one can, in any circumstance, claim for himself the right to destroy directly an innocent human being."[22] Absolute respect for the integrity of new human life follows from natural truths about the human person.

First, the human being, unlike plants and animals, is created in God's image and likeness. This means that, of all material creatures, the human being alone is rationally intelligent and free. It is the dignity of personal intelligence and freedom—that capacity of the composite human being to reveal his person through his body and bodily actions—that defines the human being as a creature who is an end in himself, a being whom God created not to be used by others merely as a means to their own ends, but someone to be valued and loved in and for himself.

It is the inherent dignity or the ontological goodness of *bios* (human life) that grounds the inviolability of the life of every human person—unique and unable to be given over completely to someone else. The human being is a subject, an "I," whose being cannot be reduced to an "it," an object of manipulation. For this very reason, *Donum vitae* defines each person's right to life as "a sign and requirement of the very inviolability of the person to whom the Creator has given the gift of life."[23] No matter their size, age, or stage of development, all human beings share equally in fundamental human rights, the first of which is the right to life.

Second, as a being whose rational soul is infused by an immediate, creative act of God, the human person stands in an irrevocable relationship with his Creator. The human per-

---

[21] John Paul II, *Evangelium vitae* (March 25, 1995), n. 39.

[22] Ibid., quoting *Donum vitae*, Introduction, n. 5.

[23] *Donum vitae,* Introduction, n. 4.

son, nuptially related to God, receives all of creation, including his or her life and embodied existence—as well as those of other persons—as gift. The covenant between the human being and God that is begun in the act of conception is destined to be consummated in "an eternal life of beatific communion with God."[24] The vocation to give self and to receive the other as gift resounds, then, in the nature of every human being who is made in the image of the person of God, the radical giver.

Correlative Norms Protecting Human Life

Three norms pertaining to infertility treatment follow from this vision of human life:

1. Infertility interventions must respect the inviolable integrity of a newly developing human life in vitro and in utero.

2. Spouses do not have a right to a child.

3. A child has the right to be conceived within marriage.

I will apply each norm, in turn, to hIVF/ET and to NPT.

Respect for the Inviolable Integrity of a
Newly Developing Human Life[25]

Applied to hIVF/ET. Donum vitae highlights the reductio ad absurdum of reproductive technologies, such as IVF, that bring life through death. The philosophy behind IVF simply tortures logic beyond all comprehension. Prior to any fertilization in the laboratory, the IVF specialist arrogates to himself the right to instruct the couple which of their embryos will be transferred, which will be surrealistically suspended through cryopreservation, which will be donated to destructive embryonic research, and which will be discarded because of developmental abnormalities. Keep in mind that all of this anti-life violence is directed toward embryos who fall outside the most popular justification for abortion, namely, "unwanted" babies resulting from so-called unplanned pregnancies. IVF embryonic human beings are specifically produced *for* reproductive purposes.

---

[24] John Paul II, "Letter on the Occasion of the 23rd National Congress of the Italian Catholic Physician's Association" (November 9, 2004), http://www.vatican.va/holy_father/john_paul_ii/letters/2004/documents/hf_jp-ii_let_20041109_medici-cattolici_en.html.

[25] *Donum vitae*, II, introduction.

Moreover, usurpation of dominion over the lives and deaths of these in vitro embryos is not limited to decisions to transfer, to cryopreserve, or to destroy. It also extends to serious endangerment of the baby's postnatal life and health. The higher number of multiple births that occur through IVF bring a commensurately higher risk for premature birth with low and very low birth weight, fetal distress, and low Apgar scores.[26] Prematurity compromises the child's chances for normal motor and mental development.[27]

As a way to defuse the unhealthy and even life-threatening situation of multiple pregnancies, the perinatal philosophy behind IVF also relies on another anti-life notion, namely, selective termination. Take the case of a mother who, as a result of IVF and ET, begins to successfully gestate triplets. Even should the woman experience second-trimester difficulties that could cause developmental compromise for all three fetuses, the responsibility of the fertility specialist in transferring three or more embryos in the first place can easily be expunged. The IVF specialist is confident that, if necessary, the woman's obstetrician or perinatologist will suggest that the mother reduce the pregnancy from triplets to twins by selecting the least healthy baby for termination.[28]

Applied to NPT. All NPT treatments for infertility respect the right to life and bodily integrity of human beings in utero. As we have seen, NPT protocols not only do nothing to deliberately destroy a newly gestating human life, they do everything to facilitate a healthy full-term pregnancy.

In the care taken to avoid high-order pregnancies in women who are given hyperovulatory drugs, there is even fur-

---

[26] Apgar scores are an assessment system for newborns developed by Virginia Apgar that quantitates the huge changes a newborn undergoes during the first few minutes of extrauterine life. The Apgar system adjudicates five features at one minute and at five minutes after birth: respiratory effort, heart rate, color, muscle tone, and motor reactions. Each factor is scored between zero and two, with a total of ten possible points. A low total of zero to three means the baby is probably not breathing well and has a slow heart rate and, therefore, needs resuscitation. A score of seven to ten indicates a well baby. Clayman, *AMA Encyclopedia*, 124.

[27] Hilgers, *Applications of NPT*, 488.

[28] Barbara Carton, "Agonizing Decision: Multiple Pregnancies Are Often Pared Back in 'Fetal' Reduction," *Wall Street Journal*, November 21, 1997.

ther demonstration of NPT's respect for the life and safety of both mother and baby. NPT's ovulation induction protocols require that, when a low-dose human menopausal gonadotropin is used, it be tracked with daily ultrasound to determine the effects of the drug on ovarian production of mature follicles. If four or more ovarian follicles mature, the couple is counseled not to have intercourse that cycle, and the dosage of the drug is decreased.[29] The statistics I presented on the low rate of multiple and premature births incontrovertibly attest to NPT's respect for the life and bodily integrity of NPT mothers and their babies.[30]

Do Spouses Have the "Right" to a Child?

Children are, and must be viewed as, a personal gift, "the supreme gift ... of marriage."[31]

Applied to hIVF/ET. Providers and users of IVF demonstrate an overtly utilitarian outlook. Infertile couples have the "right" to reproduce in any way they please and to conceive their own baby in the easiest, most expedient way they can. But the tradeoff for expedient baby-making is a devastating depersonalization. As we have seen, IVF fertility specialists reduce the parents to suppliers of fertilization material and reduce the baby to an end-product controlled by scientific technology. With this kind of objectivization, IVF's aim is straightforward: to ensure that the product it literally makes "by hand" is commensurate with the demand of consumers and conforms to the specifications of parental will and design.[32] After all, the quality and number of in vitro embryos

---

[29] Hilgers, *Applications of NPT*, 616.

[30] Ibid., 692.

[31] *Donum vitae*, II. B.8.

[32] In his inimitable way, Leon R. Kass underscores the dehumanization that incurs when life is manufactured in vitro: "With in vitro fertilization, the human embryo emerges for the first time from the natural darkness and privacy of its own mother's womb, where it is hidden away in mystery, into the bright light and utter publicity of the scientist's laboratory, where it will be treated with unswerving rationality, before the clever and shameless eye of the mind and beneath the obedient and equally clever touch of the hand. What does it mean to hold the beginning of human life before your eyes, in your hands—even for five days (for the meaning does not depend on duration)?" Kass, *Toward a More Natural Science* (New York: The Free Press, 1985), 126.

are judged by "conditions of technical efficiency" which are, ultimately, "standards of control and dominion."[33] Even the personhood of in vitro embryos awaits assignment by its manufacturers.

Applied to NPT. NPT's approach to infertility, together with the genuine humanist culture it generates, encourages couples to work cooperatively with nature, to use their reason not primarily to calculate the most expeditious way for the greatest number of infertile couples to get pregnant, but to discover and appreciate the laws of their nature and to freely cooperate with them. This dispositive attitude toward fertility begets a genuine notion of what it means to conceive a child "with the help of the Lord" (Gen.4:1). Couples who have successfully been treated for infertility through NPT, and conceive as a result, do so within their own acts of intercourse. And conceiving naturally *necessarily* requires that the parents relinquish control over their baby.

I have learned, through my eight years of experience with many NPT parents, the moral ramifications of that kind of surrender. Whether it was prenatally or postnatally, I witnessed NPT parents talking about and treating their children in a way that can only be described as profoundly respectful. Each child is a person who is cherished for his or her uniqueness, accepted as a novel life never before lived, welcomed as an "unbidden surprise"[34] for whatever specific combination of handicaps and talents he or she might have, and cherished for his or her uncharted mission in life.

In sum, what I have observed is that as a result of their openness to the possibility of parenthood within their acts of sexual union—despite problems with infertility—NPT users acquire a correct understanding of what it means to be a parent. Their good parenting translates into just relations between them and their children.

The Child's Right to be Conceived within Marriage [35]

Applied to hIVF/ET. To date, I have not found a serious discussion referencing *any* rights of an IVF child—to say nothing of whether that child has a right to be conceived in a natural

---

[33] *Donum vitae,* II. B. 4c.

[34] Leon R. Kass and James Q. Wilson, *The Ethics of Human Cloning* (Washington, DC: AIE, 1998), 33.

[35] *Donum vitae,* II. A. 1.

way. Nor do I expect to see such a work in the future. In the world of IVF and ET, the rights of the parents trump all.

However, I have a theory. The day we as a society recover our sense of the natural and the symbolic will be the day we are able to objectively evaluate the impact of depriving children of a "secure and recognized relationship"[36] to their parents' embodied love from the *first*, and *most vulnerable*, days of their life.

Applied to NPT. As already noted, NPT unambiguously helps the infertile couple conceive a child within their own acts of sexual love. Predictably, this approach to infertility also encourages NPT parents to appreciate and respect the right of their children to be conceived within, and therefore to be intimately connected to, the protection, security, and, yes, intimacy of their bodily union.

The Catholic Vision of the Value of Human Procreation

God calls a husband and wife to image his inner family life through the language their bodies speak in the act of marital intercourse. The spousal meaning of a couple's vocation to procreation—to share in the divine "mystery of Creator and Father"—is *inscribed in* the meaning of their vocation to love, "the mystery of [their] personal communion."[37]

But what does it mean for the Church to say that the act of giving life to a new human being is inscribed—that is, indelibly engraved—within the very act of giving love? To my mind, the Church invokes this powerful image to help a husband and wife better grasp how the procreative meaning of their sex acts—their vocation to parenthood—*defines, activates,*[38] and *demands* its love-giving counterpart. We might even say that in this imagery the Church is exposing infertile couples—and all of us—to a glimpse of the providential mercy of the divine design for human conception. God intends that human beings be conceived naturally so that each and every last one of us could take consolation from, and find security in, the knowledge that we *came to be out of* a personal act of our parent's *love*. Through the simple but powerful image of inscription, the

---

[36] Ibid.

[37] Ibid., Introduction, n. 3.

[38] John Paul II, *Theology of the Body: Human Love in the Divine Plan* (Boston: Pauline Books & Media, 1997), 398.

Church opens the minds of infertile couples to see why their act of sexual union is the *only* genuinely loving, and therefore human and moral, means for them to beget children.

The inseparable connection between the love-giving and life-giving meanings of marital union is not only rooted in the intrinsic structure of the marital act. It is also, and even more profoundly, anchored "in the very nature of the man and the woman," who are, at once, body and soul, gendered and generative beings.[39]

As the second creation account of Genesis teaches, male and female human beings are "halves, not wholes" of humanity. In their acts of marital union, a man and a woman are each drawn out of their incomplete, insufficient, mortal selves into a communion of persons. In their marital embrace, the couple symbolize and signify the transcendent, whole meaning—the completeness, sufficiency, and immortality—of a spousal love that imitates God's life-giving love. Bringing new human life out of their sexual act of love capacitates the infertile couple to transcend their "separateness through the children born of [their] sexual union."[40]

Correlative Norms Protecting the Value of Human Procreation

Two norms pertaining to infertility treatment follow from this view of human procreation:

1. Infertility treatments must assist, not replace, the conjugal act.
2. The dignity of conceiving a baby demands the sexual complementarity, the "two-in-one-flesh" union, of husband and wife.

I will apply each norm, in turn, to hIVF/ET and NPT.

Assistance, Not Replacement, of the Conjugal Act[41]

This is important so that "the procreation of a human person be brought about as the fruit of the conjugal act specific to the love between spouses."[42]

---

[39] Ibid., 387.

[40] Kass, *More Natural Science*, 114 and 291; *Donum vitae*, II. B. 4b.

[41] *Donum vitae*, II. B. 7.

[42] Ibid., Part II, B, n. 4.

Applied to hIVF/ET. Because fertilization of gametes takes place in a laboratory, IVF necessarily replaces the conjugal act.

Applied to NPT. Insofar as the identification and treatment of infertility's underlying pathologies facilitate natural conception, NPT's medical and surgical treatments unambiguously help the couple's act of conjugal union attain its natural end.

Conception within the "Two-in-One-Flesh" Union of Spouses

Applied to hIVF/ET. By ignoring the unitive dimension that alone makes sense out of the mystery of sexuality and human renewal,[43] IVF renders the production of new human life unintelligible. To shift conception from womb to laboratory is to jettison the personal, sexual context of transmitting human life. The price of generating new human life "sexlessly" requires us to "pay in coin of our humanity."[44] Recall Brinsden's account of the rather hapless stance and dress of the IVF father, separated from his wife by the sterile surroundings of a surgical theater. Under laboratory lights, fertilization and transfer of the human gametes take place in a series of impersonal, extra-bodily actions which relegate parents to the role of suppliers and bystanders.[45]

To proceed as if procreation can be separated from sexual union without negative consequence, as IVF does, is a flagrant canard. IVF violates the ultimate truth of human sexuality, the ultimate truth of human dignity, the ultimate mystery of beginning life within the mother's body. The sagacious wit of one of Mark Twain's maxims—"A lie can travel halfway around the world while the truth is putting on its shoes"—helps us understand why and how the deceptions of IVF have so quickly taken on a life of their own.

Applied to NPT. The NPT approach to infertility embraces the wisdom of a natural law insight: the fact that all mamma-

---

[43] Ibid.

[44] Kass, *More Natural Science*, 114. *Donum vitae* (II, Introduction) warns couples who utilize IVF that they also become the victims or patients of the same "dynamic of violence and domination" which is leveled against the child who is to be conceived.

[45] Kass calls the IVF scientist-physician the one who "presides over many creations in many patients." As such the IVF physician is not only the "sower of the seed" and the "fertilizer general" but the "matchmaker" as well. *More Natural Science*, 70.

lian reproduction is "the generation of new life from (exactly) two complementary elements, one female, one male, (usually) through coitus."[46] This insight automatically takes on the status of a moral norm when the mammals involved are human persons. Allowing the couple to responsibly respect "the language of their bodies" evidenced in their "natural generosity"[47] and desire to have their own baby is the cachet of NPT's approach to infertility.

Responsible Cooperation

In sum, there is one critical fact damning hIVF/ET as an option to family-building: it is an inherently immoral reproductive technique. First, formed by a scientific worldview that refuses to admit of the natural teleology and normative indicators of human fertility, IVF profanes the true meaning of human procreation. Second, driven by a utilitarian view of nascent human life, IVF allows, and even encourages, the deliberate destruction of human embryonic and fetal life. As such, even when hIVF/ET results in a pregnancy, it is a pyrrhic outcome. It does not and cannot present infertile couples with a good means to the good end of conceiving their own baby. It does not allow infertile couples to cooperate responsibly "with the fruitful love of God." And, from a medical standpoint, although a woman may conceive her biological baby as a result of IVF and ET, she will still be infertile after giving birth. There seems to be more than just negative medical implications from the conclusion that, as a treatment for infertility, IVF per se does nothing to treat infertility.[48]

---

[46] Kass and Wilson, *Ethics of Cloning*, 24.

[47] *Donum vitae*, II. B. 4b.

[48] IVF statistics refer to the success rate for IVF treatment of women with endometriosis or polycystic ovaries, referring to the rate at which the "treatment" gets these women with various infertility-causing diseases to respond with a pregnancy. It needs to be pointed out that the success rate attributed to IVF does not reflect how well it has treated the respective underlying disease (such as endometriosis, PCOD, tubal occlusion) directly but how well IVF gets women pregnant despite those pathologies. Women who deliver after IVF are still infertile in the sense they are still afflicted with the same pathology that caused their infertility before the conception of their IVF baby. They will still not be able to conceive naturally. In "IVF: Who's Pushing Who?" ABC Science Online reporter Anna Salleh interviewed Dr. Amin John Abboud, an Australian doctor and bioethi-

NaProTechnology, on the other hand, is an inherently moral technique for treating infertility. First, it respects the dignity of human procreation: NPT—by diagnosing and treating the pathology causing infertility—enables the infertile couple to conceive through their own acts of intercourse. Second, it respects the dignity of human life: NPT protocols support the pregnancy from day one forward, so mother and baby can be healthy throughout the forty ensuing weeks of gestation and at the time of delivery. In sum, NaProTechnology tugs parents in the direction of cooperating responsibly "with the fruitful love of God."[49] This, I hope you agree, is good news squared.

---

cist who researched the IVF industry in preparation for his address on IVF to the World Congress of Bioethics (ABC Science Online, November 8, 2004, http://abc.net.au/science/news/health/HealthRepublish_1235782.htm). Abboud concluded that couples were being offered the option of IVF before the cause of their infertility was fully established and all options were considered. This practice makes it almost impossible to get accurate effectiveness studies, since there are no standard eligibility criteria for IVF programs that are universally required.

[49] I would suggest emulation of the following educational precedent for exposing physicians, clergy and couples to NPT. In the Irish Bishops' Committee for Bioethics recommends NaProTechnology to Irish couples as a moral treatment for infertility—over IVF, ICSI, GIFT, artificial insemination by husband, intrauterine insemination, and artificial insemination by donor—because NPT "invariably involves natural (or in vivo) fertilisation. It does not, therefore, place embryos at risk to their life or bodily integrity. NaPro fosters dialogue and co-operation between the couple, with its emphasis on fertility awareness. The emphasis on respect for the natural reproductive process means that NaPro is consistent with the meaning and integrity of human sexuality." Bishops' Committee for Bioethics, *Assisted Human Reproduction: Facts and Ethical Issues* (Dublin, Ireland: Veritas, 2000), http://www.catholiccommunications.ie/pastlet/ahr.html.

POPE JOHN PAUL II ON NUTRITION AND HYDRATION FOR THE SERIOUSLY ILL AND DISABLED

Richard M. Doerflinger

On March 20, 2004, Pope John Paul II presented a clarification of Catholic teaching on a medical-moral issue that has long troubled Catholic physicians and ethicists as well as many families. He did this in the form of an allocution, or speech, near the end of a four-day conference in Rome on "Life-Sustaining Treatments and Vegetative State: Scientific Advances and Ethical Dilemmas."[1] To understand the Pope's contribution, we need to understand the situation before his speech.

---

[1] Address of John Paul II to the Participants in the International Congress on "Life-Sustaining Treatments and Vegetative State: Scientific Advances and Ethical Dilemmas" (March 20, 2004), http://www.vatican.va/holy_father/john_paul_ii/speeches/2004/march/documents/hf_jp-ii_spe_20040320_congress-fiamc_en.html (hereafter "Allocution"); reprinted in *Origins* 33.43 (April 8, 2004): 737, 739–740.

Background:
The Church's Tradition

The Catholic tradition rejects acts or omissions that are intended to bring about a patient's death. It also affirms a general obligation to sustain and support life, while judging all medical treatments in terms of what they can do *for* the human patient (in terms of benefits) and what harm they might do *to* that patient (in terms of burdens). When burdens are disproportionate to the expected benefits, even treatment to sustain life may be refused.

> Discontinuing medical procedures that are burdensome, dangerous, extraordinary, or disproportionate to the expected outcome can be legitimate; it is the refusal of "over-zealous" treatment. Here one does not will to cause death; one's inability to impede it is merely accepted.[2]

Even in such cases, one can never simply abandon the patient by denying the basic care we owe to the helpless.

> When inevitable death is imminent in spite of the means used, it is permitted in conscience to take the decision to refuse forms of treatment that would only secure a precarious and burdensome prolongation of life, *so long as the normal care due the sick person is not interrupted.*[3]

Today medicine can often sustain the life of a seriously injured patient in a state of severe mental and physical disability without curing the underlying condition. Sometimes the patient with a brain injury may survive for a long time in what many physicians call a "vegetative state," in which there are sleep/wake cycles but no sign that the patient is aware of his or her environment. In these cases, where one can impede death but perhaps not improve the patient's disabling condition, the question of basic care has become more urgent. Is continued life, even in such a state, a benefit for the patient? Where is the line to be drawn between treatment and care, especially when dealing with the medically assisted nutrition and hydration (e.g., feeding through a gastric or nasogastric tube) these patients may need to survive?

Three positions have developed:

---

[2] *Catechism of the Catholic Church*, n. 2278.

[3] Congregation for the Doctrine of the Faith, *Declaration on Euthanasia* (1980), part IV, emphasis added; reprinted in *Origins* 10.10 (August 14, 1980): 156.

1. *Food and water are basic needs of every human person, and are therefore part of the "normal care" owed to every patient, even when medical treatments have become disproportionate.* This view seems to be reflected, for example, in a 1985 statement by a study group of the Pontifical Academy of Sciences: "If the patient is in a permanent, irreversible coma, as far as can be foreseen, treatment is not required, but all care should be lavished on him, including feeding."[4]

2. *Nutrition and hydration, when provided with medical assistance, may have some aspects of a "treatment," but should still be provided unless the burdens of delivering them clearly outweigh their benefits in a given case.* They are usually "ordinary" or "proportionate" means, because they are essential for survival and can generally be provided without the risks and burdens of more aggressive treatments. This moral presumption in favor of providing nutrition and hydration also applies to the patient in a "vegetative" state. This is the position recommended by the U.S. bishops' Committee for Pro-Life Activities, in a 1992 resource paper prepared with the help of the U.S. bishops' Doctrine Committee and the Congregation for the Doctrine of the Faith. The bishops stated:

> We reject any omission of nutrition and hydration intended to cause a patient's death. We hold for a presumption in favor of providing medically assisted nutrition and hydration to patients who need it, which presumption would yield in cases where such procedures have no medically reasonable hope of sustaining life or pose excessive risks or burdens.[5]

In considering nutrition and hydration for patients in the "vegetative" state, the bishops clearly thought that such cases of excessive burden would be rare.

3. *Positions 1 and 2 are both wrong.* There is no obligation to provide any life-sustaining means, even food and fluids, to the patient diagnosed as being in a "persistent vegetative state," because such a patient has no cognitive abilities and hence cannot pursue the spiritual purposes of human life. As Father Kevin O'Rourke and Sister Jean de Blois argue: "Chris-

---

[4] Pontifical Academy of Sciences, "The Artificial Prolongation of Life," *Origins* 15.25 (December 5, 1985): 415.

[5] National Conference of Catholic Bishops Committee for Pro-Life Activities, *Nutrition and Hydration: Moral and Pastoral Reflections* (Washington, D.C.: U.S. Catholic Conference, 1992), http://www.usccb.org/prolife/issues/euthanas/nutindex.htm; reprinted in *Origins* 21.44 (April 9, 1992): 705–712.

tians acknowledge that aggressive medical care may not restore or improve a person's capacity to strive for eternal life. If
this happens, medical care may be withdrawn."[6] "In fact," writes
Fr. O'Rourke, "the presumption should be *against* the use of
ANH [artificial nutrition and hydration] for ... patients [in persistent vegetative state, or PVS] because there is no possibility of benefit for such patients once a valid diagnosis of PVS
has been made."[7] The theological basis for this stance is that
"a person in PVS cannot perform those human acts of intellect
and will that, according to Catholic tradition, are necessary to
attain the purpose of life." In short, there is no obligation to
support mere "physiological function" that cannot pursue
higher purposes, when this is all that is left in a patient in the
persistent vegetative state.[8]

Supporters of this approach cite a number of texts in support of their position—*Veritatis splendor,* the *Summa theologiae,*
even the passage from the Catechism of the Catholic Church
cited above—but none of these texts seems to be on point. To
be sure, Pope Pius XII in a 1957 allocution did say that life and
all other earthly goods are "subordinate" to the higher spiritual
good. And in light of this, he said that a life-sustaining medical
intervention that directly attacks or interferes with this higher
good (for example, by depriving the patient of consciousness or
by causing suffering that makes spiritual reflection very difficult) might be refused as unduly burdensome:

> But normally one is held to use only ordinary means—
> according to circumstances of persons, places, times, and
> culture—that is to say, means that do not involve any
> grave burden for oneself or another. A more strict obliga-
> tion would be too burdensome for most men and would
> render the attainment of the higher, more important good
> too difficult. Life, health, all temporal activities are in fact
> subordinated to spiritual ends. On the other hand, one is
> not forbidden to take more than the strictly necessary

---

[6] Sr. Jean deBlois and Fr. Kevin O'Rourke, "Issues at the End of
Life," in *Ethical and Religious Directives for Catholic Health Care Services: Seeking Understanding—A Collection of Selected Readings* (hereafter, *CHA Readings*) (St. Louis: Catholic Health Association, 2003): 33.

[7] Fr. Kevin O'Rourke, "Applying the *Directives,*" *CHA Readings,*
43.

[8] O'Rourke, "Applying the *Directives,*" 43.

[9] Pius XII, "Address to an International Congress of Anesthesi-
ologists" (November 24, 1957); reprinted in *The Pope Speaks* 4.4 (1958):
395–396.

steps to preserve life and health, as long as he does not fail in some more serious duty.[9]

But Pius XII did not say here that earthly life is solely an instrument for pursuing that higher good—or that a life already deprived of consciousness is not worth supporting even by minimal means. Rather, he was commenting on cases in which a particular burdensome means interferes with spiritual activity that could otherwise be pursued.

Yet the "spiritual purposes" standard has become a dominant view in many Catholic health-care circles in the United States. In fact, all the quotes just cited in support of this position are taken from a 2003 compendium issued by the Catholic Health Association of the United States as a guide to the U.S. bishops' *Ethical and Religious Directives for Catholic Health Care Services*, and no other position is cited in that compendium as being equally in accord with the Catholic tradition— not even the position of the U.S. bishops' Committee for Pro-Life Activities, cited in a footnote of those directives as a guide to the debate on feeding patients in PVS.[10]

Pope John Paul II's Allocution on Patients in the "Vegetative" State

In his allocution of March 2004, Pope John Paul II clearly sought to clarify and help resolve this debate. He made five major points:

1. *The inherent dignity of the human person remains intact in patients in the so-called vegetative state.* The Pope expressed great unease with the term "vegetative," which is used by some to imply that the patient has lost human value and dignity and now has the status of an animal or vegetable:

> In opposition to such trends of thought, I feel the duty to reaffirm strongly that the intrinsic value and personal dignity of every human being do not change, no matter what the concrete circumstances of his or her life. A man, even if seriously ill or disabled in the exercise of his highest functions, is and always will be a man, and he will never become a "vegetable" or an "animal." Even our brothers and sisters who find themselves in the clinical condition of a "vegetative state" retain their human dignity in all its fullness. The loving gaze of God the Father continues to

---

[10] U.S. Conference of Catholic Bishops, *Ethical and Religious Directives for Catholic Health Care Services*, 4th ed. (Washington, DC: USCCB, 2001), 42 note 39.

fall upon them, acknowledging them as his sons and daughters, especially in need of help.[11]

This is very much in keeping with the personalist message that this Pope has defended in many documents. While man's highest goods are spiritual, he is a unified being of body, mind, and spirit, and his earthly body partakes of this special dignity. Thus, however diminished or disabled, "life is always a good."[12] We cannot divide the human person into a valuable spiritual entity on the one hand and, on the other, a mere "biological existence" that serves the spiritual only as an instrument with no inherent value.[13] As the Pope says later in his allocution:

> To admit that decisions regarding man's life can be based on the external acknowledgment of its quality, is the same as acknowledging that increasing and decreasing levels of quality of life, and therefore of human dignity, can be attributed from an external perspective to any subject, thus introducing into social relations a discriminatory and eugenic principle.[14]

In short, if we reject the dualism that divides the human person this way and demeans the most vulnerable, we have to reject the "spiritual purposes" standard for sustaining life.

2. *We must acknowledge new medical evidence on the "vegetative" state.* We cannot be sure that these patients cannot

---

[11] Allocution, n. 3.

[12] John Paul II, *Evangelium vitae* (March 25, 1995), n. 34.

[13] To cite just one use of this theme in the speeches of Pope John Paul II, he said of the decision to donate organs for transplant: "It is not just a matter of giving away something that belongs to us but of giving something of ourselves, for 'by virtue of its substantial union with a spiritual soul, the human body cannot be considered as a mere complex of tissues, organs and functions ... rather it is a constitutive part of the person who manifests and expresses himself through it' (Congregation for the Doctrine of the Faith, *Donum Vitae*, 3). Accordingly, any procedure which tends to commercialize human organs or to consider them as items of exchange or trade must be considered morally unacceptable, because to use the body as an 'object' is to violate the dignity of the human person." Address of John Paul II to the 18th International Congress of the Transplantation Society (August 29, 2000), n. 3, http://www.vatican.va/holy_father/john_paul_ii/speeches/2000/jul-sep/documents/hf_jp-ii_spe_20000829_transplants_en.html.

[14] Allocution, n. 5.

feel or think to some degree, and we cannot reliably determine when all hope of recovery is lost. For example,

> we must neither forget nor underestimate that there are well-documented cases of at least partial recovery even after many years; we can thus state that medical science, up until now, is still unable to predict with certainty who among patients in this condition will recover and who will not.[15]

This simply reflects the expert medical consensus that emerged from the Rome conference itself. The papers presented at this conference included the following findings:

- Neuroimaging indicates that these patients often do have greatly reduced functional activity in the cerebral cortex, the area associated with many "higher" brain functions. In some patients there are problems with the connections between different parts of the cerebral cortex, or between the cortex and the thalamus, a brain structure that serves as a relay station from the brainstem to the cortex. But some patients have recovered from the "vegetative" state, at which time these connections seem to be restored, for reasons that are poorly understood. What seems most important in producing and maintaining the "vegetative" state is the interruption of certain *connections* between different parts of the brain, which enable the person to take in and respond to stimuli. If we restore those connections we may greatly improve the chances for recovery.[16]

- Diagnosis (even a clear and simple definition) of the "vegetative state" is notoriously difficult, in part because we cannot diagnose another person's loss of consciousness but can only infer it (make an "educated guess") on the basis of his or her response to stimuli. Thus, misdiagnosis is common. One study found that, of long-term patients in nursing homes in the United States who were diagnosed as being in a vegetative state, 18 percent were able to communicate. Another found that 37 percent of the patients with this diagnosis who were admitted to

---

[15] Ibid, n. 2.

[16] S. Laureys et al., "Residual Cerebral Functioning in the Vegetative State," in *L'Arco di Giano: Rivista di Medical Humanities*, special issue on "Life-Sustaining Treatments and Vegetative State: Scientific Advances and Ethical Dilemmas" (2004): 85–91.

one rehabilitation unit were actually aware. And a study at the Royal Hospital for Neuro-disability in the United Kingdom found that 43 percent of the patients with this diagnosis had been misdiagnosed, including several patients who had been thought to be in a "vegetative" state for several years.[17]

• Just as diagnoses are uncertain, so are prognoses for recovery. This is even more true with the rise of new techniques for stimulating these patients to respond to their environment. In one study of 134 patients diagnosed as being in a "vegetative" state for more than one month in Israel, 54 percent recovered consciousness, and half of these were able to recover complete independence in daily living; all patients who recovered after more than six months retained severe disabilities, but 40 percent of these were able to return home.[18] At the March 2004 conference in Rome, a panel of medical experts was asked: Is there any length of time in the "vegetative" state after which we can say, with moral certainty or beyond a reasonable doubt, that recovery will not occur? The experts agreed that they could not name such a period of time.

In short, in the thirty-three years since neurologists coined the term "persistent vegetative state,"[19] we have come to realize that we know far *less* about this condition than we once thought we did. Many doubt that it can be seen as one well-defined condition at all.[20] The diagnosis of "vegetative" state is an unreliable basis for setting this class of patients aside into a different moral category, especially in matters of life and death. In this regard the Pope's speech reflects the very latest medical findings.

---

[17] See the studies cited in H. Gill, "Misdiagnosis of Vegetative State," *L'Arco di Giano* special issue (2004): 94.

[18] L. Sazbon, "Rehabilitation of Patients in Vegetative State," *L'Arco di Giano* special issue (2004), 113.

[19] B. Jennett and F. Plum, "Persistent Vegetative State after Brain Damage: A Syndrome in Search of a Name," *Lancet* 1.7753 (April 1, 1972): 734–737.

[20] C. Borthwick, "Persistent Vegetative State: Usefulness and Limits of a Prognostic Definition," *L'Arco di Giano* special issue (2004), 134–138; D. A. Shewmon, "A Critical Analysis of Conceptual Domains of the Vegetative State: Sorting Fact from Fancy," *NeuroRehabilitation* 19.4 (2004): 343–347.

3. *We have an obligation to provide normal care (including food and water) to all patients, including patients in "vegetative" states.* Theologically, Pope John Paul II's most important statement is his first one, about the inherent dignity of these patients. His statements about food and fluids follow logically from this: If the person still has a right to life, then he or she still has what the Pope calls "the right to basic health care," including sustenance. But his position here is in danger of being misunderstood.

He says first, "I should like particularly to underline how the administration of water and food, even when provided by artificial means, always represents a natural means of preserving life, not a medical act."[21] Is he saying that nutrition and hydration must be provided by increasingly aggressive technical means, regardless of the circumstances? This writer thinks not, as explained further below. But the Pope is making at least two points. First, while their provision may at times require medical skill, food and water themselves are basic means by which we all care for the helpless and help them survive; their provision is not an exotic medical technology, but a basic need of everyone. Second, the provision of food and water must not be judged, as some medical treatments are, by whether it can cure or improve any medical condition, whether physical or mental. For the patient in a "vegetative" state it does exactly what it does for any of us— it simply sustains us, comforts us, and keeps us from dying of dehydration and starvation. It cannot be judged futile or without benefit because it may not enhance the patient's mental condition or produce certain kinds of mental acts. If the patient remains in a "vegetative" state, we cannot fault the food and fluids for falling short of expectations. The purpose or finality of food, in and of itself, is not to make us smarter.

Pope John Paul II then says of assisted feeding that "its use, furthermore, should be considered, in principle, ordinary and proportionate, and as such morally obligatory, insofar as and until it is seen to have attained its proper finality, which in the present case consists in providing nourishment to the patient and alleviation of his suffering."[22] This does not propose an absolute standard either, for it requires provision of these means only if, in a given case, they serve their goal or

---

[21] Allocution, n. 4.

[22] Ibid.

finality of providing life-giving nourishment and alleviating suffering. If the patient is imminently dying no matter what we do, or can no longer effectively take in nourishment, or if the efforts to provide feeding would only aggravate his suffering instead of providing comfort, the moral obligation does not apply.

Thus, when Pope John Paul II says that food and fluids are morally obligatory "in principle" [*in linea di principio*], this means "as a general rule" or "unless the special circumstances cited here apply."[23] It is a reaffirmation of the "strong presumption" in favor of feeding these patients that the U.S. bishops' Pro-Life Committee has recommended since 1992.

Even the provision of "normal care" is first and foremost at the service of the dignity and well-being of the human person, and must be judged according to what it does for the patient and to the patient. Thus, while Pope John Paul II reaffirms that medically assisted nutrition and hydration is generally to be seen as falling under the category of "normal care," he incorporates aspects of the first two theological positions I outlined above, for there is still room for judging burdens and benefits to the patient.

4. *The withdrawal of food and water may constitute euthanasia by omission.* The Pope adds:

> The evaluation of probabilities, founded on waning hopes for recovery when the vegetative state is prolonged beyond a year, cannot ethically justify the cessation or interruption of minimal care for the patient, including nutrition and hydration. Death by starvation or dehydration is, in fact, the only possible outcome as a result of their withdrawal. In this sense it ends up becoming, if done knowingly and willingly [*se consapevolmente e deliberatamente effetuata*], true and proper euthanasia by omission.[24]

Clearly, he is not saying that withdrawal of these means is euthanasia when special circumstances make them ineffective in providing nourishment or alleviating suffering. He is speaking of an intent to end the patient's life because that life is judged worthless when the prospect of recovery seems dim.

---

[23] For the Italian version of the allocution, see "Un uomo, anche se gravemente impedito non diventerà mai un 'vegetale'," in *L'Osservatore Romano* (March 20–21, 2004): 5.

[24] Allocution, n. 4.

Some might object: But death is not the *only* outcome of such withdrawal. Another outcome, and a positive one, is to save the hospital, family, and community from the costs and burdens of caring for this patient. But those goals are only served if the patient dies, so his or her death by dehydration must be chosen as the means to this end.

The cost of feeding is generally very small; what is costly is the ongoing nursing care, the hospital room, efforts at rehabilitation, and such, which are made necessary by the patient's survival. The only way to save these costs is to make sure the patient dies. This concern about the use of a "cost" standard for withdrawing food and fluids from these patients had already been raised by the U.S. bishops in their 1992 paper.[25]

So the Pope's special concern about feeding these patients is not based solely on a "slippery slope" argument— that we must insist on the value of these patients in a secular society tempted toward euthanasia (although he surely had this in mind as well). He is reaffirming a basic moral norm: In our acts *and* omissions we must not intend the death of another innocent person, even to serve other worthwhile goals. If assisted feeding is effectively providing nourishment and is consistent with the patient's comfort and physical well-being, what other reason can we have for withdrawing it?

5. *We have a social obligation to support these patients and their families.* As always, Pope John Paul II's statement here against violating human life is wedded to a positive and heroic social ethic affirming our obligation to empty ourselves in service to the most helpless. That service, worthwhile in and of itself, will also help families resist pressures to end the lives of these patients:

> It is necessary, above all, to support those families who have had one of their loved ones struck down by this terrible clinical condition. They cannot be left alone with their heavy human, psychological and financial burden. Although the care for these patients is not, in general, particularly costly, society must allot sufficient resources for the care of this sort of frailty, by way of bringing about appropriate, concrete initiatives.[26]

---

[25] NCCB Committee for Pro-Life Activities, *Nutrition and Hydration,* 4–5.

[26] Allocution, n. 6.

Here the Pope specifically mentions nursing and respite care, rehabilitation, counseling, and spiritual assistance. The cost of providing this support, in his view, is a small price to pay to remain a society that is fully human.

Reception of Pope John Paul II's Statement in Catholic Health Care

Reactions to Pope John Paul II's speech among health-care ethicists varied. The World Federation of Catholic Medical Associations, representing Catholic physicians committed to the papal magisterium, hailed the speech, and declared that patients with this condition have a right to "basic care, including hydration, nutrition, warming, and personal hygiene," as well as proper diagnosis, support, and appropriate rehabilitation.[27] In the United States, the National Catholic Bioethics Center greeted it as "a welcome clarification" of our moral obligations in this area.[28]

In Australia, Father Norman Ford, a leading proponent of the "spiritual purposes" argument, publicly reversed his position in deference to the Pope, while pointing out that there is more to be said on this issue. The allocution is authoritative, he said, without necessarily being definitive, and some questions remain: "The pope's teaching applies in principle and does not rule out the ethical use of professional judgement by doctors should other medical contraindications arise."[29]

---

[27] World Federation of Catholic Medical Associations and Pontifical Academy for Life, "Joint Statement on the Vegetative State: 'Challenges' for the Field of Health Care," in *L'Osservatore Romano,* English ed. (April 28, 2004): 2.

[28] National Catholic Bioethics Center, "Statement of the NCBC on Pope John Paul II's Address on Nutrition and Hydration for Patients in PVS" (April 23, 2004), http://ncbcenter.org/press/04-04-23-NCBCStatementonNutritionandHydration.html.

[29] Norman Ford, SDB, "The Pope on the Moral Obligation to Continue Tube Feeding for Patients in Post-Coma Unresponsiveness," in *Chisholm Health Ethics Bulletin* 9.4 (Winter 2004): 1–3. For his previous position, articulated at the March 2004 conference at which Pope John Paul II later spoke, see Ford, "Ethical Reasons Why Medically Assisted Nutrition and Hydration May No Longer Be Needed or Good for Patients Diagnosed as Permanently Unconscious," in *L'Arco di Giano* special issue (2004), 169.

The Catholic Health Association of the United States, on the other hand, has said it finds the speech puzzling, because it is in such stark contrast with what many Catholic health-care ethicists understood Church teaching to be. Until the outstanding questions are answered and the *Ethical and Religious Directives* for Catholic hospitals in the United States are revised, CHA recommends following the *current* directives.[30] As noted above, the current directives are interpreted by CHA in a way that can exclude the patient in a "vegetative" state from our moral obligation to provide feeding, because for such patients feeding provides no benefit. In line with the CHA statement, representatives of many Catholic hospitals have said they do not expect to change their protocols on withdrawal of food and fluids any time soon.[31]

One of the most interesting and troubling reactions was by Fr. John Tuohey, an ethicist at a Catholic hospital in Portland, Oregon. Writing in *Commonweal* magazine, he pretended that Pope John Paul II was a graduate theology student who had submitted his allocution as a draft proposal for a graduate thesis—and he gave the Pope a failing grade. He pointed young Wojtyla to the nuances in the *Declaration on Euthanasia*, which Tuohey called "the most authoritative statement by the church to date on the topic"[32]—apparently unaware that he was lecturing the person who, by approving the declaration in 1980, gave it that authority. Tuohey even lectured him on the Pope's own statement in 1992 against subjecting patients to "therapeutic tyranny" through overly aggressive treatment, as though that speech had been referring to efforts to feed patients.[33] In the end, Fr. Tuohey sent his student away with the admonition, "You will want to use greater care in your final project."[34]

---

[30] See "The Catholic Health Association of the United States Statement on the March 20, 2004, Papal Allocution," http://www.chausa.org/Misssvcs/Ethics/statement.asp; and Thomas A. Szyszkiewicz, "Hard to Understand?" in *The Catholic World Report* (June 2004): 50–55.

[31] For a review of early reactions to the Allocution, including reactions by Catholic hospital representatives, see Germain Kopaczynski, "Initial Reactions to the Pope's March 20, 2004, Allocution," *National Catholic Bioethics Quarterly* 4.3 (Autumn 2004): 473–482.

[32] John F. Tuohey, "The Pope on PVS: Does JPII's Statement Make the Grade?" *Commonweal* 131.12 (June 18, 2004): 10.

[33] Ibid., 11.

[34] Ibid., 12.

If it is an error to treat the Pope as just another theologian with no special authority, what word can be coined for the error of treating him as our not-very-bright theology student and assuming that he does not understand his own writings?

The genuine problem here is that many Catholic health-care ethicists had committed themselves to the third theological position described above (the "spiritual purposes" standard), and they are surprised that this is now being rejected by the Holy See. Should they have been surprised?

Continuity with Vatican Developments prior to March 2004

In fact, the Holy See has given so many indications of its thinking on this issue in recent years that it is difficult to see how theologians could have missed those signals.

As Pope John Paul II's allocution points out, several less authoritative documents already said that the *Declaration on Euthanasia*'s mandate for providing normal care to all patients applies to assisted feeding. In 1981, a document of the Pontifical Council Cor Unum said this,[35] and in 1985, as noted above, the Pontifical Academy of Sciences specifically cited an obligation to provide food and fluids to the comatose patient. The *Charter for Health Care Workers*, issued by the Pontifical Council for Pastoral Assistance to Health Care Workers in 1995, says: "The administration of food and fluids, even artificially, is part of the normal treatment always due to the patient when this is not burdensome for him: their undue suspension could be real and properly so-called euthanasia."[36]

The 1992 paper by the U.S. bishops' Committee for Pro-Life Activities, calling for a strong presumption in favor of food and fluids for the patient in "vegetative" state, has also re-

---

[35] Pontifical Council Cor Unum, *Question of Ethics regarding the Fatally Ill and the Dying*, June 27, 1981 (Vatican City: Vatican Press, 1981), n. 2.4.4; excerpt reprinted in Kevin D. O'Rourke and Philip Boyle, eds., *Medical Ethics: Sources of Catholic Teachings* (St. Louis: Catholic Health Association, 1989): 156. This document lists alimentation among "minimal" means, the interruption of which "would, in practice, be equivalent to wishing to put an end to the patient's life."

[36] Pontifical Council for Pastoral Assistance to Health Care Workers, *Charter for Health Care Workers* (Boston: Pauline Books & Media, 1995), 105, n. 120.

ceived much attention from the Holy See. Soon after publication, the paper was published in abbreviated form *in L'Osservatore Romano* as an aid to other bishops' conferences.[37] And in 1998, Pope John Paul II singled out this paper for high praise in a speech to some U.S. bishops during their *ad limina* visit, saying that the paper rightly warns against euthanasia by omission and rightly defends a "presumption in favor of providing medically assisted nutrition and hydration to all patients who need them." Here he stated that

> a great teaching effort is needed to clarify the substantive moral difference between discontinuing medical procedures that may be burdensome, dangerous or disproportionate to the expected outcome—what the *Catechism of the Catholic Church* calls the refusal of "over-zealous" treatment (n. 2278; cf. *Evangelium vitae*, n. 65)—and taking away the ordinary means of preserving life, such as feeding, hydration and normal medical care.[38]

Also significant was a statement by the U.S. bishops' Committee on Doctrine in 1996, prepared in consultation with the Congregation for the Doctrine of the Faith, which rejected a proposal for inducing premature labor for infants with anencephaly (failure of the higher brain to develop).[39] This proposal had been put forward by Father Kevin O'Rourke and Sister Jean de Blois, leading proponents of the "spiritual purposes" argument for withdrawing feeding tubes from unconscious patients, and it used the same rationale. The anencephalic child could not in any case pursue the spiritual purpose of life, so the mother had no obligation to continue providing the support of her womb; if delivered before viability the child would die sooner, but sustaining life any longer was of no benefit to the child in any case, or could be outweighed even by the mother's distress at having to continue the preg-

---

[37] Comitato "Pro-Life" dei Vescovi Cattolici Statunitensi, "Nutrizione e idratazione: considerazioni morali e pastorali," in *L'Osservatore Romano* (December 11, 1992): 5.

[38] Pope John Paul II, Ad limina address to the Bishops of California, Nevada, and Hawaii, October 2, 1988, n. 4; reprinted in *Origins* 28.18 (October 15, 1998): 316.

[39] NCCB Committee on Doctrine, "Moral Principles concerning Infants with Anencephaly" (September 19, 1996), http://www.usccb.org/dpp/anencephaly.htm; reprinted in *Origins* 26.17 (October 10, 1996): 276.

nancy of a severely disabled child.[40] While the proposal for premature induction of labor was in a different context, it used the same rationale in terms of "spiritual purposes," and its complete rejection by the Doctrine Committee should have been a warning sign. Here, too, the Doctrine Committee's report was reprinted in *L'Osservatore Romano*, with commentaries, to help other bishops.[41]

This trend became so obvious that in 2002, Fr. Kevin O'Rourke himself wrote an article in a Catholic bioethics journal expressing alarm that at various levels the Holy See had turned against his theological position, beginning with the encyclical *Evangelium vitae* in 1995.[42]

Theologians alarmed at this trend thus had ample opportunities to make their arguments to Vatican officials as to why their position had merit. These arguments were presented right up to, and during, the March 2004 conference in Rome. Obviously, they proved unpersuasive. But to say now that the Pope's allocution of March 2004 was a bolt from the blue or a one-time aberration cannot be taken seriously.

Continuity, Development, and Remaining Questions

In short, Pope John Paul II's allocution applies the Church's lasting tradition, in light of the most up-to-date medical knowledge, to a situation in which human life is especially at risk of being ignored and devalued. He clarifies and applies the tradition without in any way departing from it.

The allocution also leaves some questions unanswered. For example, it seems clear that the presumption in favor of nutrition and hydration will not apply to imminently dying patients whose ability to benefit from feeding is vanishing. But

---

[40] See Jean deBlois, "Anencephaly and the Management of Pregnancy," *Health Care Ethics USA* 1.4 (Fall 1993): 2–3; Kevin O'Rourke and Jean deBlois, "Induced Delivery of Anencephalic Fetuses: A Response to James L. Walsh and Moira M. McQueen," in *Kennedy Institute of Ethics Journal* 4.1 (March 1994): 47–53; Kevin O'Rourke, "Ethical Opinions in regard to the Question of Early Delivery of Anencephalic Infants," *Linacre Quarterly* 63.3 (1996): 55–59.

[41] *L'Osservatore Romano*, English ed. (September 23, 1998): 6–10.

[42] Kevin D. O'Rourke, "Ms. 'B' and the Vatican," *National Catholic Bioethics Quarterly* 2.4 (Winter 2002): 595–600.

what about patients with progressive chronic ailments, such as Alzheimer's disease, which involve gradually worsening dementia and will ultimately lead to death? Can anything new be said about the point at which burdens outweigh benefits in the feeding of these patients?

Questions also remain about the use of advance directives to refuse procedures such as artificially assisted feeding. The U.S. bishops' *Ethical and Religious Directives* state that a Catholic hospital "will not honor an advance directive that is contrary to Catholic teaching," and adds, "If the advance directive conflicts with Catholic teaching, an explanation should be provided as to why the directive cannot be honored."[43] Should such documents be seen as conflicting with Catholic teaching if they specify refusal of food and fluids in the case of a "vegetative" state?

It seems clear that an advance directive intended simply to ensure death when the patient falls into such a condition is not in accord with Catholic teaching. But what if a person says that he or she would see tube feeding in such a situation as an intrusion that would only aggravate his or her suffering? In this connection, Fr. Ford cites Pope John Paul II's statement that we cannot assume that a patient in a vegetative state cannot feel the suffering of starvation and dehydration. Fr. Ford asks whether this may cut both ways—that is, perhaps the patient can suffer from the perceived burdens of the feeding procedure as well.[44] The Pope's allocution is directed against discriminatory judgments about these patients imposed upon them by others, and does not directly answer this question.

A more immediate and fundamental problem, however, is that many Catholic hospitals may now have protocols based on the "spiritual purposes" standard, so that—even if families consented to assisted feeding for their loved one, or actively requested it—the hospital would deny assisted feeding to the patient in a "vegetative" state, classifying it as "futile care" that should not be provided.

Reviewing the protocols of local Catholic hospitals to ensure their compatibility with the *Ethical and Religious Directives* (as these are clarified and guided by the magisterium of

---

[43] *Ethical and Religious Directives*, 18, directive 24.

[44] Ford, "The Pope on the Moral Obligation to Continue Tube Feeding," 3.

the universal Church) is, of course, the right and duty of the Ordinary of each diocese. The *Directives* already affirm "a presumption in favor of providing nutrition and hydration to all patients, including patients who require medically assisted nutrition and hydration."[45] If a hospital protocol is already generally following that guidance, one need only make sure that the protocol now clearly includes the patient in a "vegetative" state (which for fourteen years has in any case been the recommendation of the U.S. bishops' Pro-Life Committee). Therefore, no bishop need wait for the next formal revision of the *Directives* to remind Catholic hospitals to treat these patients as people with inherent human dignity, covered by the general presumption in favor of providing food and fluids.

Are there signs of an emerging consensus on this issue that will bring all sides together? Such signs do exist in some countries. In Australia, the Catholic bishops' conference and Catholic Health Association produced a joint statement emphasizing their agreement on key features of the Pope's teaching, while noting that not all issues have been resolved.[46] Theologians and ethicists in Canada have signed a similar statement, which grew out of a dialogue conducted at the University of Toronto.[47] The idea of preparing such a consensus statement in the United States may be worth pursuing.

While questions and discussion must surely continue, the core of Pope John Paul II's teaching is crystal clear. Our support for the helpless who would die without our help must extend to all, without discriminatory "quality of life" judgments that would abandon our most mentally disabled brothers and

---

[45] *Ethical and Religious Directives*, 31, directive 58. The directive states that nutrition and hydration should be provided "as long as this is of sufficient benefit to outweigh the burdens involved to the patient." By the "spiritual purposes" standard, however, patients in PVS by definition cannot "benefit" from feeding, so the directive's reference to "all patients" is negated.

[46] Catholic Health Australia, Bishops' Committee for Doctrine and Morals, and Bishops' Committee for Health Care, "Briefing Note on the Obligation to Provide Nutrition and Hydration," http://www.cha.org.au/site.php?id=90.

[47] Colloquium of the Canadian Catholic Bioethics Institute, "Reflections on Artificial Nutrition and Hydration" (July 22, 2004), http://www.utoronto.ca/stmikes/bioethics/Documents/Reflections%20on%20ANH%2004-07-22.pdf; reprinted in *National Catholic Bioethics Quarterly* 4.4 (Winter 2004): 773–782.

sisters as though they were beyond the reach of our love and our care. In the end, the question is not whether these patients are successfully pursuing the spiritual purpose of their lives. It is whether, in order to fulfill the spiritual purpose of our own lives, we need (even at some cost to ourselves) to treat patients in this debilitated condition as our equals in human dignity. It is *our* eternal life that is at stake.

State-Mandated Immoral Procedures in Catholic Facilities

How is Licit Compliance Possible?

Peter J. Cataldo

The goal of this chapter is to examine the question of whether it is morally licit for a Catholic institution to comply with state mandates to provide health insurance for contraceptive drugs and devices, and with mandates to provide so-called "emergency contraception" to women who present in the emergency room.[1] The assumption is often made that any compliance with such mandates is ipso facto contrary to Catholic teaching. There are a growing number of states with mandates for contraception insurance coverage and for anovulatory hormonal treatment of survivors of sexual assault. This fact, together with the refusal by courts to recognize religious exemptions, behooves us to consider whether compliance with these mandates can be consistent with Catholic teaching.

---

[1] The term "emergency contraception" is not morally accurate, because use of these drugs in the treatment of survivors of sexual assault is not for the prevention of pregnancy resulting from consensual sex, as the term "contraception" implies. Rather, the anovulatory hormonal agents are used for the purpose of self-defense.

With respect to the question of contraceptive insurance mandates, it is important to note that my analysis pertains only to those situations in which a Catholic employer has no practicable alternative to avoid compliance with a mandate. This analysis will in part explore the grounds in the Catholic moral tradition for compliance with a contraceptive insurance mandate when, for example, attempts at securing a legal exemption from the mandate have failed, self-insuring is not financially feasible, and there is no option to exclude contraceptive coverage from the employer's health plan but retain other drug benefits.

Contraceptive Insurance Mandates

Within a five-year period, from 1998 to 2003, twenty states enacted laws that require employers who offer insurance coverage for drugs to include prescription contraceptives. This coverage typically includes both oral contraceptives and contraceptive devices.[2] In 1998, a federal law was enacted requiring insurance coverage of contraceptives for insurance plans that participate in the Federal Employees Health Benefits Program.[3] The state mandates that provide conscience clauses for exemption from the law range from narrowly defined to more broadly defined exemptions. The mandates typically pertain to any individual or group health plan issued or renewed in the state, and any combination of health plans, contracts between subscriber and employer, and contracts between health insurance carriers and employers issued or renewed in the state. What is mandated is coverage for contraceptive drugs and devices that have been approved by the U.S. Food and Drug Administration and, in some cases, any

---

[2] See Cynthia Dailard, "Contraceptive Coverage: A 10-Year Retrospective," *The Guttmacher Report on Public Policy* 7.2 (June 2004): 8. The states are Maryland, California, Connecticut, Georgia, Hawaii, Maine, Nevada, New Hampshire, North Carolina, Vermont, Delaware, Iowa, Rhode Island, Missouri, New Mexico, Washington, Arizona, Massachusetts, New York, and Illinois. Two additional states, Arkansas and West Virginia, enacted contraceptive mandate legislation in 2005; see Guttmacher Institute, "Contraceptive Coverage Mandates," *State Center—Monthly State Update: Major Developments in 2005* (October 2005), http://www.guttmacher.org/statecenter/updates/archive.html.

[3] Dailard, 8.

medical support associated with these drugs and devices. The mandates also apply only to fully insured employers, not to self-insured employers. Catholic employers who are self-insured may avoid cooperation in contraception all together. My analysis pertains only to fully insured Catholic employers.

The Principle of Cooperation

Does a Catholic employer engage in illicit cooperation in the evil of contraception by complying with a state mandate for insurance coverage of contraceptives? A brief sketch of the principle of cooperation will help us better understand how the principle may be applied to this question. The principle of cooperation in the Catholic moral tradition is a guide for evaluating the moral status of an action of a person who knowingly and freely assists in some specific way in the morally evil act of another person. The person who assists in this manner is called the "cooperator" and the person who receives the assistance is called the "principal agent." The cooperator and the principal agent may be individuals or corporate persons (institutions). The principle of cooperation validly applies to institutions to the extent that they act as corporate persons and engage in activity which provides assistance in the immoral acts of other institutions or individuals. There may be differences in the kind of assistance morally allowed by an individual and an institution under the principle of cooperation, but this fact reflects a difference in the nature of the cooperators, not evidence that the principle is unsuitable for evaluating institutions.

The principle divides cooperation into two major categories: formal and material. Cooperation is formal if the cooperator intends the evil act of the principal agent. Formal cooperation is explicit if the cooperator directly intends the evil act. It is implicit if the cooperator intends a good end but accomplishes that end by intending the principal agent's act as a means. Implicit formal cooperation may establish the very conditions by which the principal agent's act is possible. Institutions are particularly susceptible to this problem, for example, when Catholic health-care institutions negotiate a collaborative agreement that secures direct sterilizations at the facility of a non-Catholic partner. In this way, an institution intends the sterilizations for the sake of some good end by establishing the conditions which make the sterilizations possible. Formal cooperation in evil is never morally permissible, and institutions are particularly susceptible because their corporate actions necessarily represent an institutional intentionality.

Material cooperation, by contrast, does not intend the principal agent's act. The material cooperator's act is in itself good or morally indifferent, but the principal agent appropriates the cooperator's act in some way. Material cooperation may be morally tolerable, depending on what type it is and on the reasons for it. Immediate material cooperation is any contribution to the essential circumstances of the principal agent's act. Immediate material cooperation by an institution in direct sterilization is never morally permissible.[4] Mediate material cooperation is any assistance to the nonessential circumstances of the principal agent's act; it may be either proximate or remote. The graver the evil of the principal agent's act, the greater the good that must be achieved or the graver the evil that must be avoided, as a proportionate reason for tolerating the mediate material cooperation.

By offering health insurance plans that include coverage for contraceptives, Catholic employers contribute to the conditions that allow employees greater financial access to contraceptives. There are two ways in which a Catholic employer enables an employee or others on the employee's plan to obtain and then make use of these drugs: (1) by paying premiums to insurance carriers for drug formularies that include covered contraceptives, and (2) by making payments for contraceptives claims by employees. Without such insurance, employees might not otherwise be able to obtain contraceptives, or might be able to obtain them only with difficulty. Thus, a Catholic employer can provide a form of assistance to contraceptive acts that may be evaluated according to the principle of cooperation.

Compliance That Avoids Formal Cooperation

Is it possible for a Catholic institution to avoid formal cooperation under these circumstances? If the Catholic employer agrees to cover contraceptives in its carrier contracts and offers insurance coverage for contraceptives in its health plan literature without qualification or disclaimer, then it can

---

[4] See U.S. Conference of Catholic Bishops, *Ethical and Religious Directives for Catholic Health Care Services*, 4th ed. (Washington, DC: USCCB, 2001), n. 70.

hardly claim not to intend that to which it explicitly agrees. Moreover, if a Catholic employer establishes a rider on its health plan for the purpose of allowing its employees to pay separately for contraceptives, the employer engages in implicit formal cooperation. In order to achieve the good end of retaining employees, the Catholic employer in this instance intends the access to contraceptives secured by the rider as a means to that end.

One way for a Catholic employer to demonstrate that it does not intend the evil of contraception is to include in its carrier contracts and its health plan literature a clear disclaimer that repudiates any agreement with contraception. I have elsewhere suggested the following disclaimer language:

> Any benefits covered by this plan which are related to contraception are provided solely and exclusively by reason of legal requirement as set forth in [legislative act information]. Contraception is contrary to Catholic moral teaching and [name of employer] does not endorse, approve, or intend contraception by complying with the aforementioned legal mandate.[5]

Such a disclaimer indicates that the government is appropriating the Catholic employer's practice of offering morally appropriate health insurance as a matter of justice for purposes the employer does not intend. The employer intends justice, not contraception, and does not even implicitly intend contraception, because it is the state that establishes the conditions by which individuals are enabled to use contraceptives purchased through a health plan. However, use of a disclaimer is not alone sufficient to show that an employer does not intend contraception.

Another indicator of intent is the presence or absence of efforts to secure legal relief from a contraceptive mandate. Pursuit of a legal exemption is independent evidence that alternatives to compliance are preferable.[6] Such efforts should be legally and financially practicable, but some attempt to avoid this extrinsic coercion should be made either singly or together

---

[5] Peter J. Cataldo, "Compliance with Contraceptive Insurance Mandates: Licit or Illicit Cooperation in Evil?" *National Catholic Bioethics Quarterly* 4.1 (Spring 2004): 108.

[6] Other evidence that a Catholic employer does not intend contraception would include the implementation of policies that promote natural family planning and prohibit direct sterilization.

with other Catholic parties. If a Catholic employer refuses to include a disclaimer, establishes a rider for contraceptives, and does not pursue a legal exemption, there would appear to be grounds for formal cooperation.

It might be objected that the solution proposed here to avoid formal cooperation is not valid because it is not possible for an institution to have an intention. Because an institution is incapable of forming intentions, there is no basis on which to assess its compliance with a contraceptive mandate in terms of formal cooperation. Moreover, an institution's lack of any capacity for intentions would entail the broader conclusion that it is not legitimate to apply any part of the principle of cooperation to institutions—neither formal nor material cooperation is validly assessed. This objection does not recognize the validity of treating an institution as a legal person for the purposes of morally assessing its cooperation in evil.

A full response to this objection cannot be provided here. However, two essential points may be identified. First, acknowledging that an institution can assist in the immoral act of another institution or an individual, or that the cooperative actions of an institution may be assessed according to the principle of cooperation, presumes that an institution is a legal person as distinct from a natural person. A legal person is also called a moral, juridic, or corporate person. The legal person exists as a construct of the law (or in the case of juridic persons in the Church, legal persons exist both by law and by a special decree of a competent ecclesiastical authority[7]). There is a long history of the idea of legal personhood, which dates back to Hammurabi's code and includes Roman law, canon law, and modern civil law.[8] For example, Roman law recognized the *res publica,* or public thing, as a legal person.[9] Canon law contains separate sets of canons on physical and juridical persons respectively, and defines juridic persons in this way: "In the Church, besides physical persons, there are

---

[7] See *Code of Canon Law*, chap. II, can. 114, sec. 1 at http://www.vatican.va/archive/ENG1104/__PD.HTM.

[8] See Adam J. Maida and Nicholas P. Cafardi, *Church Property, Church Finances, and Church-Related Corporations: A Canon Law Handbook* (St. Louis: Catholic Health Association, 1984), 21–22. On p. 28, notes 1 and 2 cite Harry G. Henn, *Handbook of the Law of Corporations* (St. Paul, MN: West Publishing Company, 1970), regarding historical claims about Hammurabi's code and Roman law.

[9] Maida and Cafardi, 21.

also juridic persons, that is, subjects in canon law of obligations and rights which correspond to their nature."[10]

> Juridic persons are constituted either by the prescript of law or by special grant of competent authority given through a decree. They are aggregates of persons (*universitates personarum*) or of things (*universitates rerum*) ordered for a purpose which is in keeping with the mission of the Church and which transcends the purpose of the individuals.[11]

Canon law also divides juridic persons into many different types, including dioceses and parishes. The important canonical functioning of dioceses and parishes would not be possible if they were not treated as juridic persons.

As in canon law, the corporate person in civil law has legal obligations and duties and may, analogous to natural persons, incur liability, enter into contracts, own property, and sue and be sued, among other things. During the late nineteenth and early twentieth centuries, there was a robust debate among legal scholars about the meaning of corporate personality and its implications at law.[12] Three theories of the corporate person emerged in the debate, which are generally known as the fiction, aggregate, and real entity theories. The role of the corporate person was especially evident in torts during this period. Jonathan Kahn points out that torts increasingly "involved attributing responsibility to corporate actors just as we do to natural persons.... When applied to corporations, the law of torts implicate[d] an understanding of the corporate person as having will and volition."[13]

What the history of the idea of the corporate person indicates is that all notions of the corporate person interpret the action of a corporation or a juridic person as being analogous to human action. This is the second important point in

---

[10] *Code of Canon Law*, chap. II, can. 113, sec. 2.

[11] Ibid., chap. II, can. 114, sec. 1.

[12] For examples of recent legal scholarship on the debate, see Katsuhito Iwai, "Persons, Things and Corporations: The Corporate Personality Controversy and Comparative Corporate Governance," *American Journal of Comparative Law* 47 (Fall 1999): 583–632; and Michael J. Phillips, "Reappraising the Real Entity Theory of the Corporation," *Florida State University Law Review* 21 (Spring 1994): 1061–1123.

[13] Jonathan Kahn, "Product Liability and the Politics of Corporate Presence: Identity and Accountability in *MacPherson v. Buick*," *Loyola of Los Angeles Law Review* 35.1 (November 2001): 17–19.

response to the objection that the principle of cooperation does not validly apply to institutions and corporations.

Qualities of human action such as purposiveness, intentionality, and foresight are analogously predicated of an institution or cooperation in various ways in order to achieve either a legal or a moral evaluation of the actions associated with these entities.[14] The diversity of opinion regarding the idea of the corporate person notwithstanding, the reality is that corporations are social entities which act collectively, and in view of this fact corporate actions (made in the name of the corporation) may be assessed morally.[15] Corporations act, and insofar as they act, their actions may be evaluated as good or evil, just or unjust, for natural and corporate persons. The fact that the moral concepts and principles used to evaluate corporate actions are the same as those used to assess the actions of natural persons does not mean that those concepts and principles as applied to corporations necessarily reflect a natural significance. Thus, to determine that a Catholic health-care corporation engages in formal cooperation is to claim that there is (1) a corporate act (however defined) which (2) assists in evil, and (3) provides the assistance intentionally. The

---

[14] St. Thomas Aquinas gives an apt example in the Catholic moral tradition of how the qualities of being a man may be analogously predicated of other entities. In the course of explaining the transmission of original sin, for example, Aquinas makes an analogous predication of the term man (*homo*): "All men born of Adam may be considered as one man, inasmuch as they have one common nature, which they receive from their first parents; even as in civil matters, all who are members of one community are reputed as one body, and the whole community as one man." He proceeds to show how this analogy explains the voluntary character of original sin in each individual man. Thomas Aquinas, *Summa Theologica*, trans. Fathers of the English Dominican Province (Westminster, MD: Christian Classics, 1981), I-II, Q. 81.2, body.

[15] Even if one argues, as John Dewey did, that corporate personhood is illegitimate because the traditional idea of personality is illegitimate, one may still hold to the reality of corporate action. See, for example, "Corporate Personality" in *John Dewey: The Later Works*, 1925–1953: vol. 2, 1925–1927, ed. Jo Ann Boydston (Carbondale, IL: Southern Illinois University Press, 1984), 22–43. See also "The Public and Its Problems," 354: "A corporation as such is an integrated collective mode of action having powers, rights, duties, and immunities different from those of its singular members *in their other connections*," original emphasis.

intention is a means-end ordering which may exist to differing degrees in the minds of the natural members of the corporation, but it also exists in legal agreements of the corporation. This means-end ordering in a corporation is different from its presence in a natural person, whose intellect and will are the sources of the ordering, but it is like what is present in a natural person insofar as it *is* a means-end ordering. Recent Catholic moral teaching has recognized the reality of institutional formal cooperation. This occurred when the Congregation for the Doctrine of the Faith explicitly evaluated the cooperation by Catholic health-care institutions in direct sterilization by using the principle of cooperation.[16] The analogous application of moral principles to a corporation does not depend on viewing the corporation as a natural person. If acts can have corporate identity, there are sufficient grounds to identify assistance in evil when it occurs in corporate acts and provide a moral assessment of such assistance.

Complying with Justified Material Cooperation

We are left with the question of whether compliance with a contraceptive insurance mandate is justified on the basis of material cooperation. First, by complying with a mandate, a Catholic employer does not engage in immediate material cooperation in contraception. Offering coverage for contraceptives and paying claims for contraceptives under a health plan does not contribute the essential circumstances of an act of contraception. The essential circumstances are supplied by the physician, who writes a prescription for the correct drug and dosage, and by the pharmacist, whose actions are an extension of the physician's action.

Providing greater financial access to contraceptives through a health plan contributes a nonessential circumstance to any acts of contraception that may result from an employee using contraceptives purchased through the plan. This fact makes any cooperation mediate material. Moreover, the fact that there are numerous intervening causes between the action of the employer and the contraceptive acts of the employee makes the cooperation remote mediate material cooperation.

---

[16] See Congregation for the Doctrine of the Faith, "Reply on Sterilization in Catholic Hospitals" [*Quaecumque Sterilizatio*], March 13, 1975.

In order to understand why this mediate material cooperation is justified, several other factors must be considered.

Mediate material cooperation represents neither a positive value nor a positive obligation. Rather, it is a limiting principle, as is the whole principle of cooperation, which under the right circumstances at best allows a toleration of assisting in the evil of another. The manualists argued that material cooperation, considered in itself, simply as assistance in the evil act of another person, is illicit.[17] The evil effect which material cooperation brings about has traditionally been considered contrary to the virtue of charity and the obligation to help our neighbor do good rather than evil. The principle of cooperation ensures that the immoral effects of material cooperation are merely tolerated for proportionate reasons, not affirmed or intended. In this regard, material cooperation has traditionally been considered an application of the principle of the double effect to the cooperator.[18] The great goods proportionate to the remote mediate material cooperation resulting from compliance with a mandate include the obligations of justice.

A Catholic employer is obligated in justice to assist its employees secure health care in the only way practicable in modern society. Another good preserved is the very mission of the employer and the good work that it accomplishes in the community, which might otherwise be in real jeopardy if the employer cannot attract individuals to carry out its work because of a lack of health-care benefits. At the same time that a Catholic employer preserves these goods because of its remote mediate material cooperation, it avoids the evils of injustice and the elimination of its apostolate.

If cooperation in contraception through governmental mandates avoids formal cooperation, and is justified remote mediate material cooperation, it nevertheless remains a substantial burden on the religious belief of Catholic employers. The analysis I present here disagrees with the moral assumption of legal arguments against contraceptive mandates that compliance with a mandate ipso facto represents illicit cooperation in contraception.[19] While it is true that mandates

---

[17] See Cataldo, "Compliance," 124–126.

[18] Ibid., 126.

[19] See, for example, *Catholic Charities of Sacramento, Inc. v. Superior Court of the State of California*, no. S099822, Supreme Court of the State of California (November 13, 2001).

place a substantial burden on the religious beliefs of a Catholic employer, such a substantial burden is not exclusively associated with illicit cooperation. The fact that a Catholic institution may be able to justify remote mediate material cooperation does not necessarily entail the absence of a substantial burden in its cooperation. The burden of justified material cooperation, albeit morally tolerable, may be of such a magnitude as to ground a legal claim for an exemption from a contraceptive mandate.[20]

In fact, as we have seen, the moral permissibility of institutional cooperation is due to the substantial goods and evils that are at stake. The very nature of justified material cooperation as the toleration of evil hinges on the fact that the cooperator is substantially burdened, and without this burden, there is no justifiable reason for material cooperation. Legal arguments that equate the substantial burden of contraceptive mandates with illicit cooperation might preclude the only consistent moral grounds on which Catholic institutions may cooperate, should attempts for legal relief from the mandates ultimately fail. The moral burden on Catholic employers is not restricted to their assistance in the evil of contraception, but includes their inability to meet obligations of justice, and possibly remain in existence if they do not offer a drug benefit.

The moral burdens that Catholic institutions bear under the pressure of contraceptive mandates consist of both burdens resulting from compliance with a mandate and burdens resulting from discontinuance of drug benefits. In either case, contraceptive mandates are the cause of substantial moral burdens to the religious and moral tenets of Catholic employers. Each set of burdens in its own way justifies remote mediate material cooperation and forms the moral basis for seeking a legal exemption.

Unintentionally assisting in the evil of contraception to preserve great goods and avoid great evils does not represent illicit cooperation in this instance, but rather proportionate reasons for the mediate material cooperation. At the same time, contributing to evil, even in a mediate material way, is something that a Catholic employer would rather not do; this, together with forsaking what is just for its employees and possibly jeopardizing the continuance of Catholic health care, are all moral reasons for seeking a legal exemption. Moreover, such

---

[20] See Cataldo, "Compliance," 113–129.

legal efforts further indicate that an institution does not intend the evil of contraception, and they help avoid theological scandal. For these reasons, failure of the legal efforts does not necessitate that institutions refrain from compliance.

"Emergency Contraception" and Abortion

A related but different question of cooperation involving Catholic health-care providers concerns state mandates that health-care providers to give information about so-called "emergency contraception," or dispense these drugs on request for survivors of sexual assault who present in emergency rooms. As of April 2005, four states (California, New Mexico, New York, and Washington) had laws requiring emergency rooms both to provide information about anovulants for the prevention of pregnancy after sexual assault, and to dispense these drugs on request. Illinois required only that information about these drugs be provided, and South Carolina required only that the drugs be dispensed on request.[21]

A Catholic health-care institution does not cooperate in contraception by dispensing anovulants to survivors of sexual assault because, morally, the use of these drugs under these circumstances is an act of self-defense, not contraception. An essential component of the immorality of contraception is that the man and woman freely engage in sexual intercourse contrary to the nature of the act. Catholic moral teaching has always held that if individuals have free control over their procreative powers, then that freedom obligates them to use those powers according to their truth, i.e., according to the inseparability of their unitive and procreative meanings. The element of freedom in the use of the procreative powers is absent for the survivor of sexual assault. Therefore, to assist the survivor in preventing the unjust integration of the survivor's and attacker's fertility by using anovulants does not constitute illicit cooperation on the part of the institution.

Does a Catholic institution illicitly cooperate in any possible abortifacient effect of these drugs by either treating the survivor with these drugs under a mandate, or by transferring the patient

---

[21] The Alan Guttmacher Institute, "State Policies in Brief: Access to Emergency Contraception as of April 1, 2005," http://www. guttmacher.org/statecenter/spibs/spib_EC.pdf, updated monthly.

to another health-care provider prior to administering the drugs? This moral question is not the same as the question of the need for ovulation testing in the administration of anovulants to survivors of sexual assault. The issue of testing deserves separate consideration and is examined by Father Albert Moraczewski, O.P., in another chapter.

It is sufficient for the purposes of this article to state that reasonable efforts should be made to reduce the risk of a possible abortifacient effect resulting from the administration of a high-dose anovulant in the treatment of sexual assault survivors. Mandates that require the provision of anovulants on demand do not allow for sufficient efforts to reduce the risk of a possible abortifacient effect. Therefore, a Catholic hospital that complies with such a mandate engages in immediate material cooperation in any abortifacient effect that might occur. This is so because it contributes to the essential circumstances of an evil act, and because it has not taken measures which ensure that any possible abortifacient effect would be reasonably unforeseen.

As I have indicated, all of the current state mandates require that hospitals provide information about the use of anovulants for the treatment of sexual assault survivors. Certainly, if this information is provided in a neutral manner, then the act of conveying the information can be justified mediate material cooperation. However, if hospital personnel were to present information about the possible effect of preventing implantation in a manner that describes this effect as a benefit, the hospital would commit formal cooperation.

What if the patient is transferred to another hospital after receiving this information? Does a Catholic hospital engage in illicit cooperation in any possible abortifacient effect from the drugs used by the woman? If the hospital transfers the care of the patient to another facility and does not make a specific referral to a physician for the administration of the drug in question, then there is no illicit cooperation. The Catholic hospital would not necessarily be transferring the patient for the specific purpose of receiving the drug and would not contribute to any of the essential circumstances of a possible abortifacient act.

A final comment may be made about possible legal mandates requiring Catholic hospitals to perform direct abortions in their own facilities. The sole immediate effect of the procedure is the taking of innocent human life either before or after viability. A Catholic hospital that allows abortion un-der a mandate may be able to avoid formal cooperation but cannot avoid immediate material cooperation in the direct kill-ing of an innocent human being. The hospital contributes to some of the essential circumstances of the principal agent's act, such as providing personnel and equipment, and thereby engages in immediate material cooperation. Even if independent personnel and outside equipment were used, the proximity of involvement by the hospital staff, the fact that the Catholic facility is used, and the potential for scandal in this most grave evil would be reasons to prohibit this coop-eration. Indeed, directive 45 of the *Ethical and Religious Direc-tives for Catholic Health Care Services* states:

> Catholic health care institutions are not to provide abortion services, even based on the principle of material cooperation. In this context, Catholic health care institu-tions need to be concerned about the danger of scandal in any association with abortion providers.

Currently, forty-six states have conscience protection for institutions and individuals against providing abortions,[22] and President Bush signed a Labor/Health and Human Services appropriations bill for fiscal year 2005 which denies these funds to states that mandate the provision, payment, coverage, or referral of abortions.[23] These facts notwithstanding, Catholic health-care institutions need to remain vigilant on the issue of state-mandated provision of abortion.

Conclusion

Compliance by Catholic health-care institutions with mandates for contraception insurance and for the treatment of sexual assault survivors need not necessarily entail illicit cooperation. Measures may be taken to avoid illicit cooperation and to tolerate justified material cooperation. However, in all

---

[22] The Protection of Conscience Project, "United States Protec-tion of Conscience Laws," http://www.consciencelaws.org/Con-science-Laws-USA/Conscience-Laws-USA-01a.html.

[23] See Consolidated Appropriations Act, Public Law 108–447, Sec. 508 (d) (1), 2005: "None of the funds made available in this Act may be made available to a Federal agency or program, or to a State or local government, if such agency, program, or government subjects any institutional or individual health care entity to discrimination on the basis that the health care entity does not provide, pay for, provide coverage of, or refer for abortions."

cases, every reasonable attempt should be made to seek legal exemptions from such mandates on the basis of three factors: the nature of material cooperation, the substantial burden that toleration with the mandates creates, and the need to avoid theological scandal. It is important to note that cooperation, which has been determined to be morally licit may nevertheless be the occasion for insurmountable scandal for individuals or as a political matter.[24]

---

[24] See *Ethical and Religious Directives*, n. 71.

THE EVOLVING PRACTICE OF ORGAN DONATION

Francis L. Delmonico, M.D.

Fifty years have elapsed since the historic kidney transplantation from an identical twin performed by Dr. Joseph Murray at the Peter Bent Brigham Hospital in Boston.[1] In 1954, Richard Herrick was diagnosed with kidney failure, and his brother Ronald was found to be a genetically identical twin by a novel medical approach. Skin grafts were exchanged between the brothers as surrogate preliminary transplants to assure the Brigham team that Richard would not reject his brother's kidney. Without the kidney transplant, Richard would die, because there was no dialysis treatment at that time. Richard did eventually die within ten years of the transplant, but Ronald is still alive today. This courageous donor is the living testimony of a hero who underwent an operative procedure for the benefit of his brother that he might live.

Recent Developments

Kidney transplantation was slow to develop as a field because few people with kidney failure have identical twins who could be organ donors. Even with the introduction of immuno-

[1] M. J. Friedrich, "Joseph Murray—Transplantation Pioneer," *Journal of the American Medical Association* 292.24 (December 22, 2004): 2957–2958.

suppression, fifteen years after the Herrick transplant the initial kidney transplants performed from live donors required the donors to be genetically identical to the recipients for success to be remotely possible. Nevertheless, at some prominent medical centers in the 1970s, transplants from live donors were prohibited because of the potential donor risks (including donor death). Most transplant centers relied on kidneys obtained from deceased donors.

Over the past three decades, however, the practice of transplantation has steadily evolved to make live kidney transplantation safe and the most common organ transplant performed around the world. Reports from the United Network for Organ Sharing, the federally contracted organization that oversees the practice of transplantation in the United States, show that in the year 2001, the number of live organ donors surpassed that of deceased donors in this country.[2] There have not been a sufficient number of deceased donors to meet the ever-increasing need of patients requiring a transplant. Today, there are more than eighty thousand people on the waiting list.

With this continuing need for organs, it is no surprise that patients on the list for a kidney transplant are asking spouses and friends to be donors. The survival of kidney transplants from so-called unrelated donors is now known to be just as good as the outcome achieved from a genetically matched sibling, parent, or child. The percentage of donors who are unrelated to recipients—spouses, friends, and even strangers—has increased to more than 20 percent. In other words, one in five donors is unrelated to the recipient; the donor and recipient have no genetic identity between them whatsoever, and yet the outcome is excellent. Transplant programs are aware of the change in the acceptance of live-donor transplantation, and as a result the following standard has been realized: anyone who is medically suitable and properly motivated can be a live kidney donor.

The other advance in transplantation that has propelled live donation is the surgical technique of laparoscopic nephrectomy. Thirty years ago, physicians embarking on this field would not have contemplated the donor operation performed in this way. This innovation has made the procedure much more acceptable to living donors. Surgeons who perform laparoscopic nephrectomy watch their dissection on a television screen.

---

[2] Based on data from the Organ Procurement and Transplantation Network/UNOS Registry as of October 28, 2005.

The abdominal cavity is filled with gas, so that the viscera come away from the abdominal wall, allowing the kidney to be seen more clearly. The operative dissection is made with instruments passed through tiny holes made in the abdominal wall. Once the kidney has been separated from its attachments, it is passed through a small incision, large enough to accommodate the size of the kidney being removed.

The advantage of the laparoscopic procedure is that the donor may go home the day after kidney removal and should be able to return to daily life within a week. The laparoscopic method is a marked improvement over the nephrectomy procedure that involves removal a portion of a rib. By the classical approach, kidney donation used to take three to four weeks for the donor to recover and return to work. The advances in this technical procedure and the improvements in immunosuppression are the key developments that have enabled successful transplantation from unrelated donors and have propelled live-donor transplantation to the extent it is practiced today.

Some Extraordinary Examples

Organ transplantation is not limited by the gender of the donor or the donor's ethnicity. A modern-day example is the case of Warren Brown, a black man, who received a kidney from his friend Martha McNeal Hamilton, a white woman, who had worked with him at the Washington Post for many years.[3] The disparities of gender and ethnicity are quite evident, and yet the transplant was successful.

In another example of extraordinary goodness, Harold Mintz gave his kidney to Gennet Belay, who had been on the waiting list for ten years.[4] He came forward and said he would like to give his kidney to anybody who needed it. This transplant was possible because there is no longer any requirement for genetic identity between the donor and recipient, as there was in 1954 with Dr. Murray and the Herrick twins. Harold gave a kidney to a stranger whom he had never met before in his life.

---

[3] See Martha McNeil Hamilton and Warren Brown, *Black and White and Red All Over: The Story of a Friendship* (New York: Perseus Books, 2002).

[4] Juliet Crichton and Courtney Clarke, "Altruistic Hokies: Making a Motto Meaningful," *Virginia Tech Magazine* 25.2 (Winter 2003), http://www.vtmagazine.vt.edu/winter03/feature2.html.

Kidney transplantation has every likelihood of success as long as the donor and recipient are blood-type and immunologically compatible. "Immunologically compatible" denotes the absence in the recipient of antibodies to the donor that would be detected in a test-tube crossmatch. The crossmatch mixes the recipient's serum with the donor's white blood cells. If antibodies that are reactive with the HLA antigens of the recipient (antibodies that can arise after a blood transfusion or pregnancy) are detected in the crossmatch, the transplant is not performed, because the recipient would immediately reject the kidney.

Until recently, transplant centers have not permitted a live donor to give a kidney to a blood-type incompatible recipient. But blood-type incompatibilities are no longer contraindications to successful kidney transplantation, because protocols have been developed to enable paired live donations or exchanges of kidneys from live donors who are compatible with the recipients. So, for example, if donor A wishes to give his kidney to his wife B and cannot because they are blood-type incompatible, donor A can request that he give his kidney to a compatible person—for example, recipient D—if donor C (who is incompatible with recipient D) is willing to donate a kidney to recipient B.

Such an exchange of kidneys has been endorsed by the medical community via publication in the *New England Journal of Medicine*.[5] Robin wanted to give a kidney to her husband, Tracy. She is an A blood type, he is a B blood-type—a biological obstacle that would cause Tracy to reject Robin's kidney. Susanna wanted to give her kidney to her husband, Rosario. She is a B, he is an A—the reverse incompatibility. What if Susanna and Robin each simultaneously gave a kidney to the other's husband? That is what they did, and the transplants were successful.[6]

---

[5] Francis L. Delmonico, M.D., "Exchanging Kidneys—Advances in Living-Donor Transplantation," *New England Journal of Medicine* 350.18 (April 29, 2004), 1812–1814, and de Klerk et al., "Donor Exchange for Renal Transplantation," *New England Journal of Medicine* 351.9 (August 26, 2004), 935–937.

[6] Scott Allen, "Cross-Donor System Planned for Region's Kidney Patients," *Boston Globe*, June 5, 2004, http://www.boston.com/news/nation/articles/2004/06/05/cross_donor_system_planned_for_regions_kidney/.

This kind of exchange can be successful in transplants performed at different institutions, where each donor is in an operating room adjacent to the recipient and the transplants take place simultaneously. These transplants can even defy social and cultural obstacles. In the Middle East, a live-donor exchange has occurred between Arab and Israeli families.

Live-donor transplantation is not restricted to kidneys. The liver has become another organ for live transplantation, in the absence of livers recovered from deceased donors. The liver is a bi-lobed organ with left and right lobes. A lobe of a donor's liver can be removed and transplanted to a recipient, if a sufficient mass of liver is transplanted to the recipient in need and a sufficient mass of liver is retained in the donor to survive. Right-lobe and left-lobe liver transplants are being done from deceased and from live donors. In general, a left-lobe transplant is done for a child, because not as much mass is needed for the transplant, but for an adult a right-lobe transplant is done.

Problems with live-donor liver transplants are challenging the transplant community to make the procedure safe for donors. There have been three deaths among living liver donors in the United States, and fourteen around the world.[7] Because live organ donors are perfectly healthy, the death of a donor is a tragedy of incomprehensible dimension. Nevertheless, live organ donation will continue despite the dangers, because there are not enough deceased-donor organs.

Buying and Selling Organs

The success of live kidney donation has created an international scandal of immense proportions. The fact that a donor no longer needs to be a family member has led to the creation of markets in kidney sales. Poor people in developing countries are selling their kidneys to affluent recipients through brokers in distant locations such as the Middle East. An industry has developed that promotes a "transplant tourism," attracting recipients from the United States to the Philippines, Pakistan, and South Africa for their transplants. For example, a woman from Brooklyn went to Durban, South Africa, to receive a kidney from a Brazilian man through a broker in Tel

---

[7] Denise Grady, "Death of Donor Halts Some Transplants," *New York Times*, January 16, 2002.

Aviv.[8] Not all governments agree that vendor kidney sales are unethical. In Iran, the government has a regulated market for kidney sales.

In the United States, it is against the law to buy and sell kidneys. In June 2003, there was a congressional hearing about financial incentives to increase organ donation, chaired by James Greenwood (R-Pa). Some members of Congress wanted to add a financial motivation to encourage deceased organ donations. Testimony on behalf of the National Kidney Foundation before the Greenwood panel may have influenced Congress to preserve the National Organ Transplant Act,[9] which prohibits any person from knowingly acquiring, receiving, or otherwise transferring "any human organ for valuable consideration for use in human transplantation."

Despite this direction from Congress, the availability and use of the Internet in everyday life have added a more complex dimension to the potential sale of organs. Vendors can be identified via market brokers on the Internet, to enable the purchase of a kidney in South Africa, Pakistan, the Philippines, and South America. The field of organ transplantation has become a victim of its own success, since vendors no longer have to be genetically related to the recipients who purchase the kidneys for transplantation.

At the Web site matchingdonors.com, anyone who needs a kidney can place his name on the site for thirty days for $295. Potential donors can then go to the Internet site and offer their kidneys. Matchingdonors.com is not fundamentally unethical. Society cannot legislate how we develop relationships. But an opportunity for vendors to come forward is created by Internet sites, and it poses an additional burden on transplant centers to assess the motivations of donors to determine whether they are altruistic. In October 2005, a Colorado man connected over the Internet with a donor from Tennessee.[10] On the surface, the intentions of the donor seemed altruistic, but a subsequent media report revealed that the

---

[8] Larry Rohter, "Tracking the Sale of a Kidney on a Path of Poverty and Hope," *New York Times*, May 23, 2004.

[9] National Organ Transplant Act of 1984, Public Law 98-507, *U.S. Statutes at Large* 98 (1984): 2339–2348.

[10] Laurie Barclay, M.D., "Brokering Organ Transplants on the Internet Raises Ethical Issues," *Medscape Medical News*, October 25, 2004, http://www.medscape.com/viewarticle/491837.

kidney donor was wanted for child support.[11] This news story illustrated the potential hazards for recipients whose live donors are identified through the Internet. The psychosocial evaluation of all live donors has become an important standard of live-donor assessment.

Deceased Organ Donation

To promote deceased organ donation, a uniform definition of death that is legally accepted in every country is most needed. Not all cultures accept the concept of determining death by neurological criteria. Death can be pronounced either by the irreversible cessation of all functions of the entire brain, including the brain stem, or by the irreversible cessation of circulatory or respiratory function.

At the International Congress of Transplantation in 2000, Pope John Paul II read a statement to congress participants that affirmed the practice of deceased organ donation and the concept of determination of death by neurological criteria:

> Acknowledgement of the unique dignity of the human person has a further underlying consequence: *vital organs which occur singly in the body* [e.g., heart, liver] *can be removed only after death,* that is from the body of someone who is certainly dead. This requirement is self-evident, since to act otherwise would mean intentionally to cause the death of the donor in disposing of his organs. This gives rise to one of the most debated issues in contemporary bioethics ... I refer to the problem of *ascertaining the fact of death.* When can a person be considered dead with complete certainly?[12]

The Pope responded directly to that question with the following:

> In this regard, it is helpful to recall that *the death of the person* is a single event, consisting in the total disintegration of that unitary and integrated whole that is the personal self. It results from the separation of the life principle (or soul) from the corporal reality of the person. The death of the person, understood in this primary sense, is

---

[11] Associated Press, "Kidney Donor Wanted for Child Support," *USA Today*, October 23, 2004, http://www.usatoday.com/news/nation/2004-10-23-internet-kideney-cs_x.htm.

[12] John Paul II, "Address to the International Congress on Transplants," August 29, 2000, n. 4, original emphasis.

an event which *no scientific technique or empirical method can identify directly.*

Yet human experience shows that once death occurs, *certain biological signs inevitability follow,* which medicine has learned to recognize with increasing precision. In this sense, the "criteria" for ascertaining death used by medicine today should not be understood as the technical-scientific determination of the *exact moment* of the person's death, but as a scientifically secure means of identifying *the biological signs that a person has indeed died.*[13]

Pope John Paul II subscribed to the concept of brain death when he noted:

it is a well-known fact that for some time certain scientific approaches to ascertaining death have shifted the emphasis from traditional cardiorespiratory signs to the so-called *"neurological"* criterion. Specifically, this consists in establishing, according to clearly determined parameters..., the complete and irreversible cessation of all brain activity (in the cerebrum, cerebellum, and brain stem).[14]

Death by neurological criteria is determined by not only the loss of cortical function but also the loss of brain stem function. Someone has to have suffered irreversible loss of cortical function and the capacity to breathe spontaneously in order to be declared brain dead. When death is declared by the irreversible absence of brain function, organs can be recovered even though the heart is still beating.

As to support for the recovery of organs from non-heart-beating donors, the Pope noted in his statement that death can be determined by traditional cardiorespiratory assessment. There can then be donation after cardiac death. In this instance, organs are recovered after the heart has stopped and the person is no longer breathing.

Last year, there were approximately seven thousand brain-dead donors in this country. The practice of recovering more organs from donors after cardiac death is developing rapidly, and we might anticipate over five hundred of these donors in 2006 in the United States.

The shortage of deceased donors, the need for live donors, and the selling of organs, may be resolved in the future only if scientists can someday develop a replaceable line of

---

[13] Ibid., original emphasis.

[14] Ibid., n. 5, original emphasis.

organs from pigs, that is, by xenotransplantation.[15] The research in this field has made good progress. Some pigs have been cloned to "look" human, that is, to have no distinctive pig marker on their blood vessels. At the Massachusetts General Hospital, pig-to-baboon kidney and heart transplants have been performed with genetically manipulated pigs. The sugar molecule on the pig blood vessels that would be rejected by human antibodies is knocked out of the genetic repertoire of the pig so that the blood vessel does not look like that of a pig but rather like that of a human being. If a line of such pigs could be widely developed, then perhaps we could apply xenotransplantation clinically.

I hope we can go in that direction in the future to solve this crisis of the ever-expanding need for organs, which has resulted in live donation being the prominent form of transplantation that we now have around the world. Live organ donation cannot be the final testimony of medicine in resolving this crisis.

---

[15] Sheryl Gay Stolberg, "Breakthrough in Pig Cloning Could Aid Organ Transplants," *New York Times*, January 4, 2002.

VACCINES AND THE RIGHT OF CONSCIENCE

Edward J. Furton

As a father of five, I have been confronted with the question of whether to vaccinate my children against rubella (German measles). As many now know, this vaccine is currently produced from a cell line that had its origin in abortion.[1] Two other vaccines are similarly implicated in the tragedy of

---

This paper was originally published in the *National Catholic Bioethics Quarterly* 4.2 (Spring 2004): 53–62.

[1] The rubella vaccine, produced by the pharmaceutical manufacturer Merck & Co., uses WI-38 cells. There are two hepatitis A vaccines, one produced by Merck, the other by Glaxo SmithKline, both of which use MRC-5 cells. The varicella vaccine, again produced by Merck, uses both WI-38 and MRC-5 cells. For the scientific details on WI-38 cells, see L. Hayflick and P. Moorehead, "Serial Cultivation of Human Diploid Cell Strains," *Experimental Cell Research* 25 (1961): 585–621. For MRC-5 cells, see J.P. Jacobs, C.M. Jones, and J.P. Baille, "Characteristics of a Human Diploid Cell Designated MRC-5," *Nature* (London) 227 (July 11, 1970): 168–170. Also of interest are L. Hayflick et al., "History of the Acceptance of Human Diploid Cell Strains as Substrates for Human Virus Vaccine Manufacture," *Development of Specifications for Biotechnology Standards* 68 (1987): 9–17; and S.A. Plotkin et al., "Attenuation of RA27/3 Rubella Virus in WI-38 Human Diploid Cells," *American Journal of Diseases of Children* 118.2 (August 1969): 178–185.

abortion: the hepatitis A and the new varicella (chicken pox) vaccines. As unfortunate as these facts are, an analysis of the problem, using traditional Catholic moral principles, does not seem to indicate that there is any obligation on the part of parents to avoid the use of these products. For my own part, therefore, I have not hesitated to have my children protected against these diseases.

Nonetheless, there are many parents who have come to the opposite conclusion. They believe that it would be immoral to inoculate their children with these products. They hold that a vaccine with even the most remote connection to abortion is forbidden to them, and thus, they refuse immunization on the grounds of conscience. What is the status of this refusal? Can it be supported by Catholic teaching? We have a moral obligation to follow the light of conscience. Indeed, this duty is so fundamental that, even if one's judgment is in error, conscience must still remain the standard of our conduct. To argue otherwise would be to say that we should do what we personally judge to be immoral.

From a theoretical standpoint, therefore, the path would seem to be clear. Parents who reject all association with abortion should feel free to refuse vaccination for themselves and for their children. Nonetheless, when this approach is put into practice, many difficulties arise. For example, objectors often face a problem when they attempt to place their children into a school system, whether public or private. School administrators, who have both a moral and legal obligation to protect the health and well-being of their students (as well as their teachers, school administrators, and all who work there), routinely prohibit attendance by children who have not been vaccinated against rubella and other contagious diseases. Many states offer exemptions from immunization requirements; some do not or do only for very specific reasons. Thus, a state may accept a religious exemption, but may refuse one based on medical concerns if they are deemed unjustifiable. In cases where an exemption is denied, parents find themselves with very few options.

The difficulty is heightened for Catholics because there is no official teaching of the Church on the question of whether the use of these vaccines is permissible. There are, it is true, various "probable opinions" issued by respected Catholic theologians and Catholic organizations, but the Church itself has taken no position. Thus, Catholic parents who object to immunization with vaccines implicated in abortion can make no appeal to official church teaching, and if they attempt to do so, they are likely to be shown a statement from some recognized Catholic authority that contradicts their views. Can an appeal to conscience serve as a ground for an exemption to vaccination when there is no Catholic teaching on this matter? To explore this question is the purpose of this essay.

The Danger of These Diseases

Let us first be clear about the seriousness of these diseases—because sometimes opponents to vaccination argue that these diseases are minor. Take rubella as an example. This disease is indeed usually mild in children, causing a rash on the face and neck that usually lasts two or three days. Teenagers and young adults may also experience swollen glands in the back of the neck and some swelling and stiffness in the joints. Most people recover quickly and without any aftereffects following infection. The primary danger of harm from this disease, however, is to unborn babies. A woman who contracts rubella in the early stages of pregnancy has a chance of giving birth to a deformed baby. This risk is estimated at 20 percent by the Centers for Disease Control.[2] Defects range from deafness, blindness (atrophic eyes, cataracts, chorioretinitis), and damaged hearts to unusually small brains. Mental retardation is a possibility. Miscarriages can also occur among pregnant women who contract rubella.

The purpose of vaccinating young children, therefore, is not simply to protect them personally from the discomfort of a fairly mild disease, but also to prevent the unborn children of pregnant women from suffering through contact with infected children. Children who are immune to rubella cannot spread it to others. A girl who attains adulthood will also be protected against contracting this disease and transmitting it to her unborn child, although it is important to realize that one who is properly vaccinated can still sometimes become infected.[3] This shows

---

[2] See the Centers for Disease Control and Prevention, "Rubella—In Short," http:www.cdc.gov/nip/diseases/rubella/vac-chart.htm.

[3] Daniel A. Salmon et al., "Health Consequences of Religious and Philosophical Exemptions from Immunization Laws: Individual and Societal Risk of Measles," *Journal of the American Medical Association* 282.1 (July 7, 1999): 47–53. This study indicates that as the number of exemptions to vaccination increases, the incidence of infection among those who have been properly vaccinated also increases.

that the closer society comes to universal compliance against rubella, the smaller the danger will be of an outbreak of this disease. Thanks to the efforts of primary care physicians and public health officials, rubella has been nearly eradicated in the United States. The last large-scale outbreak occurred in 1964, when almost twenty thousand babies were born with severe birth defects. This is something we all hope will never happen again.

Thus, the primary reason why we should use the rubella vaccine is to protect the unborn. The issue, in essence, is one of justice, which, as Catholic theologians have defined it, is the one virtue that is directed toward the good of others. Justice implies a type of equality among human beings, St. Thomas Aquinas says, and he states, by way of example, that "a man's work is said to be just when it is related to some other by way of some kind of equality, for instance, the payment of the wage due for the service rendered."[4] In the present case, however, we have the equality of our common human nature, which obliges each of us to respect the right to life and health that belongs to every human being. We live in a world, of course, in which many claim that human beings are not equal by nature and that some should be accorded greater value than others. The Catholic tradition sees this as a denial of our inherent human dignity, and if it recognizes any such distinction at all, it is that preference ought to be given to the weakest and most vulnerable among us. Those who are unborn and who are subject to the possibility of contracting a serious and debilitating disease within the womb are members of this class.

The Right of Conscience

Most people tend to think of conscience as a mental faculty, but for Aquinas conscience is the act of arriving at a correct moral conclusion about what is to be done, and John Paul II says the same thing.[5] The principles that ought to guide us in our conduct toward each other are not inborn, but are

---

[4] Thomas Aquinas, *Summa theologiae*, II-II, Q. 57.1. As Aquinas states at Q. 58.2, "Since justice by its name implies equality, it denotes essentially relation to another, for a thing is equal, not to itself, but to another."

[5] "For conscience, according to the very nature of the word, implies the relation of knowledge to something: for conscience may be resolved into *cum alio scientia*, i.e., knowledge applied to an individual case. But the application of knowledge to something is done by some act. Wherefore from this explanation of the name it is clear

acquired over time through experience and education; hence, we must first acquire a moral code before we can exercise conscience.[6] Once we have a grasp of the principles of morality, we can apply these to our daily life. One "sees" that doing such-and-such a thing would be good (or evil) and thus concludes that this ought (or ought not) to be done. This understanding of conscience is reflected in the *Catechism of the Catholic Church*.

The dignity of the human person implies and requires *uprightness of moral conscience*. Conscience includes the perception of the principles of morality (synderesis); their application in the given circumstances by practical discernment of reasons and goods; and, finally, judgment about concrete acts yet to be performed or already performed. The truth about the moral good, stated in the law of reason, is recognized practically and concretely by the *prudent judgment* of conscience. We call that man prudent who chooses in conformity with this judgment.[7]

The exercise of conscience, therefore, is a type of rational decision making. Given that no one else can carry out this task for me (another can offer me moral guidance, but I must accept or reject that advice according to the light of conscience), the Church recognizes that "man has the right to act in conscience

---

that conscience is an act." Ibid., I, Q. 79.13. "The judgment of conscience is a *practical judgment*, a judgment which makes known what man must do or not do, or which assesses an act already performed by him." John Paul II, *Veritatis splendor* (Boston: St. Paul Books & Media, 1993), n. 59, original emphasis.

[6] Aquinas, *Summa theologiae*, I, Q. 79.12. Aquinas follows Aristotle on this point. "Now, the first speculative principles bestowed on us by nature do not belong to a special power but to a special habit, which is called 'the understanding of principles,' as the Philosopher explains." See Aristotle, *Nicomachean Ethics*, bk. VI, ch. 6 (1140 b3–1141 a8). The same view is again present in John Paul II: "But whereas the natural law discloses the objective and universal demands of the moral good, conscience is the application of the law to a particular case; this application of the law thus becomes an inner dictate for the individual, a summons to do what is good in a particular situation. Conscience thus formulates *moral obligation* in the light of the natural law: it is the obligation to do what the individual, through the workings of conscience, *knows* to be a good he is called to do *here and now*." John Paul II, *Veritatis splendor*, n. 59, original emphasis.

[7] *Catechism of the Catholic Church*, 2nd ed., trans. U.S. Catholic Conference (Vatican City: Libreria Editrice Vaticana, 1997), n. 1780.

and in freedom so as personally to make moral decisions." Quoting Vatican Council II's document, *Dignitatis humanae*, the *Catechism* adds, "He must not be forced to act contrary to his conscience. Nor must he be prevented from acting according to his conscience, especially in religious matters."[8]

This would seem to indicate that those who sincerely believe that it would be wrong to vaccinate their children against rubella should be permitted to refuse immunization on the grounds of conscience. One might also appeal here to the priority of the family. The rights of parents in the care and education of their children should take precedence over any duty owed to the state. Under the principle of subsidiarity, decisions about the moral good should be left under the care of those who have the most immediate responsibility and should not be usurped by higher authorities. Thus, the decisions of the parents have priority over those made by the state.

But let us suppose that those who refuse vaccination are mistaken in their judgment. Let us say that the Church issues a directive stating that there is no illicit cooperation with abortion in the case of these vaccines. Nonetheless, the obligation to follow an erroneous conscience remains.[9] We cannot oblige a person to violate his conscience, but we must respect that decision even if we ourselves are convinced that it is wrong. On all of these grounds, therefore, one can argue forcefully that parents who do not want to have any association with the practice of abortion, and who refuse to have their children vaccinated, should be free to do so.

Certainly, it would be wrong to force parents to vaccinate their children. We cannot compel anyone to act against his will except as punishment for a crime. Beyond this, however, it is difficult to know what more can be said about the refusal to vaccinate on the basis of conscience. Catholic teaching holds

---

[8] Ibid., n. 1782.

[9] "A human being must always obey the certain judgment of his conscience. If he were deliberately to act against it, he would condemn himself. Yet it can happen that moral conscience remains in ignorance and makes erroneous judgments about acts to be performed or already committed." Ibid., n. 1790. Sometimes that ignorance is blameworthy, namely, when we are responsible for our own lack of knowledge. Ibid., n. 1791. At other times that ignorance is not, and "the evil committed by the person cannot be imputed to him. It remains no less an evil, a privation, a disorder. One must therefore work to correct the errors of moral conscience." Ibid., n. 1793.

that there is an objective moral order that ought to guide the activity of conscience. Obviously, we are not free to decide whatever we wish—every moral person will agree on this point. The moral order that ought to guide our conduct does not depend upon the judgment of Church officials, but exists independently of all human decision. The mind must conform to reality in order to know the truth, but in the absence of any announced position by the Church, one can only appeal to the authority of one's own conscience, which will, it is hoped, be well grounded in observation and sound thinking. The more our appeal takes its bearings from a knowledge of the facts and the true principles of morality, the more likely it will be that our exercise of conscience will successfully choose the good.

One of the facts of this case concerns whether we should identify the right not to violate one's own conscience with the demand for an exemption to a duly established public policy. One might easily argue that these two are not the same. Parents who refuse to vaccinate their children are not compelled to act contrary to their consciences under the law. If they are refused an exemption under some established public policy, then they will suffer the consequences of their refusal. Their children will not be permitted to enter the local school system or some other public facility. This not a violation of conscience, but is a denial of an exemption. The case is not comparable to that of a Catholic health-care facility which is obliged by the state to dispense contraceptives, because there is no compulsion to vaccinate one's children. If one wants to appeal to conscience in order to justify a decision not to vaccinate one's children, then the freedom not to violate one's own conscience is all that can rightly be expected by the parent. The further claim that the exercise of conscience demands that the state must cede to the wishes of the parent for an exemption does not follow—at least, not as the right of conscience is understood by the Catholic Church.

Why There Is No Illicit Cooperation

As a Church which professes a definite body of doctrine, the appeal to conscience is not enough to satisfy the demand for an exemption from the law. There must also be a teaching to which the Catholic can appeal as evidence that he is being deprived of some good on the basis of his religious beliefs. For example, in the case of Catholic hospitals which are being compelled by state law to provide contraception and abortion, the administrators can appeal to the *Ethical and Religious Di-*

rectives for Catholic Health Care Services. The states that are forcing Catholic facilities to violate their own consciences do not care about these teachings; in fact, it is precisely because of these teachings that these states wish to harm Catholic health-care facilities. This is a violation of conscience not merely on the subjective grounds of personal belief, but on the objective grounds of doctrinal teaching. In the case of these implicated vaccines, however, there is no teaching. Nor is it at all clear that the Church will agree with those who claim that they should be exempt from state laws mandating vaccinations because of a perceived association between present use and the original abortions.

My own views on the question of whether there is any inappropriate association have been expressed elsewhere.[10] There certainly seems to be abundant evidence to suggest that there was a high degree of cooperation between those who began the cell lines WI-38 and MRC-5 and those who carried out the abortions.[11] Regardless of what kind of coop-

---

[10] See my "Levels of Moral Complicity in the Act of Human Embryo Destruction," in *Stem Cell Research: New Frontiers in Science and Ethics*, ed. Nancy E. Snow (Notre Dame, IN: University of Notre Dame Press, 2003), 100–120. The article applies my earlier reasoning on vaccines grown in the descendant cells of an abortion ("Vaccines Originating in Abortion," *Ethics & Medics* 24.3 [March 1999]: 3–4) to products that might arise from research on embryonic stem cells taken from destroyed human embryos. Similar, though not identical, views are expressed by the Secretariat for Pro-Life Activities, U.S. Catholic Conference, "Embryonic Stem Cell Research and Vaccines Using Fetal Tissue," June 3, 2003, http:www.usccb.org/prolife/issues/bioethic/vaccfac2.htm; Dan Maher, "Vaccines, Abortion, and Moral Coherence," *National Catholic Bioethics Center* 2.1 (Spring 2002): 51–67; and John D. Grabenstein, "The Social Benefits of Vaccination," *Ethics & Medics* 25.8 (August 2000): 1–3; among others.

[11] I had previously said in my writings (see the preceding note) that the activity of the tissue researchers who produced WI-38 and MRC-5 was wrong because it constituted immediate material cooperation in the intrinsically evil action of abortion. A more detailed review of the evidence (see note 1 above) suggests that the tissue researchers played a much more direct role in the culture of abortion than I had realized. Hence, I revise my view to say that those tissue researchers were engaged in immoral formal cooperation with abortion. The activity of those who established these cell strains should be distinguished from that of the researchers who used them to invent the new vaccines. The latter, I continue to hold, were engaged at the level of immoral proximate material cooperation.

eration it was, it was profoundly wrong. Aborted fetuses do not form a proper subject matter for use in scientific research.[12]

Once these cell strains were established, however, a new question arose, concerning whether scientific researchers (e.g., vaccine researchers) might work with these cells in the hopes of finding cures for serious diseases. Clearly, these researchers did not intend that abortions take place, and given the fact that they would be working with descendant cells, we cannot say that their actions would involve any intrinsically evil activity. The cells found in WI-38 and MRC-5, for example, are not those of the deceased child, but have an independent existence. There is, nonetheless, some reason to think that even this type of research would be too closely associated with the evil of abortion, for it is possible that, supposing that the research is successful, others would be led to believe that the use of aborted fetuses is justifiable in view of the good that it can produce. Although the researchers would have no intention of cooperating with abortion, their work could still encourage the practice of using aborted fetuses in research programs.[13]

The same concern would seem to apply to those pharmaceutical firms that use these established human cell lines to manufacture vaccines. This concern is heightened by the fact that, even though there are some very specific requirements necessary for the growth of particular vaccines, other media have been successfully used in this process.[14] Once a particular

---

[12] An exception to this rule would be the use of fetal material from indirect or spontaneous abortions, such as that recommended by Maria Michejda, M.D., in "Spontaneous Miscarriages as Source of Fetal Stem Cells," *National Catholic Bioethics Quarterly* 2.3 (Autumn 2002): 401–411.

[13] Moral theologians generally recognize that illicit material cooperation occurs not only when one cooperates with an intrinsically evil act, but also "according to its circumstances ... if by reason of its adjuncts, it is wrong, as when it signifies approval of evil, gives scandal to others, or violates a law of the Church." John A. McHugh, O.P., and Charles J. Callan, O.P., *Moral Theology: A Complete Course Based on St. Thomas Aquinas and the Best Modern Authorities*, vol. 1 (New York: Joseph F. Wagner, 1929, 1958), n. 1517.

[14] Thus, in the case of rubella, there is a Japanese product, not approved for use by the U.S. Food and Drug Administration, that is grown in rabbit kidney cells. The Chiron Corporation is currently exploring the possibility of licensing and marketing this vaccine in the United States.

method of manufacture has been set up, however, it is very expensive and time-consuming to alter it. Thus, the executives at these companies did not act prudently when they originally approved the manufacturing process. Other media should have been used, but were not. The companies that made use of the WI-38 and MRC-5 human cells should have known of their association with abortion. As with any individual who finds himself in a compromising situation but who has obligations that must be fulfilled to others, I do not think that these pharmaceutical companies should immediately cease to produce these products. These vaccines are needed to protect society against serious diseases. These companies should, however, begin to explore other possible avenues of production for existing implicated vaccines and, certainly, for new vaccines that may be developed in the future. The larger scientific community should also consider what it will do when the current batches of WI-38 and MRC-5 are exhausted. Although these lines replenish themselves in culture, they are not immortal. What is to replace them in the future? Will new human cell strains be started that once again have their origin in aborted fetal material?[15]

A Proxy Right of Conscience?

Having considered the previous cases, we arrive at the question of what kind of cooperation with abortion obtains when a parent decides to immunize a child against rubella. The parent has no intention of participating in abortion and, living in the present, has no connection whatsoever to the abortions performed in the past. Neither does the parent make use of the cells taken from an abortion, but makes use of a vaccine that was grown in descendant cells. The capacity of these cells to duplicate in culture shows that their use applies little to no pressure on others to perform abortions. There is an abundant supply.

---

[15] Prospects do not look good. The biotechnology company Crucell N.V. and Aventis Pasteur S.A. are seeking approval from the U.S. Food and Drug Administration to introduce PER-C6, a cell strain made from a fetus aborted at eighteen weeks. Even more disconcerting are the efforts of biotechnology companies to produce new drugs and therapies from embryonic stem cells. Some U.S. states have recently passed laws encouraging this research. Any new products made from these strains will be even more controversial than the implicated vaccines.

If there were some remaining level of cooperation here, it could only be remote. This cooperation would be completely permissible because (1) parents have no choice but to use these products if they wish to protect their children and society from these serious diseases, and (2) the good that parents are seeking to secure through vaccination exceeds any harm that might be caused by that use.[16] Thus, it would represent a very harsh judgment, in my opinion, to say that unborn children must face the risks of serious birth defects or even death because others feel an obligation to make a strong statement against the evil of abortion. The fault surely lies with the original tissue researchers and, less directly, with the pharmaceutical companies or those who made imprudent decisions at the time these products were first manufactured. The fault does not lie with the parents and surely not with the children who suffer the risk.[17]

If the above reasoning is correct, and there is no immoral cooperation with abortion in the use of these vaccines, then we are led back to the problem of conscience from an entirely new perspective. One who properly exercises conscience will recognize that he has a moral obligation to protect the life and health of his neighbors and that he must therefore ensure that he and his children are vaccinated as a correct means to

---

[16] Thus, McHugh and Callan argue that "a grave reason for cooperation exists when, if one refuses it, a great good will be lost or a great evil incurred. A day's wages or income is generally a great good; a severe or long-continued pain, great anger of an employer or other superior, things that bring on notable annoyance, shame, repugnance, etc., are examples of great evils." McHugh and Callan, *Moral Theology*, n. 1520. Serious disease justifies this use.

[17] No one should suppose that the position advanced lends any support to the claim that scientists should be free to work with fetal tissue in research. It should be obvious that those who set up arrangements with Planned Parenthood or other abortion facilities to receive the remains of aborted children, so that the remains can be used in programs of experimental research, are doing something that cannot be justified under any principle of Catholic teaching. The direct cooperation between the parties in this matter sullies the hands of those who receive the fetal materials and makes them cooperators in the evil of abortion. In the case at hand, I am talking about the use of the *cells* that descend from an abortion, cells which replicate themselves in culture, from which vaccines are made. That product is then made available for use by physicians. The level of cooperation in the two cases is radically different, as the above brief rehearsal should make plain.

that end. He will recognize that there is a moral question at issue in the use of vaccines, but he will also see that there can be no justification for risking the health and life of unborn children who have had absolutely no hand in the original wrongdoing. He will bear in mind that his own children will learn from his decision and that the occasion presents him with an opportunity to explain to them how to think about difficult moral problems. The formation of conscience is a responsibility that a parent has toward his child throughout his time in the home.[18] What will the child learn from a parent who refuses to vaccinate him out of an exaggerated concern that the use of these vaccines is immoral? Hopefully, the entire event will pass without his notice.

Let us suppose that the child who is not vaccinated contracts rubella while his mother is pregnant. Let us also suppose that the unborn child is then infected and born with birth defects. This is not an unreasonable scenario, especially for those who tend to have larger families. The most likely transmission is from a born child to one who is unborn. What will be the lesson that the child learns as he sees his brother or sister born with such defects? Will he say to himself, "Yes, we must suffer even this, in order to show our strong opposition to abortion"? Or will he say, "No, this cannot be right. How does the suffering of my brother or sister advance the cause of abolishing abortion?" This question would be especially troubling for a child who realizes that his sibling has suffered this calamity because he himself contracted the disease and passed it on. The child should understand, of course, that what happened was not his fault, but it may not prove easy for him to distinguish between his role as the source of the disease and his innocence of any moral responsibility. And if he is not to blame, who will the child hold responsible for this tragedy?

There is an even more fundamental question at stake. Can a parent exercise a right of conscience for a child? How can *I* risk *your* health in order that I might make a strong stand against abortion? This, in fact, is impossible, because it is contrary to the very nature of conscience, which is always the

---

[18] "The education of conscience is a lifelong task. From the earliest years, it awakens the child to the knowledge and practice of the interior law recognized by conscience." *Catechism of the Catholic Church*, n. 1784.

personal act of a particular individual.[19] I cannot carry out an act of conscience for you. Only you can do that for yourself. But someone will say, "In this case the child is not old enough to decide for himself; therefore, the parent must decide on his behalf." Exactly, and that is all the more reason to act for the sake of the child's health. That is the moral principle that ought to govern all decisions in this area. Just as the demand for an exemption to a law mandating vaccination seems unjustifiable, so does the appeal to the right of conscience. No one can exercise the right of conscience for someone else—not even for one's own child. All one can do is act for the sake of the child's life and health. Hence, an adult is free to appeal to the right of conscience in order to justify his own refusal to vaccinate himself, but he cannot appeal to the right of conscience in order to justify his decision not to vaccinate those who are under his supervision and who rely on him for their medical care. We should not allow the one who carried out an abortion in the past to hold our children hostage in the present.

---

[19] "Conscience makes its witness known only to the person himself. And, in turn, only the person himself knows what his own response is to the voice of conscience." John Paul II, *Veritatis splendor*, n. 57.

BIOETHICAL CHALLENGES FOR THE CATHOLIC CHURCH

A LATIN AMERICAN PERSPECTIVE

Oscar J. Martínez-González

The advance of knowledge and technology in biomedical science has generated a degree of moral questioning similar to what occurred after the Second World War in response to the use of nuclear energy to destroy entire populations.

In the 1970s, a new discipline emerged in the field of biomedicine: that of bioethics. Bioethics first surfaced in the United States in academic debate about the ethical repercussions of the increasing use of technology in the health sciences. The overriding concern was the ever-increasing dehumanization among health-care professionals and administrators.

In 1970, the U.S. government established the National Commission for the Protection of Human Subjects. A few years

---

This chapter is based on Dr. Martínez-González's original presentation in Spanish, which appears in Appendix B of this volume, on p. 323. The English translation is by Come Alive Communications, Inc., West Grove, Pennsylvania, www.comealiveusa.com.

later, the President's Commission for the Study of Ethical Problems in Medicine and Biomedical and Behavioral Research was established.

With advances in science and technology, health care has become an effective as well as a costly reality. Controversies, both moral and legal, over public policies have started to occur, and there is doubt about the proper ethics that should guide health-care and biomedical decision making.

Principlist bioethics, which is currently the most widely used, proposes four principles: autonomy, beneficence, non-maleficence, and justice. These four principles are used to analyze and substantiate the majority of bioethical questions. H. T. Englehardt, Jr., explains that

> as the field of bioethics was taking shape, it was greatly influenced by a volume authored by a rule utilitarian and a deontologist [T. L. Beauchamp and J. F. Childress], who, despite their theoretical differences, were able to craft middle-level principles through which they could come to common resolution of controversial cases.[1]

This method of solving ethical problems evolved into a type of practice that even those with no formal training in philosophy could use to resolve controversial cases in bioethical decision making. This helps us understand why hospital ethics committees have adopted principlism as a methodology, since it offers those who have little education in philosophy and who lack a firm moral viewpoint a way to approach bioethical problems and arrive at consensus.

In response to principlist bioethics, *personalist bioethics* is emerging. Two important principles are attributed to it: The first principle is based on an integral perception of man; the second recognizes that moral truth can be attained by using human reason. By definition, ethics seeks goodness, and goodness is attained when truth is known and respected. Therefore, truth is one of the foundations of ethics.

These days, it seems as if everything matters, everything is equal, and it is fine for everyone to make his or her own truth, since there is no hierarchy of values. This cannot be

---

[1] H. Tristam Englehardt, Jr., "Consensus Formation: The Creation of an Ideology," *Cambridge Quarterly of Healthcare Ethics,* vol. 11.1 (2002), 15, referring to Beauchamp and Childress's *Principles of Biomedical Ethics* (New York: Oxford University Press, 1979).

true; if it were, we could rightfully declare that nothing is worth anything at all.

Faced with the irrefutable certainties offered by technical science, *moral* certainties currently seem more fragile and refutable than ever. Many feel that "reasonable" applies only to what can be indisputably verified, such as mathematical formulas or techniques; on this basis, knowledge is limited to what can be measured and proved.

It can be observed that the current moral debate is concerned principally with finding substitute solutions that, in a relative world such as ours, might somehow guarantee the fundamental framework of the *ethos.*

With the exception of personalism, most philosophical viewpoints regarding bioethics—such as consequentialism, principlism, and utilitarianism—assume that it is impossible for us to identify norms that are derived from man's very essence and from the things around him. If such norms were identifiable, these viewpoints hold, then it would be impossible to behave in any way that opposed them. Moral action in these cases would be determined not by the content of an act in itself, but rather by its ends and its foreseeable consequences. From this perspective, good and evil would not exist; the only things that would exist are those that are *better* and those that are *not so good.*

In this regard, it is necessary to remember that every man is, by his very nature, a being with fundamental rights that no one can take away from him, since no human act has granted these rights to him. They are inherent in his nature as a human being.

If we take a look around and consider the current living situation in civilized society, and the degree of discernment society possesses to distinguish between good and evil, we might conclude that we are in a crisis, in the most dangerous crisis of all: that of confusing good and evil, thus making it impossible to build and preserve moral order.

We know well that, from an ethical perspective, science and advanced technology are neither good nor evil in themselves. It is only in their application that an ethic necessarily emerges.

The application of science and technology in the field of health sciences in contemporary society motivates us to ask ourselves the following question: Are science and technology really being used to benefit mankind?

For science and technology to promote true human development, they must always be at the service of mankind. Despite scientific progress, many scientists have limited themselves to explaining and accepting only what they can physically perceive, quantify, or measure; therefore, in not knowing how to explain the intangible in man, they prefer to deny it, thus also denying his dignity.

The Meaning of Every Person's Human Existence

When asked about the meaning of a human life, most scientists and technicians do not know how to answer. There are some, however—those who have cultivated their science from philosophy and theology—who have discovered answers to this question.

The search for meaning in one's personal existence is a concern for most people. This search is rewarded only through religious experience, since science in itself offers no guarantee that its results will contribute to human development or to man's spiritual progress.

Neither science nor technology in itself can create meaning for human existence. We know well that progress in science and technology has not always promoted the good of mankind; indeed, it has often resulted in humanity's regression.

Science and technology should always favor human progress, since they would be meaningless otherwise. Science lacks meaning if it is not based on the principle of humanism. Therefore, all scientific activities must be oriented toward respect for human life and human dignity as a supreme value, since it is the human being who gives meaning to science.

The Catholic Church and Life

In the *Apostolic Constitution on Catholic Universities*, His Holiness John Paul II tells us that

> scientific and technological discoveries create an enormous economic and industrial growth, but they also inescapably require the correspondingly necessary *search for meaning* in order to guarantee that the new discoveries be used for the authentic good of individuals and of human society as a whole.... For, "What is at stake is the *very meaning of scientific and technological research, of social life*

and of culture, but, on an even more profound level, what is at stake is *the very meaning of the human person."* [2]

These words are directed especially to Catholic universities— the academic centers that should promote science and technology in the service of human beings. In *Evangelium vitae,* which this year celebrates the tenth anniversary of its promulgation, Pope John Paul II states further that

> with the new prospects opened up by scientific and technological progress there arise new forms of attacks on the dignity of the human being. At the same time a new cultural climate is developing and taking hold, which gives crimes against life a new and—if possible—even more sinister character, giving rise to further grave concern: broad sectors of public opinion justify certain crimes against life in the name of the rights of individual freedom, and on this basis they claim not only exemption from punishment but even authorization by the State ... The end result of this is tragic: not only is the fact of the destruction of so many human lives still to be born or in their final stage extremely grave and disturbing, but no less grave and disturbing is the fact that conscience itself, darkened as it were by such widespread conditioning, is finding it increasingly difficult to distinguish between good and evil in what concerns the basic value of human life.[3]

He says later:

> Decisions that go against life sometimes arise from difficult or even tragic situations of profound suffering, loneliness, a total lack of economic prospects, depression and anxiety about the future. Such circumstances can mitigate ... the consequent culpability of those who make these choices which in themselves are evil. But today the problem goes far beyond the necessary recognition of these personal situations. It is a problem which exists at the cultural, social and political level, where it reveals its more sinister and disturbing aspect in the tendency ... to interpret ... crimes against life as legitimate expressions of individual freedom, to be acknowledged and protected as actual rights.[4]

---

[2] John Paul II, *Apostolic Constitution on Catholic Universities* [*Ex Corde Ecclesiae*] (August 15, 1990), n. 7, original emphasis.

[3] John Paul II, *Evangelium vitae* (March 25, 1995), n. 4.

[4] Ibid., n. 18.

The Holy Father's words help us better understand the magnitude of the problem. Attacks against life have taken on a dimension that should not only *preoccupy* us, but also *occupy* us, as we use our greatest talents in the aim of establishing the "culture of life" of which His Holiness spoke so insistently.

Current Challenges in Bioethics

If we look at the biomedical practices that currently provoke the most serious attacks against life and the dignity of the human person, we find that the most controversial relate to the beginning and the end of human life. These issues include:

· *In genetics:* the possible use of information obtained by the Human Genome Project to identify individuals who show alterations in their genomes; therapeutic cloning through the attempted use of embryonic stem cells; and prenatal screening that often results in death sentences for babies via eugenic abortion

· *In artificial reproduction:* low rates of success; the deaths of thousands of human embryos; the preservation of frozen embryos; the use of gametes and "donated" embryos; and surrogate pregnancy

· *In birth control:* the indiscriminate endorsement of birth control by public and private institutions; the use of abortifacient contraceptives, such as the intrauterine device and "emergency" contraception; and the tacit acceptance of suggestions made in developed countries to halt population growth in developing countries, which even go so far as to propose the legalization of abortion in all circumstances so that it may be used as a method of birth control

· *In scientific research on human subjects:* continual human rights violations, which are particularly notable in developing countries

· *In the doctor-patient relationship:* the effects of technology that "gets between" the two parties, so that a doctor has little direct contact with his patients; the intervention of third parties who are responsible for the payment of fees; unjust fee schedules; the unfair distribution of resources in socialized medicine, which undermines mutual confidence between doctor and patient; and attempts by some doctors to "get rich quick"

- *In diagnosis:* the influence of certain minority groups on medical decisions, which has led, for example, to the assertion by certain medical associations that homosexuality is not an illness and therefore must not be treated

- *In organ transplantation:* a drastic change in the traditional definition of death

- *In the treatment of persons with handicaps:* discrimination and a frequent failure to regard handicapped persons as individuals whose dignity must always be respected

- *In the allocation of health-care resources:* the expenditure of large amounts of money on non-priority health issues, with few or no resources devoted to areas that should be considered priorities

- *In the management of terminal illness:* proposed legislation that seeks to legalize euthanasia, on the basis that people have a right "to die with dignity"

We could continue with this list of assaults against life, but as His Holiness John Paul II states, "Perhaps it is better to say no more than this about such a painful subject."[5]

How Have We Arrived at This Situation?

In *Evangelium vitae,* His Holiness John Paul II describes how we arrived here:

In the background there is the profound crisis of culture, which generates skepticism in relation to the very foundations of knowledge and ethics, and which makes it increasingly difficult to grasp clearly the meaning of what man is, the meaning of his rights and his duties. Then there are all kinds of existential and interpersonal difficulties, made worse by the complexity of a society in which individuals, couples and families are often left alone with their problems. There are situations of acute poverty, anxiety or frustration in which the struggle to make ends meet, the presence of unbearable pain, or instances of violence, especially against women, make the choice to defend and promote life so demanding as sometimes to reach the point of heroism.

---

[5] John Paul II, *Crossing the Threshold of Hope* (New York: Alfred I. Knopf, 1994), 206.

All this explains, at least in part, how the value of life can today undergo a kind of "eclipse," even though conscience does not cease to point to it as a sacred and inviolable value.[6]

He adds:

In seeking the deepest roots of the struggle between the "culture of life" and the "culture of death," we ... have to go to the heart of the tragedy being experienced by modern man: the eclipse of the sense of God and of man.... When the sense of God is lost, there is also a tendency to lose the sense of man, of his dignity and his life.[7]

A Recent Experience

In November 2001, the conference "Unwanted Pregnancy and Unsafe Abortion: Public Health Challenges in Latin America and the Caribbean" took place in Cuernavaca, Mexico, organized by the Population Council and the Alan Guttmacher Institute (both based in New York). More than 300 researchers from twenty-four countries attended. It was decided that the two main challenges that institutions face in legalizing abortion in Latin America and the Caribbean are:

· The influence of the Catholic Church and, above all, the influence of devotion to Our Lady of Guadalupe. This has made it difficult to spread a pro-abortion ideology in countries that have primarily Catholic populations.

· The influence of bioethics on health-care professionals, since bioethical debate is changing doctors' minds and leading them to defend a culture that favors life.

Regarding strategies, the organizers of the meeting proposed to the participants, primarily the women, that they try to approach the priests and bishops of the Catholic Church in their own countries—especially those who agree with the principles of sexual equality and women's rights—to help the priests and bishops make women see the benefits of legalizing abortion.

Regarding bioethics, organizers mentioned that it was important that the bioethics they supported be based on a liberal ideology, which defends women's rights and is not deeply rooted in an anthropology that recognizes the irreplaceable nature of the human being.

---

[6] *Evangelium vitae*, n. 11.

[7] Ibid., n. 21.

Conclusion

The pastors of the Catholic Church in Latin America, together with us, lay persons dedicated to training health-care professionals in the ethics of personalism, have a doubly difficult mission.

First, we must fight to establish a "culture of life" amid the moral relativism in our countries—above all when scientific and technological applications in the health sciences present us with bioethical challenges that are increasingly difficult to solve.

Second, our efforts must stand up to the pressure exerted by institutions that seek to impose birth control through abortive methods of contraception and to legalize abortion, euthanasia, techniques of artificial reproduction, and research using embryonic stem cells. These institutions have great influence on public policy and on the powers-that-be in our countries, and they influence the management of public debt according to compliance with their proposed projects.

I conclude by quoting Father Marcial Maciel, founder of the Legion of Christ and of Anáhuac University, whose words help us have hope amid these difficulties:

> If one wishes to enter the encounter with mankind, he must get on the road, endure the sun, the wind and the cold of the journey.... The daily reality of an apostle is dimmer than one might imagine. He waits for multitudes to come, and only a few appear. He imagines shining success and only manages small accomplishments.... It is necessary to learn to read the history of the world and one's personal history with eyes of faith. As we read in the Book of Revelation, the battle with the powers of evil will reach cosmic proportions.... But Christ has crushed the devil's power with the cross.... Your mission is to go out into the world in Christ's name, not in your own name. If he has sent you, he will give you the necessary grace to fulfill your mission.[8]

---

[8] Marcial Maciel, L.C., *Apóstoles de la Nueva Evangelización* [*Apostles of the New Evangelization*] (Hamden, CT: Circle Press, 1993), quotation translated from the Spanish by Come Alive Communications, Inc.

Appendices

Desafíos actuales de la bioética para la Iglesia Católica en Europa

Rev. Gonzalo Miranda, L.C.

Hace algunos años un grupo de médicos católicos visitaba los domingos las parroquias de Roma promoviendo la donación de órganos. Al pedir a un párroco si podían alentar en su iglesia el trasplante de órganos, el sacerdote reaccionó muy seriamente: «Ese órgano lleva ahí tres siglos y no se mueve más».

Cuando pienso en los desafíos actuales de la bioética para la Iglesia Católica me viene a la memoria esa anécdota. Los problemas que el progreso y la práctica de la medicina, y de las ciencias biológicas, presentan hoy día a nuestra sociedad constituyen auténticos desafíos para la Iglesia Católica. Y, desgraciadamente, no siempre los pastores, sacerdotes y agentes de pastoral estamos suficientemente preparados para afrontarlos. Por ello mismo, la convocación periódica a este curso destinado a los obispos de los Estados Unidos responde a una importante necesidad de la Iglesia y merece el más caluroso aplauso.

Se me pide que comente los desafíos actuales de la bioética para la Iglesia Católica *en Europa*. Por una parte, los problemas afrontados por la bioética tienen un claro carácter universal, válido para todos los países y para las iglesias de todas las regiones: el respeto por la vida naciente, el respeto por el paciente como persona, el respeto por el medio ambiente, etc. son valores que afectan a todo ser humano, de cualquier latitud. Además, el proceso de creciente globalización hace que determinados problemas, quizás en un primer momento localizados en una región, se conviertan enseguida en problemas que sienten otras partes del planeta, incluso en regiones donde la práctica problemática específica no se presenta como posibilidad real. Éste es el caso, por ejemplo, de la clonación. En muchos países no se plantea todavía, ni por asomo, la posibilidad de llevarla a cabo; y sin embargo, la clonación se ha convertido también en esos países en tema de encendido debate, por la sencilla razón de que toca la raíz de la comprensión y el respeto de la vida humana y suscita perplejidad ética en la conciencia de todos los seres humanos, independientemente de su cultura o religión.

Por otra parte, cada región geográfica y cultural presenta algunas características específicas que conviene tener en cuenta cuando se consideran los desafíos de la bioética para la Iglesia Católica. El análisis de la situación europea puede ayudar a comprender mejor los desafíos que enfrenta la Iglesia en los Estados Unidos. Hay que tener en cuenta, además, que el flujo de ideas, ideologías y estilos de vida entre estos dos continentes es singularmente significativo; por lo tanto, debemos tener en cuenta lo que sucede al otro lado del Atlántico para orientar mejor nuestras opciones pastorales.

Problemas específicos de bioética en Europa

Durante la reunión del Consejo de las Conferencias Episcopales de Europa celebrada en junio de 2001, el secretario general Aldo Giordano explicó que el tema de la bioética había sido incluido entre los temas a tratar como respuesta a la preocupación de los obispos de muchos países.[1] Es un hecho que los pastores de muchas diócesis de diversos

---

[1] Cfr. Aldo Giordano, «Themes in the Agenda of the European Bishops' Conferences», reunión anual de los secretarios generales del Concilium Conferentiarum Episcoporum Europae (CCEE), Prague, Czechoslovakia, junio 21–25, 2001, http://ccee.ch/english/press/segretarifinale.htm.

países europeos están muy preocupados y, a veces, perplejos ante las circunstancias culturales, legales y prácticas que se presentan de manera cada vez más problemática en sus diócesis o en sus países. A veces se trata también de medidas, resoluciones o proyectos legislativos que se plantean en el ámbito de la comunidad europea en cuanto tal (en alguna de sus múltiples instancias como la Comisión Europea, el Parlamento Europeo, etc.) y que influyen en mayor o menor medida sobre la realidad de cada uno de los lugares que componen el mosaico de Europa.

El mismo Giordano recordó en su ponencia algunos de los problemas más urgentes en Europa. Mencionó, por ejemplo, las iniciativas europeas en materia de manipulación genética, la ambigüedad y confusión de muchos códigos legales sobre el estatuto jurídico del embrión humano, la legalización de la eutanasia en algunos países europeos, la esclavitud de la prostitución de mujeres y niños así como el concepto de familia, que «en algunos países se ha ampliado hasta incluir dos realidades contradictorias».[2]

Giordano comentó: «Conscientes de que estos problemas determinarán el futuro de Europa y de la humanidad, las conferencias de obispos sienten la responsabilidad de salvaguardar la vida y actuar en el ámbito cultural, pastoral y legislativo».[3]

Sería interesante analizar juntos algunos de estos desafíos concretos y actuales en el campo de la bioética, en términos de cómo se están viviendo en Europa. Pero también llevaría demasiado tiempo y, fácilmente, se convertiría en una crónica de hechos que no nos ayudaría mucho a entender los problemas de fondo. Por eso me limitaré a describir sólo algunos aspectos de la situación europea. Podemos considerar, por ejemplo, que la práctica del aborto ya ha sido legalizada en la mayoría de los países europeos; de hecho, sólo Irlanda y Malta quedan fuera de la lista.

Las prácticas de reproducción asistida también han sido legalizadas en muchos países del continente. Sin embargo, las leyes europeas en ese campo varían ampliamente de un país a otro. Inglaterra y España cuentan con leyes sumamente

---

[2] *Ibidem.*

[3] *Ibidem.*

anarquistas, en las que casi todo está permitido. En varios países del norte de Europa, en cambio, se ha regulado esas prácticas de manera más restrictiva. También Alemania tiene una ley bastante rigurosa y, en Italia, se aprobó por fin una ley en febrero de 2004. El artículo 1 de la ley italiana reconoce que el embrión concebido es una persona con derechos y los artículos subsiguientes prohíben las prácticas imprudentes no fundamentadas. Se prohíbe la producción de más de tres embriones y todos estos deben ser implantados en el útero de la madre; además se prohíbe tanto la congelación de embriones como la experimentación con ellos.

La equiparación de la unión de personas homosexuales con el matrimonio, incluido el derecho a la adopción, se ha concretado legalmente en Holanda y Dinamarca y, recientemente, el gobierno español ha dado pasos firmes en esa dirección, queriendo demostrar al mundo que España, bajo la batuta del gobierno socialista, es un país moderno.

Respecto a los problemas bioéticos que se refieren al final de la vida, tristemente Europa ocupa otro primer lugar: la eutanasia ha sido legalizada, por primera vez en el ámbito nacional, en dos países: Holanda y Bélgica. El movimiento a favor de la eutanasia sigue luchando por su legalización en varios países. Actualmente, el gobierno de España está promoviendo un cambio cultural que podría llevar a su legalización.

Basten estos ejemplos para darnos cuenta de que la situación europea es verdaderamente dramática y sufre una fuerte y casi continua aceleración. Es más interesante ahora, como decía, hacer un análisis de los desafíos *de fondo* para la Iglesia en Europa: un análisis del *sustrato cultural* en el que se alimentan y florecen esos procesos.

Algunas características socioculturales de la situación europea

El surgimiento y desarrollo de muchos de los problemas actuales en la bioética están relacionados con determinadas características sociales, culturales y religiosas de nuestro tiempo, como el fruto se relaciona con la raíz de la planta. Por ello mismo, conviene que nos detengamos un momento a considerar algunas de las características de la Europa moderna. En el fondo, los desafíos actuales de la bioética para la Iglesia Católica en Europa se juegan en este plano.

Secularización progresiva

Desgraciadamente, no hace falta detenerse demasiado para demostrar que en Europa se sigue dando un grave y paulatino proceso de secularización. Son múltiples los estudios sociológicos que indican con claridad el avance de ese fenómeno.

En algunos países (como en los Países Bajos, Inglaterra y Francia), buena parte de la sociedad en general no se reconoce ya en la fe y en la cultura cristiana. En otros (como Irlanda, España e Italia) persiste un profundo sustrato de identidad católica pero se nota también el avance de una cultura sin Dios y una práctica de vida cada vez más indiferente a los principios morales evangélicos propuestos por la Iglesia Católica. En otros países (como Polonia y Croacia), el viento de la secularización europea ha soplado fuerte desde la caída del muro de Berlín.

En realidad, los estudios y la observación atenta muestran situaciones muy contradictorias. A veces se tiene la impresión de vivir en el desierto espiritual. Los medios de comunicación social, las declaraciones de buena parte de los políticos, los planteamientos de muchos de los más conocidos y reconocidos líderes culturales (literatos, filósofos, personajes del espectáculo, por ejemplo), dan la impresión de que la fe y la religión han desaparecido casi por completo de la escena.

Sin embargo, cuando menos lo esperamos, saltan sorpresas que contradicen esa impresión. Ha sucedido, por ejemplo, siempre que se ha celebrado en Europa la jornada mundial de la juventud con el Santo Padre: seiscientos mil jóvenes en Santiago de Compostela, un millón de jóvenes en la laica París, dos millones de jóvenes en la celebración del jubileo del año 2000 en Roma. Después de cada uno de estos encuentros sociólogos, analistas políticos y comentaristas de todos los colores se devanan los sesos durante varias semanas tratando de interpretar, cada uno a su modo y según su ideología o sus intereses, ese sorprendente fenómeno. Se diga lo que se diga, esos jóvenes no son hongos que surgieron de repente a causa de un poco de humedad. Pocos se dan cuenta o quieren reconocer que esos jóvenes «ya estaban ahí»: en el grupo parroquial, en esa pequeña comunidad cristiana, participando con entusiasmo en el ideal de ese movimiento laical o formándose en aquella escuelita dirigida por las monjas. A estos observadores les sorprende, también, el hecho de que un altísimo porcentaje de familias opten por clases de religión para sus hijos menores y que un alto número de contribuyentes señala la casilla de la Iglesia Católica para destinar a ella un porcentaje fijo de sus ingresos que marca la ley.

Posiblemente tengamos que reconocer, a partir de la mención de estas contradicciones, que las raíces profundas del cristianismo en Europa siguen vivas, pero que, por otra parte, se las sigue despreciando sobre todo entre los líderes que más influyen en la cultura, las leyes, la política y la opinión pública. Evidentemente, la débil presencia de la identidad cristiana en esos niveles provoca su paulatino debilitamiento en *todos* los niveles sociales.

A mi entender, existe una estrecha relación entre la secularización y la pérdida del sentido de la dignidad universal del ser humano. Esto provoca, como consecuencia, la aceptación y promoción de prácticas gravemente contrarias a esa dignidad como el aborto, la destrucción de embriones humanos y la eutanasia.

En principio, los valores y las normas que nos ayudan a entender la obligación moral de respetar siempre a todo ser humano, de cualquier condición, raza, sexo, religión o edad (también si todavía no ha nacido) son de carácter racional y están profundamente arraigados en nuestra naturaleza humana. Por lo tanto, deberían ser entendidos y aceptados por todos los seres humanos y no sólo por los creyentes en un Dios creador o en Jesucristo. Pero, de hecho, en muchas partes da la impresión de que los cristianos o los católicos tuviéramos una especie de monopolio, no buscado ni deseado, sobre el respeto por la vida humana.[4]

Cualquiera puede entender, si es que se abre a los datos actuales de la embriología, que el embrión humano es un individuo humano desde el primer momento de su existencia; y cualquiera puede llegar a entender, con un razonamiento puramente natural, que todo ser humano debe ser respetado en su derecho a la vida. Sin embargo, apenas uno afirma esas verdades científicas racionales, se le identifica como católico y se le acusa de querer imponer a la sociedad su propia ideología religiosa.

Da la impresión de que el cristiano, que no ha encontrado en la sagradas escrituras detalles específicos sobre la condición

---

[4] Cfr. Juan Pablo II, *Evangelium vitae* (25 de marzo de 1995), n. 21

del embrión humano o sobre la condena moral asociada con la clonación humana tuviera una tremenda disposición natural a la comprensión de ciertas verdades científicas y naturales y a sacar sus conclusiones a partir de ella. No es que el cristiano vea más porque posea luces especiales; es que *quiere* ver y mira las cosas como son.

Da la impresión también de que, por el contrario, quienes no creen en Dios no logran ver lo que la ciencia demuestra claramente o, tal vez, no pueden entender verdades que se basan en la simple razón natural. Puede tratarse, a veces, de una actitud que tiende a justificar determinadas prácticas ya asumidas y a promover ciertos intereses; y, a veces, lo mejor para justificar la propia conciencia es no ver y, para no ver, lo mejor es no mirar.

Pero hay algo más de fondo en este fenómeno. Lo explica Juan Pablo II en la *Evangelium vitae*:

> Es necesario llegar al centro del drama vivido por el hombre contemporáneo: *el eclipse del sentido de Dios y del hombre,* característico del contexto social y cultural dominado por el secularismo, que con sus tentáculos penetrantes no deja de poner a prueba, a veces, a las mismas comunidades cristianas. Quien se deja contagiar por esta atmósfera, entra fácilmente en el torbellino de un terrible círculo vicioso: *perdiendo el sentido de Dios, se tiende a perder también el sentido del hombre,* de su dignidad y de su vida. A su vez, la violación sistemática de la ley moral, especialmente en el grave campo del respeto de la vida humana y su dignidad, produce una especie de progresiva ofuscación de la capacidad de percibir la presencia vivificante y salvadora de Dios.[5]

Estas consideraciones nos llevan a concluir que el mejor modo en que la Iglesia de Europa puede promover la dignidad humana y el respeto por la vida es empeñarse con renovado entusiasmo a la tarea de la nueva evangelización del continente. En la medida que los ciudadanos y los pueblos de Europa redescubran el Evangelio serán capaces de descubrir el Evangelio de la vida.

Pero también acontece lo opuesto: en la medida que descubran el Evangelio de la vida estarán mejor dispuestos a recibir el Evangelio de la salvación. Lo dice el Papa al final del texto citado anteriormente: la violación de la moral,

---

[5] *Ibidem.*

especialmente en el campo del respeto por la vida humana, ofusca el corazón y la mente y dificulta la percepción de la presencia de Dios. Dicho positivamente, si con nuestra labor paciente en el campo de la bioética logramos que los hombres y las mujeres de Europa estén mejor preparados para recibir y respetar la vida humana, estarán más dispuestos a recibir al Señor de la vida. La bioética, correctamente implementada, se presenta, en ese sentido, como una labor de «pre-evagelización».[6]

Relativismo y libertarismo

Europa no está perdiendo sólo la fe, esté perdiendo también la razón. Si la primera fue rechazada por la cultura moderna, hija de la Ilustración, la segunda está muriendo en la cultura postmoderna. Da la impresión de que la razón, elevada sobre un pedestal que no era el suyo, forzada a jugar el falso papel de «diosa razón», se hubiera desgastado excesivamente y no creyera ya en sus propias fuerzas. Es lo que se denomina en Europa «pensamiento débil».

En buena parte, la pérdida de la confianza en la razón proviene del alejamiento de Dios. Como dice Juan Pablo II en la encíclica *Veritatis splendor*,

> ...el hombre es tentado continuamente a apartar su mirada del Dios vivo y verdadero y dirigirla a los ídolos (cf. *1 Tes* 1, 9), cambiando «la verdad de Dios por la mentira» (*Rom* 1, 25); de esta manera su capacidad para conocer la verdad queda ofuscada y debilitada su voluntad para someterse a ella. Y así, abandonándose al relativismo y al escepticismo (cf. *Jn* 18, 38), busca una libertad ilusoria fuera de la verdad misma.[7]

El Papa Juan Pablo II denunció claramente la tendencia al relativismo absoluto en el discurso pronunciado durante su histórica visita al parlamento italiano.[8] Como continuando su

---

[6] Puede ser emblemático el conocido caso de Bernard Nathanson. De ser un judío no creyente y vigorosamente dedicado a la práctica y la legalización del aborto, se convirtió primero al respeto y la defensa de la vida y, a partir de ahí, recorrió un largo y profundo camino de conversión humana y religiosa que le llevó a las mismas puertas de la Iglesia Católica, en la que llegó a recibir el bautismo.

[7] Juan Pablo II, *Veritatis splendor* (6 de agosto de 1993), n. 1.

[8] Juan Pablo II, «Discurso durante su histórica visita al Parlamento italiano (Palazzo Montecitorio)», (14 de noviembre de 2002), http://

mensaje, el presidente del Senado italiano, Marcello Pera (filósofo y no creyente) dedicó recientemente uno de sus discursos, pronunciado en la Pontificia Universidad Lateranense de Roma, a analizar y denunciar ese fenómeno corrosivo del relativismo.[9] Lo presenta en su dimensión axiológica: «...la idea de que no existen fundamentos a nuestros valores y que no se pueden aducir pruebas o argumentos sólidos para establecer que algo es mejor o vale más que otra cosa».[10]

En su análisis, Pera identifica sobre todo dos modalidades en el relativismo actual: el contextualista y el deconstructivista.[11] El primero sostiene que todo concepto o valor debe ser considerado solamente y necesariamente dentro del contexto cultural en el que opera, por lo que no puede ser comparado con un concepto o valor perteneciente a otro ámbito cultural. De ese modo todo es relativo, dependiente del ámbito de referencia, y no puede decirse que algo sea mejor o peor.

El segundo, el deconstructivista, cuyo maestro principal fue Nietzsche, busca mostrar, sobre todo recurriendo a los casos limite, que los conceptos supuestamente absolutos y universales son intrínsecamente aporéticos (sujetos a la duda) y contradictorios. De este modo, lo que algunas (o muchas) personas piensan que es en sí bueno, se revela contrario a la bondad, con lo cual se concluye que el bien y el mal son siempre relativos.

El cardenal Joseph Ratzinger, ahora Papa Benedicto XVI, ha escrito que «el relativismo se ha convertido de algún modo en la verdadera religión del hombre moderno»[12] y constituye «el problema más grande de nuestra época».[13] Tanto él y el Papa Juan Pablo II como Marcello Pera han tenido que constatar la penetración de la mentalidad relativista incluso entre los creyentes y hasta en la misma teología.

---

www.vatican.va/holy_father/john_paul_ii/speeches/2002/november/documents/hf_jp-ii_spe_20021114_italian-parliament_sp.html.

[9] Marcello Pera, «Il relativismo, il cristianesimo e l'Occidente», en *Senza radici, Europa, relativismo, cristianismo, islam,* por Marcello Pera y Joseph Ratzinger (Milano, Italia: Mondadori, 2004), 5–45.

[10] *Ibidem,* 14.

[11] *Ibidem,* 14-23.

[12] Joseph Ratzinger, *Fede, verità, tolleranza* (Siena, Italy: Cantagalli, 2003), 87.

[13] *Ibidem,* 75.

También en la bioética el relativismo se ha extendido como la gangrena. El filósofo italiano Uberto Scarpelli, maestro entre los definidos «laicos» en ese país, afirma que no es posible, no es correcto desde el punto de vista lingüístico, hablar de verdad en el terreno de la ética,[14] como trató de mostrar en un libro titulado «*L'etica senza verità*».[15] En otro texto dice explícitamente:

> Quien creyera que haya una ética verdadera, de forma que las otras sean falsas, podría, aún más, debería tomar partido por la ética verdadera y de ella, o en ella, deducir una bioética, descalificando toda otra ética o bioética. Pero en la ética no hay verdad. Los valores de verdadero y falso convienen a las preposiciones del discurso descriptivo-explicativo-predictivo, no convienen a las preposiciones del discurso descriptivo-valorativo.[16]

Esta mentalidad, ampliamente extendida entre los cultores de la bioética pero también muy presente entre la gente común, lleva a justificar cualquier tipo de comportamiento. El relativismo lleva así a una mentalidad y a una práctica libertaria: no existiendo la verdad ética, queda sólo el valor de la propia libertad, la que se convierte en una especie de autojustificación: mi acto es bueno por el hecho de ser libre. La autodeterminación se convierte así en el único criterio moral en relación, por ejemplo, con la práctica y la legalización de la eutanasia.

Soy de la opinión de que en muchos casos, ese relativismo es una excusa cómoda, una pantalla o un velo que permite que cada uno tenga las opiniones que más le gusten, sin tener que dar cuenta siquiera a la propia razón. De ese modo, se dice por ejemplo que cada uno debe decidir en qué momento del desarrollo del embrión o el feto considera que tiene suficiente valor como para merecer respeto.

Durante un debate en un congreso de medicina, un filósofo italiano, exponente también él de la así llamada «bioética laica» se lamentaba diciendo: «Para ustedes, los

---

[14] Uberto Scarpelli, «Giovanni Paolo e la Centesimus annus», en *Bioetica Laica* (Milano, Italia: Baldini & Castoldi, 1998), 58.

[15] Uberto Scarpelli, *L'etica senza verità* (Bologna, Italia: Il Mulino, 1982).

[16] Uberto Scarpelli, «La Bioetica. Alla ricerca dei principi», *Biblioteca della Libertà,* vol. 99 (1987), 227.

católicos que creen en la verdad, todo es más fácil. Piensan que han encontrado la verdad y se sienten seguros; nosotros, en cambio, estamos siempre en la búsqueda, vivimos el drama [la tragedia] de saber que nunca la encontraremos». A esta reflexión, un tanto romántica, respondí: «Nosotros, los católicos que creemos en la posibilidad de encontrar alguna verdad, sentimos la obligación de buscarla; ustedes, en cambio, no tienen que buscar algo que piensan que no se puede hallar. Nosotros tenemos miedo de equivocarnos; ustedes no deben temer: si no existe la verdad tampoco existe el error. Nosotros tenemos que forzarnos para ser coherentes con las verdades conocidas; ustedes no. En realidad, la tragedia de ustedes es que saben que, en el fondo, la afirmación de que la verdad no existe es falsa».

La Iglesia, esposa de Aquel que es «Camino, Verdad y Vida», debe, como Él y con Él, dar testimonio de la verdad y servir a cada hombre en su búsqueda dramática. Ésta es quizás una de las mayores contribuciones que los católicos podemos ofrecer hoy al mundo con relación al respeto por la vida humana: la construcción de una reflexión bioética que no se reduzca a la justificación de lo útil o placentero, o de ciertos intereses creados.

Laicismo excluyente e intolerante

La secularización y el relativismo, tan difundidos en Europa, están relacionados con otro movimiento en el continente: el laicismo (secularismo) excluyente e intolerante que tiende a dominar todo el ámbito público.

La actividad del actual gobierno de España, que se ha dado en llamar «zapaterismo» (por José Luis Rodríguez Zapatero, recientemente elegido primer ministro de España), es un claro ejemplo de la virulencia que anima a ciertos grupos de la sociedad europea. Apenas llegados al poder [en 2004], el partido propuso un nuevo programa social que contempla, entre otras, las siguientes «conquistas»: equiparación de las uniones de personas homosexuales con el matrimonio, incluido el derecho de adopción, modificación de la ley de divorcio para favorecer el así llamado «divorcio exprés» que permite la disolución de un matrimonio en pocas semanas, ampliación de las condiciones permitidas para realizar un aborto, modificación de la ley sobre reproducción asistida, retocada recientemente por el gobierno anterior en noviembre de 2003, para permitir la experimentación con embriones humanos, incentivación del debate social con respecto a la legalización de la eutanasia.

La actitud de esos grupos, ahora en el poder, se distingue por una explícita repulsión hacia todo lo que sea expresión de la religión; o más precisamente, de la fe cristiana o católica. De hecho, mientras que por una parte pretenden limitar la enseñanza de religión en las escuelas, por otra, han decidido que el Estado financie la enseñanza, en las mismas escuelas, de la religión islámica. El eslogan utilizado por el Sr. Zapatero en su campaña electoral, «más gimnasia y menos religión», ayuda a entender su solemne respeto por la fe de la mayoría de los españoles.

No podemos engañarnos creyendo que se trata solamente de un fenómeno español. El rechazo de la Unión Europea por la mención de las raíces judeocristianas de Europa en el preámbulo de la Constitución Europea fue una clara manifestación de la obstinación con que ciertos grupos dominantes pretenden excluir la fe cristiana del horizonte público.

El reciente «caso Buttiglione» ha reverberado fuertemente en el centro mismo de Europa. En octubre de 2004 se negó a Rocco Buttiglione, ministro de Asuntos Europeos de Italia, el acceso al cargo de Comisionado de la Unión Europea a causa de sus opiniones acerca de la homosexualidad. No se trataba de que el ministro italiano anunciara medidas discriminatorias en relación con los homosexuales; ni siquiera de que hubiera hecho quién sabe qué declaraciones de carácter despectivo hacia esas personas. Simplemente, en sus agotadoras sesiones de confirmación, los miembros del Parlamento Europeo insistieron hasta lograr que Buttiglione dijera (tras haber insistido que una cosa es el *pensamiento moral personal* y otra la *política pública*, que no debe nunca permitir la discriminación de nadie), que «podría pensar que el comportamiento homosexual es pecaminoso».[17] De hecho, apenas se presentó su nombre como candidato para la Comisión Europea, ciertos grupos en Italia y otros países europeos protestaron porque se proponía a una persona «demasiado católica».

En 2004, el cardenal Ratzinger presentó un interesante análisis del fenómeno del laicismo fanático e intolerante

---

[17] Una transcripción de las audiencias está disponible en el http://www.acton.org/press/special/buttiglione.php#3.

europeo, contraponiéndolo a la situación de los Estados Unidos. Dice:

> Aunque en América la secularización proceda a ritmo acelerado ... allí se percibe, mucho más claramente que en Europa, un reconocimiento implícito de las bases religiosas y morales que surgen del cristianismo y que sobrepasan las diversas religiones. Europa —contrariamente a los Estados Unidos— está rumbo a una colisión con su propia historia y se hace, a menudo, portavoz de un rechazo casi visceral en todas las posibles dimensiones públicas de los valores cristianos.[18]

El análisis de las causas de ese fenómeno me parece por demás esclarecedor. En los Estados Unidos, la separación de la Iglesia y el Estado nació como exigencia de la misma experiencia religiosa de sus fundadores, que deseaban practicar su fe sin estar sometidos a la iglesia dominante de sus países europeos de origen. Por esta misma razón, esa separación busca permitir a la religión tener su propia naturaleza, respeta y protege su espacio vital distinto del estado y sus ordenamientos; es una separación concebida positivamente.

En Europa, en cambio, el Iluminismo (que proclamaba la autonomía de la razón y su emancipación de la fe tradicional) y el catolicismo (fuertemente aferrado a su patrimonio de fe) «se vieron contrapuestos el uno al otro en un conflicto insanable».[19] Desde entonces la separación entre católicos y laicistas se convirtió en algo típico de los países europeos latinos.

> Ser «laicista» indica pertenencia ... al movimiento espiritual del iluminismo y, desde ese momento, no parece que exista ningún puente que conduzca a la fe católica; los dos mundos parecen haberse convertido en mutuamente impenetrables. Y dado que «laicismo» significa también libre pensamiento y libertad de toda constricción religiosa, ello comporta también la exclusión de los contenidos y valores cristianos de la vida pública.[20]

---

[18] Joseph Ratzinger, «Lettera a Marcello Pera», en *Senza radici, Europa, relativismo, cristianismo, islam,* por Marcello Pera y Joseph Ratzinger (Milano, Italia: Mondadori, 2004), 99.

[19] *Ibidem,* 104.

[20] *Ibidem,* 105.

A la luz de estas causas históricas se comprende mejor la actitud beligerante de muchos grupos «laicistas» europeos. *No se trata* de una expresión del «laicidad» entendida como la separación complementaria entre la esfera política y la religiosa, sino que *es* una expresión del «laicismo» entendido como la exclusión intolerante de todo lo religioso. Los laicistas [o «laicos», como ellos mismos prefieren llamarse], pretenden así negar a la Iglesia el derecho a pronunciarse sobre las cuestiones públicas, acusándola de querer imponer a la sociedad su propio punto de vista y su propia moral. Hasta el punto de que, como acaba de suceder otra vez en España, se denuncie ante un juez a un obispo por haber recordado en una carta pastoral la doctrina del *Catecismo de la Iglesia Católica* sobre la homosexualidad.

En esta situación, los pastores de la Iglesia Católica europea sufren una enorme presión pública que puede provocar en ellos la tentación de condescender y callar. Y dejar de ser la luz del mundo y la sal de la tierra. Pero es interesante notar que frecuentemente son las mismas personas que protestan cuando el Papa o un obispo se pronuncian sobre cuestiones morales o sociales quienes protestan porque, según ellos, el Papa Pío XII no se pronunció con suficiente firmeza contra los atropellos del régimen nazi. ¿En qué quedamos? ¿No eran también aquéllas cuestiones morales y sociales?

De hecho, por más que muchos lo nieguen, las sociedades europeas siguen interesadas en saber qué opina la Iglesia sobre las principales cuestiones morales y los temas más debatidos en el campo de la vida y la familia. Recientemente, un conocido director de cine italiano lamentaba, desde las columnas de un periódico de gran difusión, que se viera tan frecuentemente a religiosos y sacerdotes en los debates y programas de televisión. Según él, esas personas no deberían presentarse cuando se tratan temas de interés público porque no representan más que a una minoría de la población. Pero el hecho es que, efectivamente, los medios de comunicación social asiduamente buscan la presencia de algún eclesiástico porque saben bien que gran parte de la población está interesada en saber qué piensa y dice la Iglesia sobre los temas más candentes y vitales.

Esto se ha demostrado otra vez recientemente. Una breve declaración del secretario y portavoz de la Conferencia Episcopal Española sobre el uso del condón como protección contra el SIDA recibió un eco fuerte. La noticia dio la vuelta al mundo en unas horas y se multiplicaron los comentarios de todo género por parte de todo tipo de personas: desde teólogos de diversas tendencias a representantes de grupos de homosexuales ¿Por qué tanto revuelo? ¿No se trata, al fin y al cabo, de la opinión de un religioso sobre un tema público en el que la Iglesia no debería entrometerse? ¿En qué quedamos?

Conclusiones

Podríamos seguir analizando otros aspectos significativos de la situación europea. Algunos de ellos son muy específicos, como la enorme complejidad de la red institucional que constituye la realidad sociopolítica, todavía no bien definida, que denominamos Europa. El parlamento europeo responde a ciertos problemas de bioética con resoluciones que no son normativas pero pueden influir más o menos en las legislaciones nacionales. Otras veces se trata de decisiones de la Comisión Europea o del Consejo de Ministros que, en realidad, son expresiones de los diversos ministerios nacionales. Etcétera, etcétera.

Pero creo que las características de la cultura actual europea analizadas aquí, secularización progresiva, relativismo y libertarismo, y laicismo exclusivo e intolerante, nos ayudan a comprender el derrotero que están tomando en los últimos tiempos los problemas de la bioética. Y nos ayudan también a comprender los desafíos que esos problemas y esas características culturales significan para la Iglesia en Europa.

Para cada una de las características he presentado una descripción, sus repercusiones en el campo de la bioética y, al final, una breve alusión a las posibilidades y oportunidades que presenta a la Iglesia Católica en una situación difícil.

Una de las primeras conclusiones de este análisis, en efecto, debería ser que la Iglesia no puede escapar en retirada, esconderse, encerrarse en el silencio. La Iglesia en Europa (y en otros continentes) debe preguntarse sobre la fuerza, claridad e inteligencia con que ha afrontado y afronta estos problemas que son tan decisivos para el bien de la humanidad y tan centrales para la aceptación del evangelio.

A veces se tiene la impresión de que buena parte de los pastores y agentes de la pastoral se ocupan demasiado poco de estos problemas, no están suficientemente preparados y no se pronuncian públicamente sobre ellos. La anécdota del inicio (sobre los trasplantes de órganos) es sólo un ejemplo de esa situación. Creo que las cosas van mejorando en este sentido; se van multiplicando las iniciativas orientadas a la formación y acción en este campo entre los obispos, sacerdotes y laicos católicos.

Es importante tomar conciencia de que, como señalaba anteriormente, la sociedad secularizada, relativista y laicizada de nuestros días, sigue atribuyendo grande importancia al pensamiento de la Iglesia. Por ello mismo, unos están atentos a lo que dice la Iglesia y otros están preocupados cuando habla. Recientemente, un grupo de miembros del Partido Popular español pidió a los pastores, en una reunión con representantes de la Iglesia, que se pronuncien en forma más clara y enérgica sobre estos temas. A decir verdad, en los últimos meses muchos obispos españoles lo han hecho y suscitaron la ira de los laicistas más fanáticos. Sin embargo, los católicos activos en el campo de la política piden todavía más presencia de la Iglesia.

Es importante también renovar la confianza en la real eficacia de las intervenciones inteligentes, respetuosas y firmes de la Iglesia en este campo. Podemos tener la impresión de que la sociedad no escucha y que pronunciarse sobre estos temas en la arena pública no es más que una pérdida de tiempo o, peor todavía, un modo de alejar más a la gente de la Iglesia y del Evangelio. Sin embargo, no faltan ejemplos que muestran que si la Iglesia (sus sacerdotes, sus agentes de pastoral y sus laicos) se movilizan de modo inteligente, prudente y, al mismo tiempo, con firmeza y claridad, es posible lograr resultados importantes.

Uno de esos ejemplos es la ya mencionada ley 40 que regula en Italia la reproducción asistida, desde febrero de 2004. Se trata de una ley que, aunque con algunos defectos, es un verdadero «milagro» en una sociedad europea como la italiana. Los grupos que pretenden una mayor liberalización de las prácticas de fecundación asistida han protestado porque, dicen, la ley fue aprobada gracias a la influencia de la Iglesia Católica. Y tienen razón: detrás de esa ley hay años de intenso trabajo por parte de varios grupos católicos muy activos en la sociedad. Detrás de ellos estaba el apoyo y, a veces, la participación directa de algunos miembros del clero, bien conscientes de la importancia de lo que estaba en juego.

Juan Pablo II, plenamente consciente de los graves y urgentes desafíos que la Iglesia encuentra en el campo de la defensa de la vida en Europa y en todo el mundo, llama a los obispos a encarar con entusiasmo esos desafíos. En

Evangelium vitae, refiriéndose a los obispos, dice: «...somos los primeros a quienes se pide ser anunciadores incansables del *Evangelio de la vida*». Y luego continúa:

> Al anunciar este Evangelio, no debemos temer la hostilidad y la impopularidad, rechazando todo compromiso y ambigüedad que nos conformaría a la mentalidad de este mundo (cf. *Rm* 12, 2). Debemos estar *en el mundo,* pero no ser *del mundo* (cf. *Jn* 15, 19; 17, 16), con la fuerza que nos viene de Cristo, que con su muerte y resurrección ha vencido al mundo (cf. *Jn* 16, 33).[21]

---

[21] Juan Pablo II, *Evangelium vitae,* n. 82.